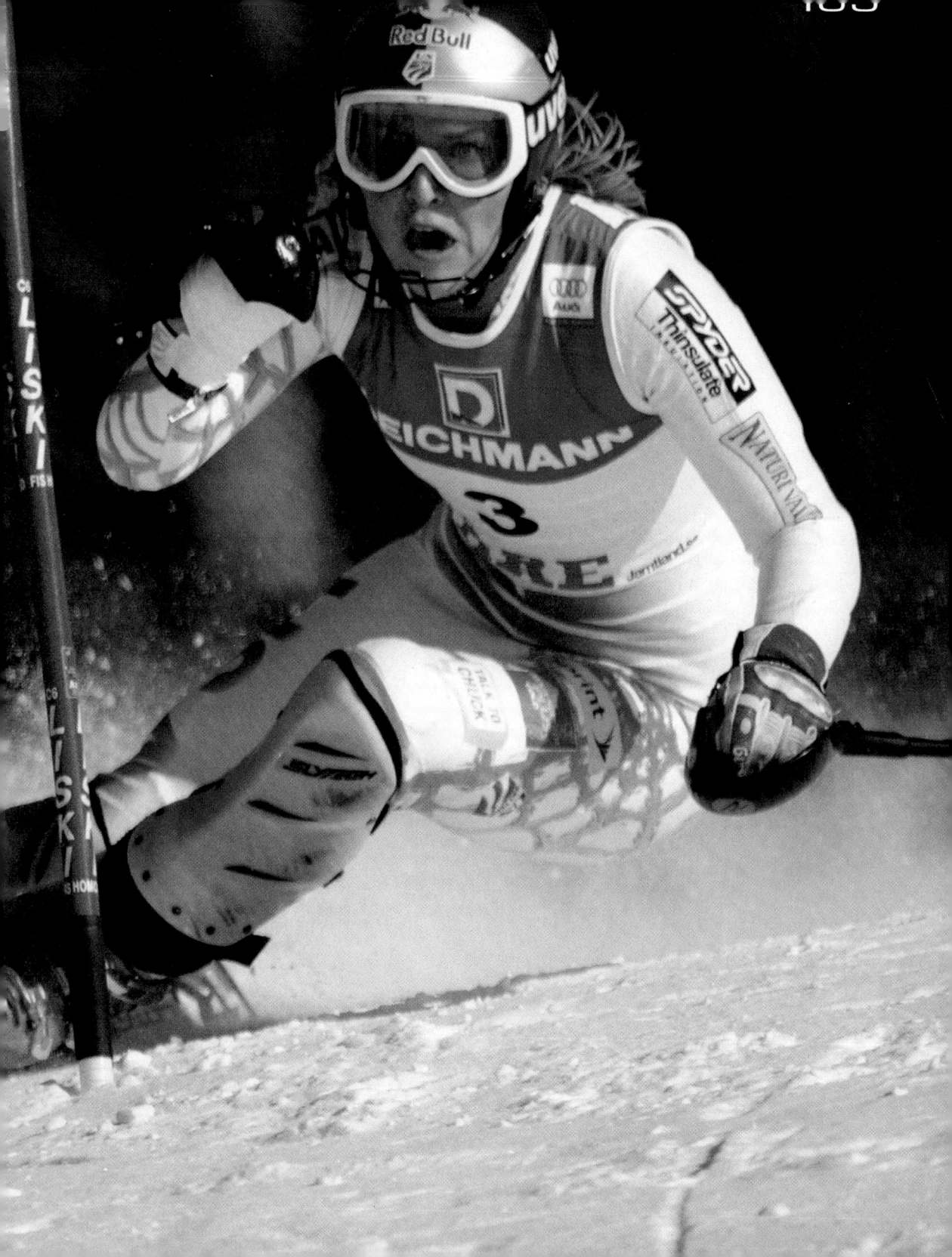

WINTER SPORTS

Speed Skating

Trevor Marsicano was a world-record holder . . . for a few hours. Then his teammate, Shani Davis, shaved four hundredths of a second off of Trevor's time in the 1000 meters. At the World Championships a week later, Marsicano earned four medals, including gold in the 1000 meters, while Davis, who already holds two Olympic gold medals, captured the 1500-meter title. As the sport's top stars gather in Vancouver in February, will it be the young hero or the veteran star who skates to gold? The battle between these two will be fun to watch.

In short-track skating, 2006 Olympic hero Apolo Anton Ohno won his amazing eighth U.S. championship in the 500 meters. At the World Championships, he was not as successful, but he did anchor the gold-medal-winning relay team.

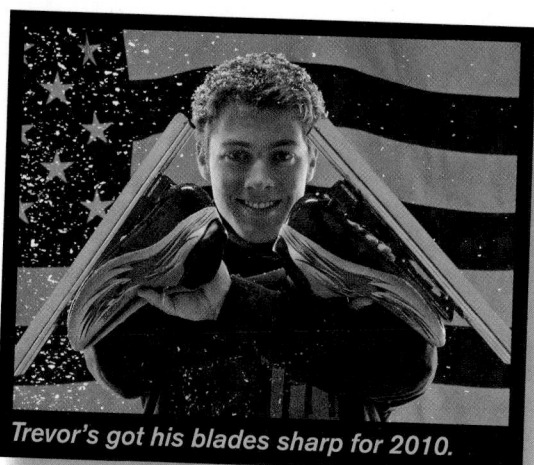

Trevor's got his blades sharp for 2010.

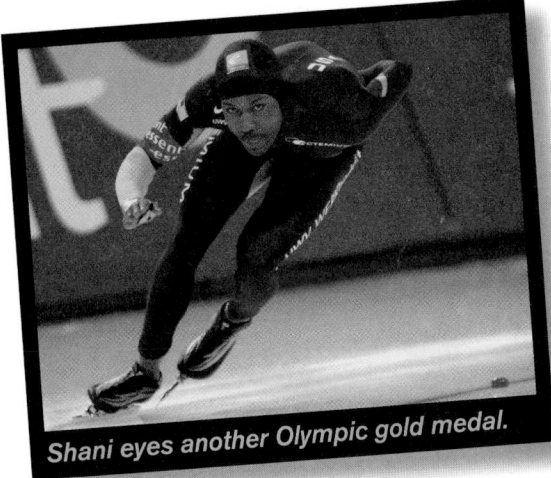

Shani eyes another Olympic gold medal.

WINTER WONDERLAND Watch all the excitement of the 2010 Winter Olympics. The "snow-and-ice" Games run from February 12 to 28, in locations in and around Vancouver, Canada. This will be Canada's third time hosting the Winter Games. Plus, the rockin', rollin' sport of ski cross will make its Olympic debut.

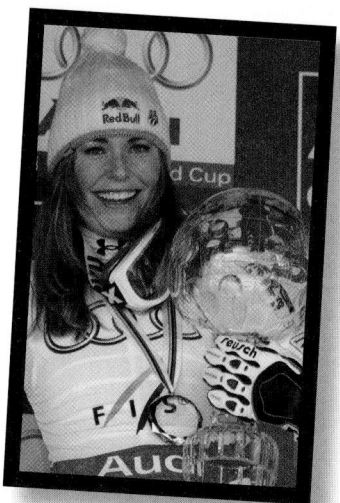

Skiing

With the Winter Olympics looming in February 2010, an American skier finds herself on top of the world. Minnesota native Lindsey Vonn has won the past two World Cup overall titles. The World Cup is the annual points championship. Skiers need to be outstanding in all the different types of ski racing to capture the overall title. Vonn's specialty is the dangerous downhill, and she's the defending world champ in that category.

She's already a two-time Olympic participant. However, for all her World Cup success, she hasn't done well at the Winter Games . . . yet. With the momentum of her back-to-back world titles, gold at the Olympics is the next goal on her snowy radar screen.

Figure Skating

There's a new world champion in figure skating, and he's a Lakers fan! Evan Lysacek became the first American male to capture the world title in 14 years, with a graceful and athletic performance at the 2009 Worlds in Los Angeles. The Chicago native (he moved to L.A. to train) has been a national champion at every level. Wearing a tuxedo-like suit and leaping and spinning beautifully, Lysacek thrilled the pro-American crowd by winning the big event over competitors from Canada and France.

The women's champion was South Korea's Yu-Na Kim. A former junior champion, she finished third in the 2008 Worlds. A move to a new coach, Canadian world champ Brian Orser, expanded her routines. In 2009, she set a new record for most points awarded in the final and set herself up as the gold-medal favorite in 2010.

While no American pairs skaters "figure" in the 2010 mix, ice dancers Tanith Belbin and Ben Agosto might climb the podium. They won silver at the 2006 Olympics and have several high finishes in recent world competitions.

HORSE RACING

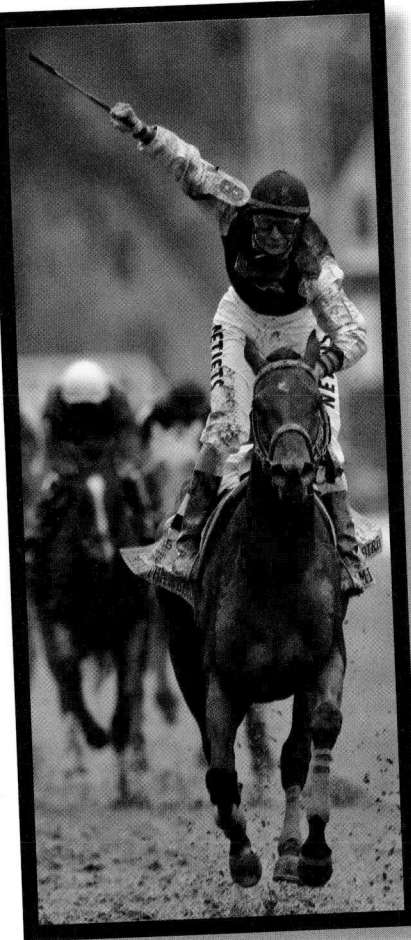

Miracle at the Derby!

The Kentucky Derby has seen a lot of racing since it started in 1875. The 2009 edition of the "Run for the Roses," as the race is nicknamed, featured one of the biggest upsets in the history of horse racing's most famous event.

How big was it? In horse racing, each horse has "odds" put on it. High numbers mean that most people do not expect a horse to win. Long odds might be 10–1 or 20–1. Heading into the start of this Derby, Mine That Bird was listed as a 50–1 "long shot."

Stunning just about everyone except her jockey, Calvin Borel, Mine That Bird became the second-biggest long shot to win the Derby in its 135 years. (The longest was a 91–1 winner named Donerail way back in 1913!) The racing world was shocked.

The Triple Crown (see box) is made up of three famous races. Normally, it's the horse that goes for the Triple Crown. In 2009, it was the jockey. Borel rode Mine That Bird in the Derby and switched to a horse named Rachel Alexandra for the running of the Preakness . . . and he won again!

With the win, Borel had a shot at becoming the first jockey ever to win the Triple Crown on different horses. In the Belmont Stakes in June, however, back aboard Mine That Bird, Borel could not complete the unprecedented sweep. Summer Bird won the long race, with Mine That Bird coming in third. It was nonetheless a very memorable summer for Borel and Bird!

2009 Triple Crown Winners

RACE	TRACK	HORSE	JOCKEY
KENTUCKY DERBY	Churchill Downs	Mine That Bird	Calvin Borel
PREAKNESS	Pimlico	Rachel Alexandra	Calvin Borel
BELMONT STAKES	Belmont Park	Summer Bird	Kent Desormeaux

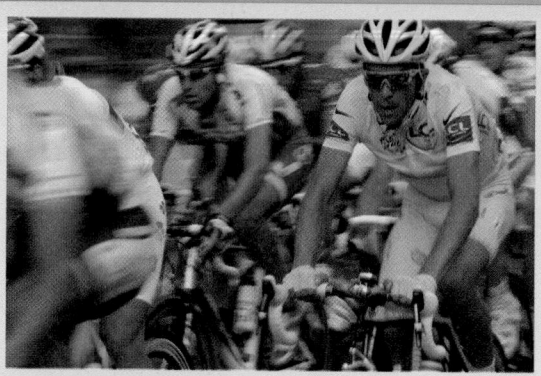

Spaniard Wins Tour de France . . . Again

For the fourth consecutive year, a rider from Spain won cycling's prestigious Tour de France. Alberto Contador (at right, in the leader's yellow jersey), who also was the champion in 2007, beat second-place finisher Andy Schleck of Luxembourg by a comfortable margin in the famous 21-stage race. American Lance Armstrong was third.

Although Contador won for the second time, Armstrong's presence was the big story. The 37-year-old cancer survivor had not competed since winning his seventh Tour de France in 2005. Amstrong held the lead in the early part of the 2009 competition, but Contador pulled away after the race entered the grueling mountain stages.

Contador and Armstrong both raced for the Astana team. That was a unique situation, because most teams have only one dominant rider whom the other cyclists help try to win.

ANOTHER RACE OF ANIMALS

While horses run in the dirt and grass for about two minutes, the animal racers of the Iditarod plod through snow and ice for days! Since 1973, the Iditarod has challenged dogsled teams—dogs and drivers—on a winding track through the Alaskan wilderness. It takes stamina, bravery, daring, and a lot of dog food to make it through the event.

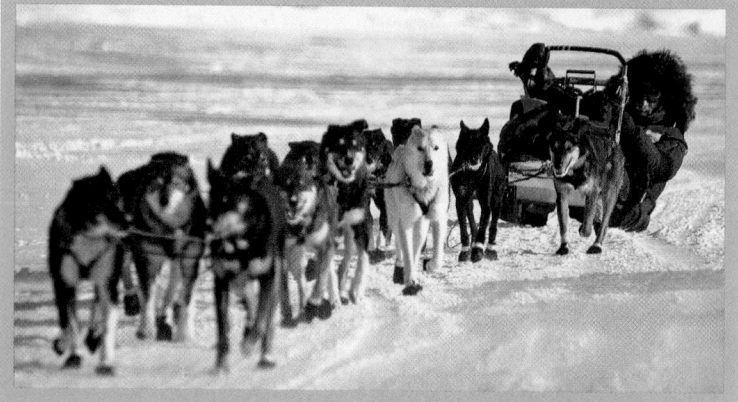

In 2009, a familiar face graced the medal stand at the end: Lance Mackey won his third straight Iditarod. He was following a family tradition—Lance's dad won in 1978.

TRACK AND FIELD

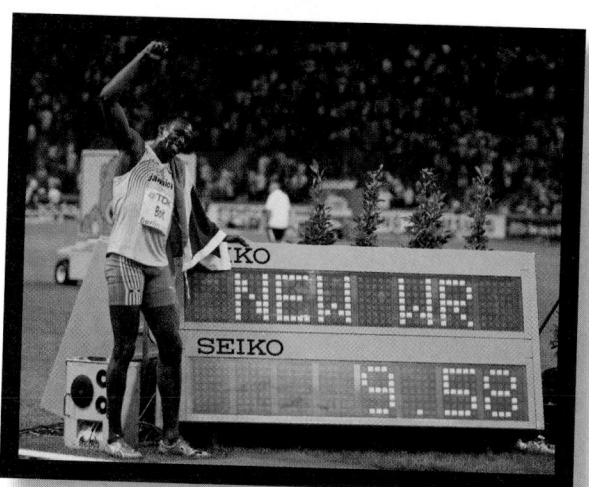

TWO MORE BOLTS!

On the list of amazing things that happened this past year in sports, perhaps nothing was more amazing than what Usain Bolt did in less than 10 seconds in August in Berlin. At the World Track and Field Championships, the 2008 Olympic gold medalist from Jamaica shocked the world—again!—by running the 100 meters in a world-record 9.58 seconds. Seriously. 9.58 seconds. He beat his "old" record by more than 1/10 of a second. That might not seem like a lot, but no one had lowered the world mark by that much in 88 years! To top it off, he then set a new world record in the 200 meters at 19.19 seconds, lowering the old mark by 0.11 seconds.

"Lightning" Bolt has staked a pretty solid claim to the title of "world's fastest man." Meanwhile, Shelly-Ann Fraser won the women's 100 meters, making Jamaica home to both of the world's fastest people.

Tyson Gay set a new American record in the 100-meter final, with a time of 9.71 seconds. No one will remember that great feat, however, in light of the Bolt from Jamaica.

In other results, Americans earned some gold: Trey Hardee became the "world's greatest athlete" by winning the decathlon; Sanya Richards captured the 400 meters; and Christian Cantwell won the shot put competition.

REMEMBERING A HERO

The championships were held in Berlin, which was also the site of the 1936 Summer Olympics. Before the competition, organizers honored the great American athlete Jesse Owens, who stunned the world by winning four gold medals (100, 200, 4x100, and long jump) at the 1936 Games. What made Owens's feats more remarkable is that he did them in the face of outright racism from the Nazi-run German government. His bravery in the face of evil has made him an American legend.

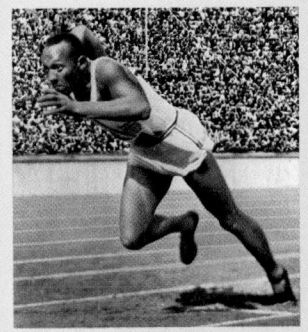

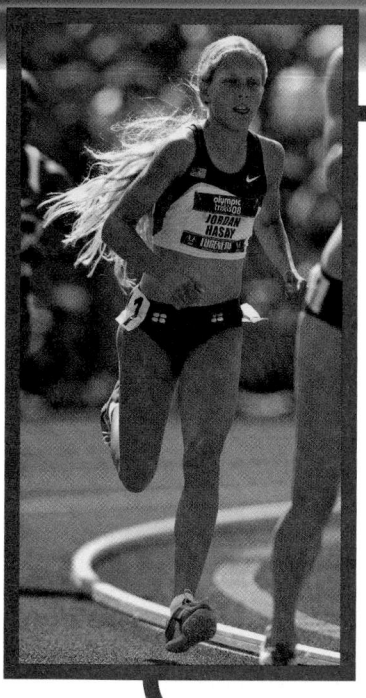

ONE TO WATCH... if you can catch

her! Since she was 12 years old, Jordan Hasay of California has been breaking records at just about every running distance. If she keeps up the pace, she could have a golden future.

In 2008, she was named the top high school track athlete in the country by USA Track and Field. She excels on the track in the mile, the 1,500 meters, and the 3,000 meters, but she's also a star in the cross-country events. She won the 2008 national title in the 5,000-meter cross-country event.

"My aim isn't to be remembered as the best high school runner ever, but as one of the better U.S. distance runners in the future."

Ironman (and Woman!)

Some call it the hardest race in the world. It certainly calls for an enormous amount of strength, endurance, skill, and courage. Any one of the three parts of the famous Ironman Triathlon would be enough to tire out top athletes. Yet the racers in this event do all three, back to back. First, they swim 2.4 miles in choppy ocean waters. They climb out and immediately jump onto a bike for a 112-mile ride. As if that was not enough, they top it off by running a marathon: 26 miles, 385 yards.

In 2008, Craig Alexander of Australia (right) won the men's race, while Chrissie Wellington from Great Britain won the women's. It was the first Ironman win for both racers. Craig took just over 8 hours and 17 minutes to finish, while Chrissie hustled home in just over 9 hours.

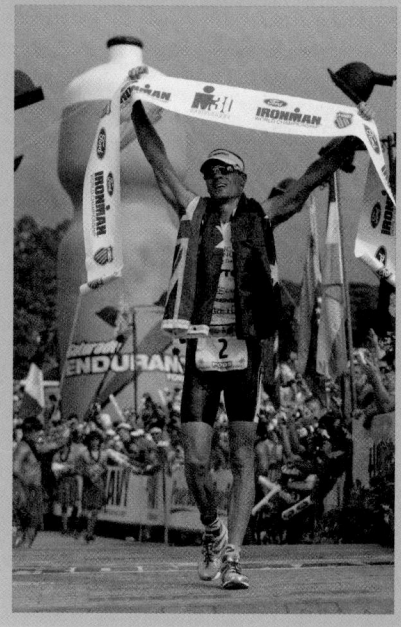

BEACH VOLLEYBALL

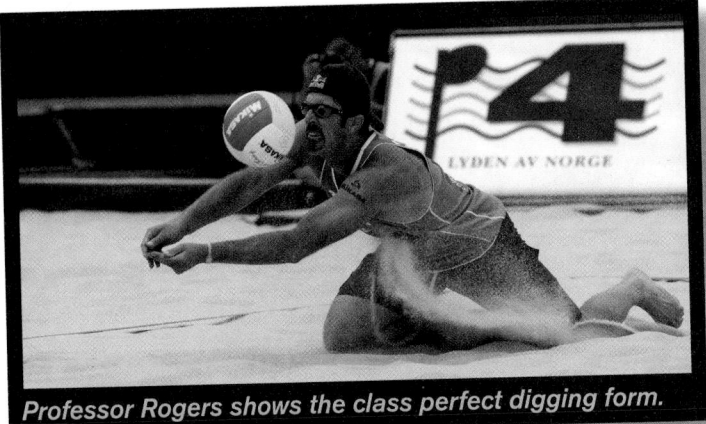

Professor Rogers shows the class perfect digging form.

A DOOR OPENS

On the women's side of the beach, the 2008 season was a mirror of the men's game. The mighty team of Misty May-Treanor and Kerri Walsh also took home Olympic gold, and they also won 12 of 15 pro touraments. They even wrapped up an all-time record of 112 straight match wins. May-Treanor was named the MVP, Best Offensive Player, and even Best Defensive Player.

However, unlike the men's side, the 2009 season has been a very different story. Walsh missed the summer when she became pregnant. She and her husband Casey Jennings welcomed a baby boy in May. She aims to return in 2010.

TWO FOR THE SHOW

What do you do after you win a gold medal? Simple: You come home and keep winning! In 2008, along with capturing beach volleyball gold, Todd Rogers and Phil Dallhauser won 11 of 15 tournaments to capture the annual Association of Volleyball Professionals (AVP) title. The duo dominated the sport, winning every postseason award. Dallhauser is known as "The Thin Beast," and he was named the season MVP and Best Offensive Player. Rogers, called "The Professor," was named Best Defensive Player. That's a pretty good combination! It was Rogers's fifth straight honor for "best digger."

The duo continued their success in 2009, leading the AVP Tour tournament wins through midsummer. Looks like these golden beach boys still have a lot of wins in them!

May-Treanor missed 2009, too, but it wasn't such good news. While filming the *Dancing with the Stars* TV show, she hurt her Achilles tendon. The serious injury ended her volleyball season. With that team out, Elaine Youngs and Nicole Branagh jumped up to take advantage. Through midsummer, they led the tour with nine victories, more than twice as many as any other team.

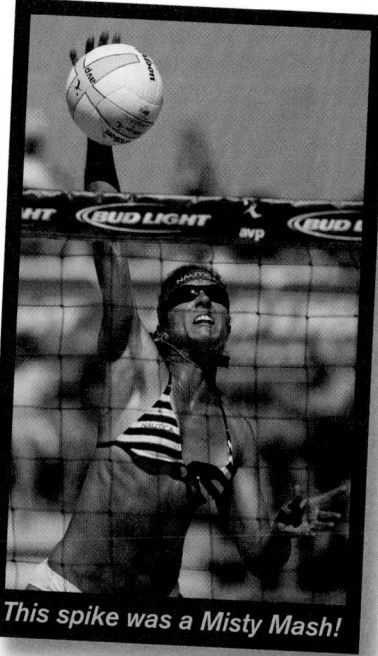

This spike was a Misty Mash!

BOXING

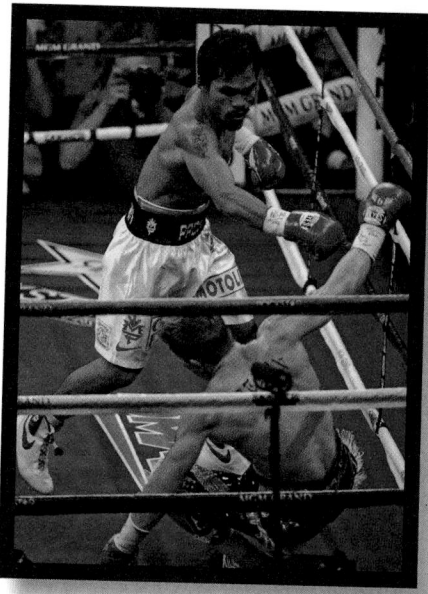

The Big Fight

The most anticipated fight of the past year was between Manny Pacquiao, a slender man from the Philippines, and Ricky Hatton, a fiery fellow from Great Britain. These two foreign fighters met in Las Vegas in May 2009. Thousands of Hatton fans flew "across the pond" to cheer on their lad. It was a long trip . . . but a short fight. Hatton was down and out by the second round, whipped by Pacquiao's devastating right hand and superb quickness. "Magic Manny" retained the 140-pound title and cemented his reputation as perhaps the finest boxer around in any weight class.

GOODBYE, GOLDEN BOY
One of boxing's most celebrated careers came to an end in early 2009. Oscar de la Hoya decided to hang up his gloves not long after losing to Manny Pacquiao. De la Hoya was at one time perhaps the most popular fighter in the world. His smiling face, easy personality, and intense fighting style made him the hero of the boxing world. He held a total of 10 championships in 6 weight classes, and his fights against Bernard Hopkins, "Sugar" Shane Mosely, and Floyd Mayweather were classics. He also won the 1992 Olympic gold medal. He already has a statue outside the Staples Center in Los Angeles. De la Hoya hopes to keep entertaining people, but in movies and music, not the ring.

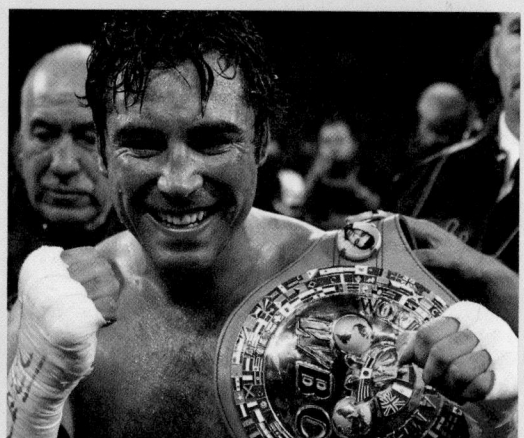

OTHER SPORTS

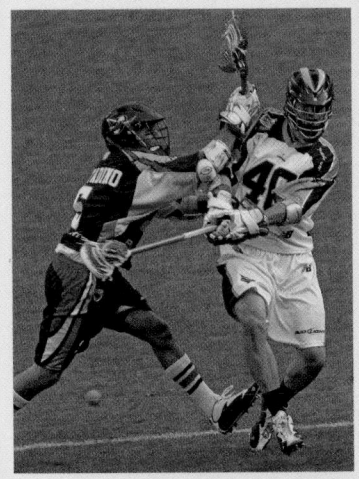

LACROSSE

Two pro leagues compete for the attention of lacrosse fans in the U.S. The sport is actually one of the fastest growing in the nation, with more and more schools adding it to the choices they offer students.

More than 13,000 people watched the indoor National Lacrosse League's championship game in May. The Calgary Roughnecks earned their second title by knocking off the New York Titans 12–10. Indoor lacrosse is played on a hockey-sized rink. Tight spaces make for hard-hitting action and great stickwork.

On the outdoor side, Major League Lacrosse (action at left) is the pro level of the sport. The league boasts six teams. Other than Denver, most are in the East. In August, MLL held its championship game. The Toronto Nationals defeated the Detroit Outlaws in a close game, 10–9.

Bowling

There's a new King of Bowling, and he earned his crown in style! In May, Wes Malott had a pair of perfect-score 300 games during the nationally televised World Championships of the Professional Bowlers Association (PBA). Bowlers had to finish in the top 10 in a series of events to qualify for a shot at the crown. Malott's championship 300s were the first on TV, too.

Let's also give a special tip of the bowling shoe to Emma Hendrickson, who took part in the U.S. women's championships. Emma bowled a 107 in her best game. So what's the big deal? Well, she is 100 years old. Emma became the oldest participant ever, but it was not that big a surprise, since she's been bowling in the event for 50 years! She's signed up to hit the lanes again in 2010.

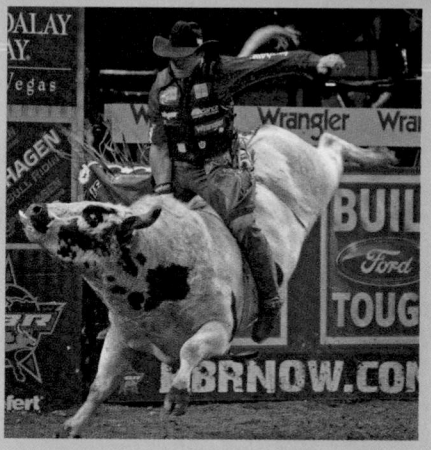

RODEO

Famed in song and story, celebrated by cowboys and cowgirls from all over, rodeo combines traditional Western jobs with action-packed sport. There are two major pro circuits of rodeo competition.

The Professional Bull Riders (PBR) tour spends almost as much time promoting the bulls as the riders. However, it's the brave and talented riders who take home the trophies . . . and the bruises. Bull riders have to spend at least eight seconds atop a massive, powerful bull that is jumping and bucking to flip the poor rider off. Believe it or not, during all that, the rider is judged on style, too! The 2008 champion, Guilherme Marchi (above), came all the way from Brazil to easily win the season title.

In the all-around Professional Rodeo Cowboys Association (PRCA), Texas's own Trevor Brazile was the 2008 Top Cowboy. Trevor didn't win any of the individual events (barrel riding, steer wrestling, bull riding, and bronco busting), but he finished high enough in all of them to earn the gold belt buckle.

GYMNASTICS

Bridget Sloan (pictured below) squeaked out a victory in the Visa Championships, held in August, making her the U.S. national champ. Sloan won the uneven parallel bars and the floor exercises, and beat balance beam winner Ivana Hong by only 0.3 points!

In the men's championships, Jonathan Horton from Houston won the rings and tied for first on the horizontal bar. Those titles gave him enough points to slip by Tim McNeill for the all-around championship.

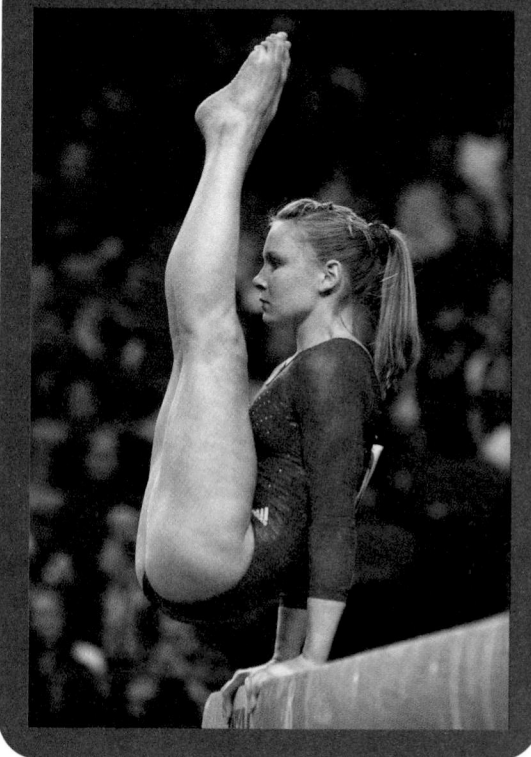

A WORLD OF SPORTS

Just because some sports don't get nightly mention on SportsCenter doesn't mean that millions of people aren't following every bounce of the ball. Here's a quick look at some sports news from around the world that was (almost) as big as the World Series or the Super Bowl.

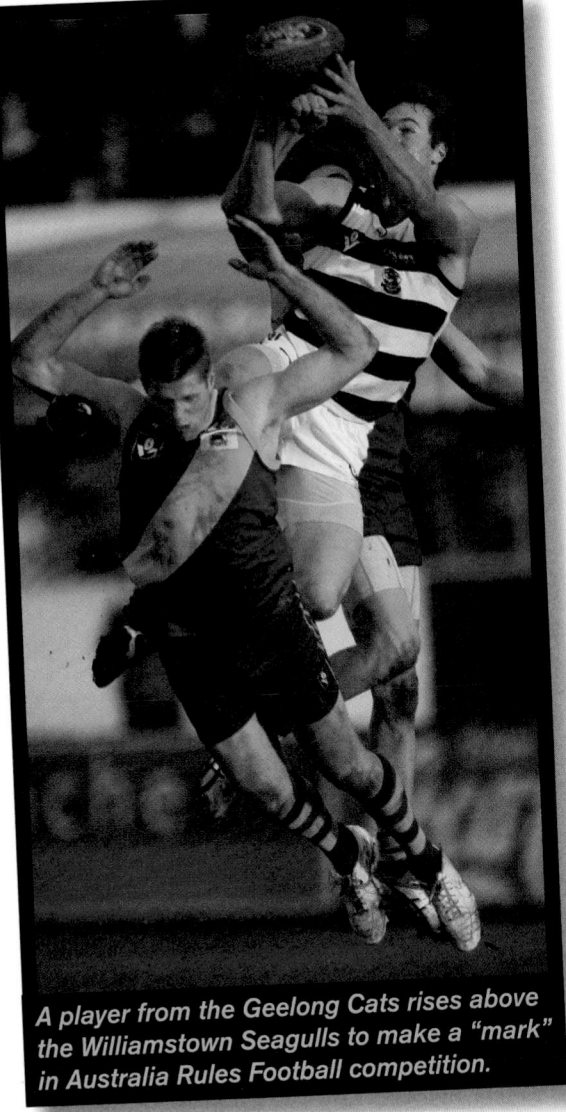

A player from the Geelong Cats rises above the Williamstown Seagulls to make a "mark" in Australia Rules Football competition.

◀◀◀ AUSTRALIAN RULES FOOTBALL

Combining the kicking skills of soccer, the catching abilities of NFL football, and the hitting power of rugby, Australian Rules football is an exciting, action-packed sport. Players, often tall and lean, kick the ball long distances with great accuracy. If they catch the ball—often having to battle and outleap opponents—they get a free kick to a teammate or toward the goal. In the 2008 Grand Final (the sport's Super Bowl), the Hawthorn Hawks defeated the Geelong Cats 115-89 as a packed house in Melbourne watched.

FIELD HOCKEY

In lots of countries outside the United States, field hockey—played by both men and women—is a super-popular sport. When the men's World Cup is played in India in 2010, millions will tune in to the big matches. India is one of the favorites, along with the Netherlands, Germany, and Pakistan. Dutch star Teun de Gooijer might be the key to bringing gold back to Europe.

The best female player in the world is Argentina's Luciana Aymar, a five-time world player the year. Known as "La Maga" (The Magician) for her ability to elude defenders, she has led her team to many high finishes, including a gold medal at the 2002 World Cup.

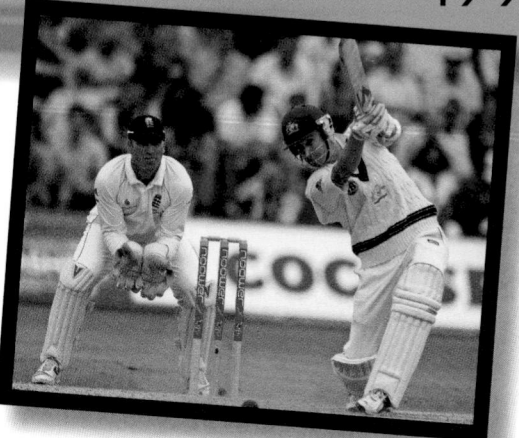

RUGBY ▼ ▼ ▼

Rugby is similar to football, with hard hitting, long kicks, and speedy runs. However, there's one big difference: no pads! Rugby teams normally have 15 players to a side. Among the top international teams are New Zealand, Australia, South Africa, England, and Fiji. The Rugby World Cup will be held in 2011 in New Zealand and will draw the attention of millions of fans of hard-hitting action.

In 2009, a smaller, faster game called rugby sevens, played with smaller teams, held its own World Cup. Wales beat Argentina 19–12 in an action-packed finale.

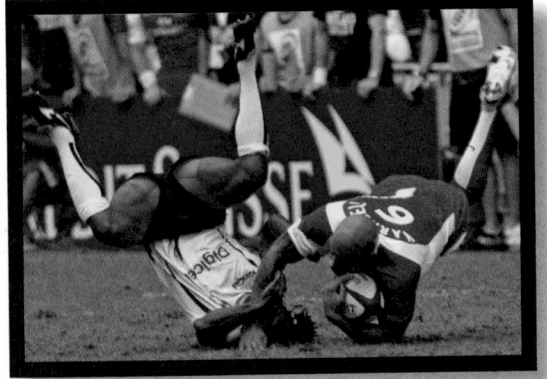

▲ ▲ ▲ CRICKET

If you live in Britain or in a country that Britain once controlled, you probably know cricket. Although it incorporates some baseball-like elements such as batting (above) and pitching (though they call it "bowling"), it's still very much its own sport. Cricket matches, or tests, can last for days.

One of the biggest international cricket events is known as The Ashes. It is played every two years or so between the national teams of Great Britain and Australia. The prize is, literally, an urn filled with ashes. (What? And you don't think an old oaken bucket or an axe isn't sort of silly, too? College football teams play for those!) In 2009, England captured the coveted urn for the second straight time.

A faster, more exciting version of the sport is called Twenty20, after the number of turns each team gets at bat. A world championship was held in the summer of 2009. England won the women's championship, while Pakistan won the men's title.

THE WILD AND WEIRD

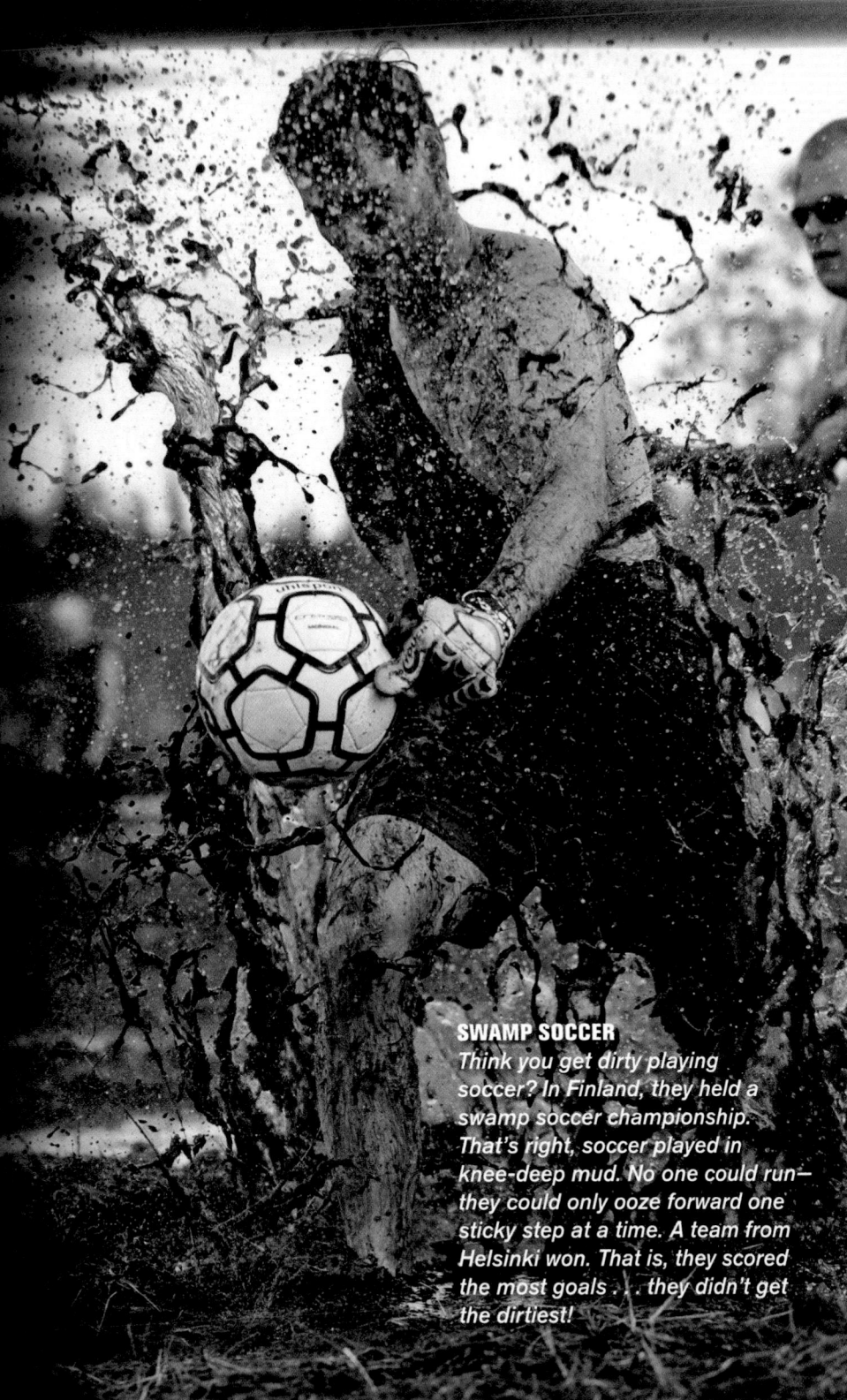

SWAMP SOCCER
Think you get dirty playing soccer? In Finland, they held a swamp soccer championship. That's right, soccer played in knee-deep mud. No one could run— they could only ooze forward one sticky step at a time. A team from Helsinki won. That is, they scored the most goals . . . they didn't get the dirtiest!

The world of sports is not just wins, losses, championships, and titles. It's also a place where odd things happen, people do strange things, and life is just plain weird. Here are a few examples of the wild and woolly from the world of sports, 2008–2009.

Golf or Pool?

At the Canadian Open, Leif Olson hit a shot that landed beyond the hole and then rolled back down the green. Along the way, it bounced off another ball that was already on the green. And then, like a perfect pool bank shot, Olson's ball rolled right into the cup for a hole in one! For making that once-in-a-lifetime shot, he won a fancy new car!

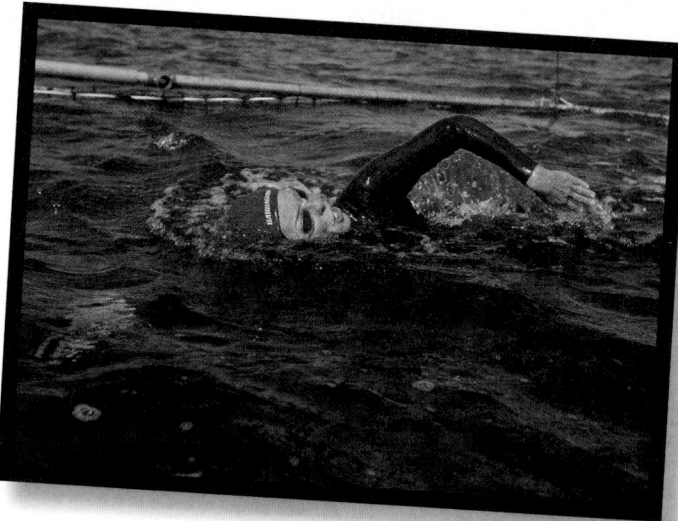

STRANGE INJURIES

It's not nice to laugh at someone who is injured. However, in sports, players can miss games due to some pretty bizarre ways of getting hurt.

◆ Jose Guillen of the Kansas City Royals hurt his knee while putting on a plastic shin guard.

◆ Atlanta Braves shortstop Yunel Escobar hurt his stomach muscle jumping up and down in the on-deck circle.

◆ Cubs pitcher Ryan Dempster missed a start after hurting his toe jumping over the dugout railing to celebrate a win.

◆ Detroit Lions wide receiver Bryant Johnson got bumps and bruises in an off-season golf cart accident.

Fact Check ▲

In February 2009, news agencies reported that Colorado's Jennifer Figge became the first woman to swim across the Atlantic Ocean. It turned out that Figge did cross the Atlantic . . . but most of it was in a boat. Figge supposedly swam from the west coast of Africa to the Caribbean in 25 days, but the story didn't hold water. Several astute readers took out their atlases and calculators and figured that she would have had to swim about 80 miles a day to make it in that time frame.

Sports Is for the Birds, Part I

In June of 2009, the Cleveland Indians and the Kansas City Royals were tied at 3–3 in the

bottom of the 10th inning when Cleveland's Shin-Soo Choo came to bat with runners on first and second and no one out. Choo lined a ball toward Royals center fielder Coco Crisp. But before Crisp had a chance to make a play on it, the ball struck a seagull. The ball ricocheted past Crisp, and Mark DeRosa easily trotted home from second base for the winning run. For the record, the dazed seagull soon flew away, unhurt.

Sports Is for the Birds, Part II ▼

The Atlanta Hawks–Miami Heat NBA play-off game in April of 2009 was interrupted in the first quarter by a real hawk. "Spirit," Atlanta's

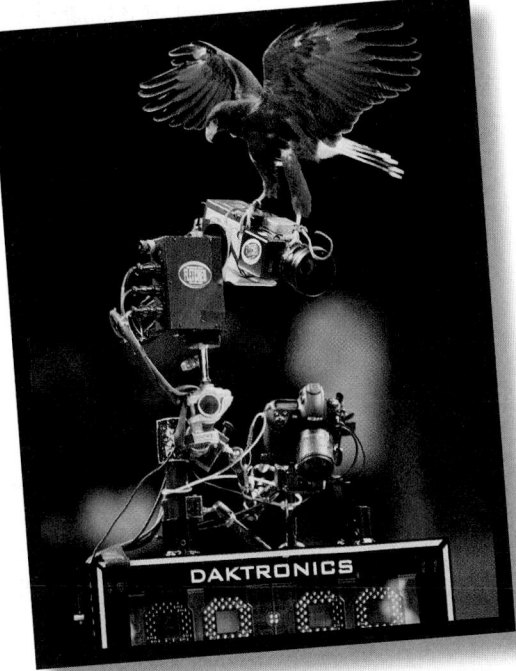

DAKTRONICS

What the . . . ?

✳ A large number of school near Athens, Georgia, had to close one Friday last fall. Too many teachers had called in sick to go to Saturday's Florida–Georgia football game!

✳ The Minnesota Timberwolves had a special night to celebrate the importance of reading. They passed out posters for the kids. One problem: On the poster, the team nickname was spelled W-O-V-E-S. Guess someone didn't read it first!

✳ The New York Mets gave each fan at their July 14 game a bag of potato chips. During the second inning, all 39,203 people crunched at once. They set a world record for the most people eating potato chips at the same time.

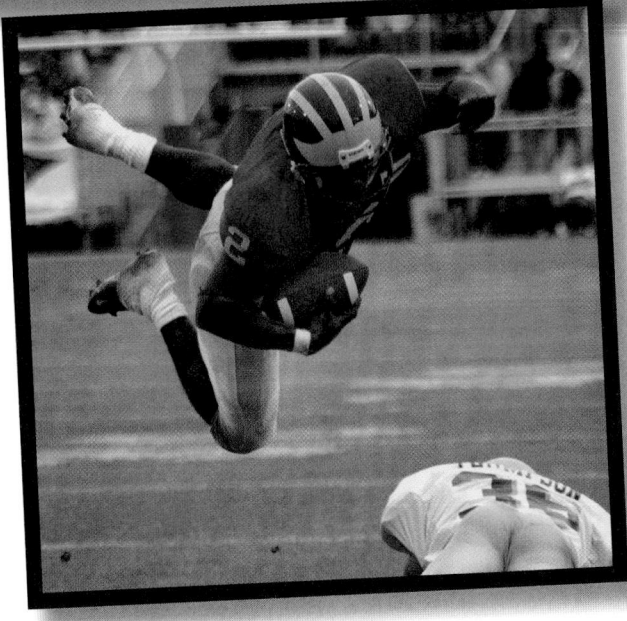

team mascot, swoops from the rafters during pregame introductions. But on this night, it decided it wanted a bird's-eye view from one of the basket supports. Then it buzzed the crowd before landing on a camera above the shot clock. That was enough to make the crowd jittery and have players ducking for cover. Play was stopped until the bird's handler coaxed it down. Spirit failed to scare the Heat: Miami won 108–93.

Yer Out!
Yer All Out!

More than 100 fans were on hand for a high school baseball game in West Burlington, Iowa, in June of 2009. None of them saw the end of West Burlington's 12–11 victory over Winfield-Mount Union—because they were all ejected. Umpire Don Briggs took the unusual step of throwing out all the spectators after they became unruly. Police were called in and the game was delayed for 40 minutes before continuing . . . with 18 players on the field and no one in the stands.

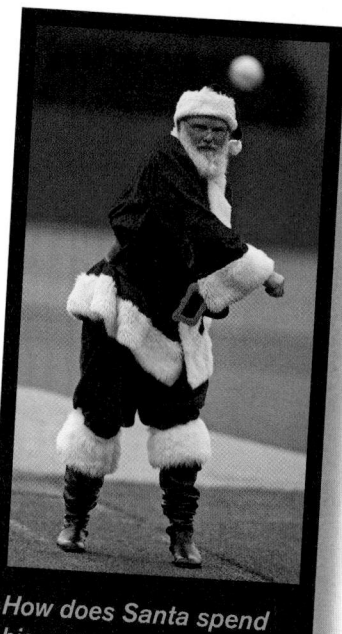

How does Santa spend his summer vacation? Throwing out the first pitch at a Tigers game.

Tough Start ▲

Delaware State opened the 2009 college football season with a loss . . . four months before its first scheduled game. In May, the Hornets accepted an offer to play at Michigan on October 17. The only trouble was, Delaware State was already scheduled to play North Carolina A&T on that day. When those two schools couldn't agree on another date, the Hornets were forced to forfeit to A&T. The big pile of money the Hornets were guaranteed for playing (and most likely losing) at the "Big House" in Ann Arbor helped take the sting out.

THE MEGA-AWESOME SPORTS INTERNET LIST!

MAJOR SPORTS WEBSITES

These are the "Big Five" of professional sports leagues. Each of these websites includes links to the individual websites of the teams in the league, plus bios of top players, video clips, schedules of games, even how to find tickets!

Major League Baseball
www.mlb.com

National Football League
www.nfl.com

Major League Soccer
www.mlsnet.com

National Hockey League
www.nhl.com

National Basketball Association
www.nba.com
www.wnba.com

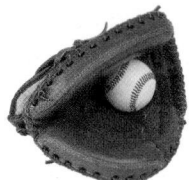

OTHER SPORTS LEAGUES

Check out these websites for schedules, results, and info on athletes in your favorite sports featuring individual competitors.

Action Sports
www.asptdewtour.com

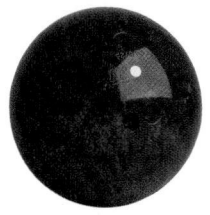

Bowling
www.pba.com

Drag Racing
www.nhra.com

Golf
www.pgatour.com
www.lpga.com

Editor's Note for Parents and Teachers: These websites are for information purposes only, and are not an endorsement of any program or organization over others. We've made every effort to include only websites that are appropriate for young sports fans, but the Internet is an ever-changing environment. There's no substitute for parental supervision, and we encourage everyone to surf smart . . . and safe!

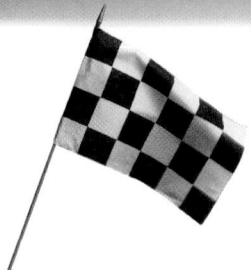

Ice Skating
www.usfigureskating.org

Indy Car Racing
www.indycar.com

Motocross/ Supercross
www.supercross.com

Stock Car Racing
www.nascar.com

Surfing
www.aspworldtour.com

Tennis
www.atpworldtour.com

www.sonyericsson wtatour.com

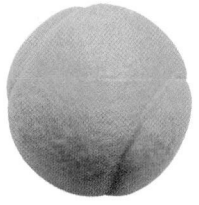

COLLEGE SPORTS

Follow your favorite team's road to the football BCS championship or the basketball Final Four with these major college sites. You can find links to the schools that are members of these conferences.

Bowl Championship Series
www.bcsfootball.org

Atlantic Coast Conference
www.theacc.com

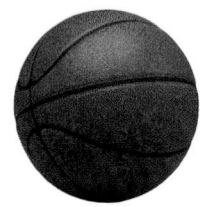

Big East Conference
www.bigeast.org

Big Ten Conference
www.bigten.org

Big 12 Conference
www.big12sports.com

Conference USA
http://conferenceusa .cstv.com

Mid-American Conference
www.mac-sports.com

Mountain West Conference
www.themwc.com

Pac-10 Conference
www.pac-10.org

Southeastern Conference
www.secsports.com

Sun Belt Conference
www.sunbeltsports.org

Western Athletic Conference
www.wacsports.com

National Collegiate Athletic Association
www.ncaa.com
(This site features information about all the college sports championships at every level and division.)

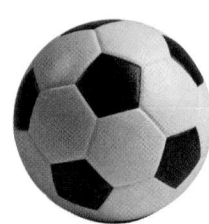

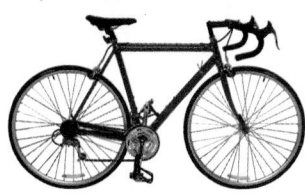

MAJOR SPORTS EVENTS

You'll find links to most big-time events—like the Super Bowl, the World Series, or the NBA Finals—on those sports' league websites. But here are several more worldwide sporting events that are worth a bookmark.

Little League World Series
www.littleleague.org/ worldseries

The Masters
www.masters.com

Pan Am Games (2011)
www.guadalajara2011 .org.mx/eng

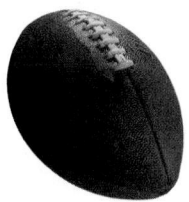

Summer Olympics (2012)
www.london2012.com

Summer X Games
http://espn.go.com/ action/xgames

Tour de France (English version)
www.letour.fr/us

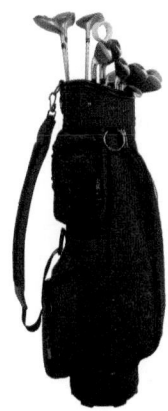

Winter Olympics (2010)
www.vancouver2010.com

Winter X Games
http://espn.go.com/ action/xgames

World Cup (Soccer)
www.fifa.com/ worldcup

YOUTH SPORTS ORGANIZATIONS

Rather play than watch? These websites can help get you out on the field!

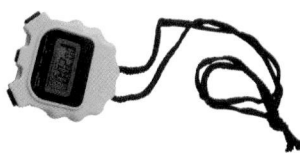

Baseball
www.littleleague.org

Basketball
www.njbl.org

Football
www.usafootball.com

Golf
www.juniorlinks.com

Ice Hockey
www.usajuniorhockey.com

Soccer
www.ayso.org

Tennis
www.usta.com

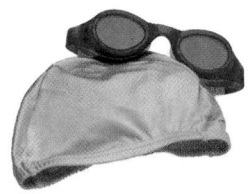

MEDIA SITES

If you're looking for the latest scores or news about your favorite sport, try some of these websites run by sports cable channels or sports publications.

CBS Sports
www.cbssports.com

ESPN
http://espn.go.com

FOX Sports
http://msn.foxsports.com

Sporting News
www.sportingnews.com

Yahoo! Sports
http://sports.yahoo.com

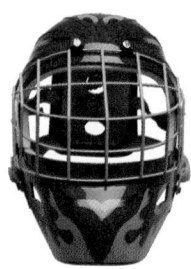

SPORTS HISTORY

It seems like big fans know all there is to know about the history of their favorite sport. Learn more about yours at any of these websites that take you back in time.

Hickok Sports
www.hickoksports.com

Retrosheet (Baseball)
www.retrosheet.org

Sports Illustrated **Vault**
http://vault
.sportsillustrated.cnn
.com/vault

Sports Reference Family of Sites
www.baseball-reference.com

www.basketball-reference.com

www.pro-football-reference.com

www.hockey-reference.com

www.sports-reference.com/olympics

PLAYERS ASSOCIATIONS

You're probably a little young to think about making money playing a sport. But if you're interested in the business side of things or want to discover more about what it's like to be a pro athlete, these sites may help.

MLB Players Association
http://mlbplayers.mlb.com

MLS Players Union
www.mlsplayers.org

NBA Players Association
www.nbpa.com

NHL Players Association
www.nhlpa.com

NFL Players Association
www.nflplayers.com

GAMES

Finally, check out these sites for some rainy-day sports fun and games on the computer.

www.nflrush.com

www.sikids.com

NCAA DIVISION I CHAMPS

MEN'S SPORTS
(2008–2009 School Year)

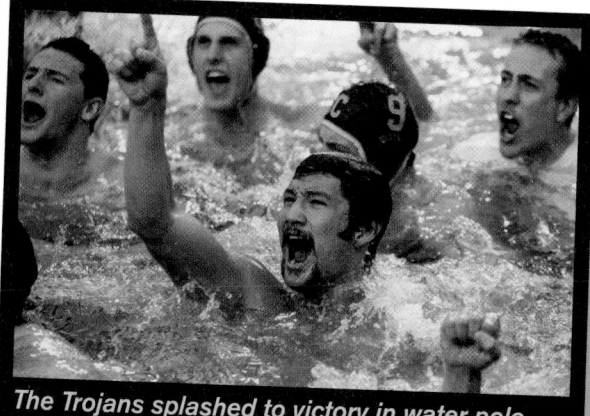
The Trojans splashed to victory in water polo.

ICE HOCKEY
Boston

LACROSSE
Syracuse

RIFLE (CO-ED TEAM)
West Virginia

SKIING (CO-ED TEAM)
Denver

SOCCER
Maryland

BASEBALL
LSU

SWIMMING AND DIVING
Auburn

BASKETBALL
North Carolina

TENNIS
USC

CROSS COUNTRY
Oregon

TRACK AND FIELD (INDOOR)
Oregon

FENCING (CO-ED TEAM)
Penn State

TRACK AND FIELD (OUTDOOR)
Texas A&M

FOOTBALL (BCS)
Florida

VOLLEYBALL
UC Irvine

GOLF
Texas A&M

WATER POLO
USC

GYMNASTICS
Stanford

WRESTLING
Iowa

WOMEN'S SPORTS
(2008–2009 School Year)

BASKETBALL
Connecticut

BOWLING
Nebraska

CROSS COUNTRY
Washington

FIELD HOCKEY
Maryland

GOLF
Arizona State

GYMNASTICS
Georgia

ICE HOCKEY
Wisconsin

LACROSSE
Northwestern

ROWING
Stanford

SOCCER
North Carolina

SOFTBALL
Washington

SWIMMING AND DIVING
California

TENNIS
Duke

TRACK AND FIELD (INDOOR)
Tennessee

TRACK AND FIELD (OUTDOOR)
Texas A&M

VOLLEYBALL
Penn State

WATER POLO
UCLA

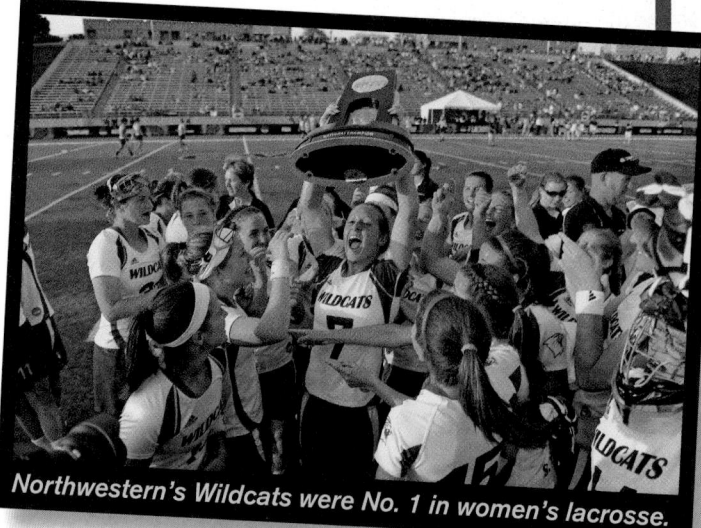

Northwestern's Wildcats were No. 1 in women's lacrosse.

THE BIG EVENTS CALENDAR

September 2009

6 Cycling
Mountain Bike World Championships, Canberra, Australia

9–13 Gymnastics
Rhythmic Gymnastics World Championships, Mie, Japan

10 NFL
Regular season begins

12–13 Tennis
U.S. Open final matches, New York City, New York

21–27 Wrestling
World Championships, Herning, Denmark

24–27 Golf
PGA Tour Championship, Atlanta, Georgia

TBA* NBA
WNBA finals

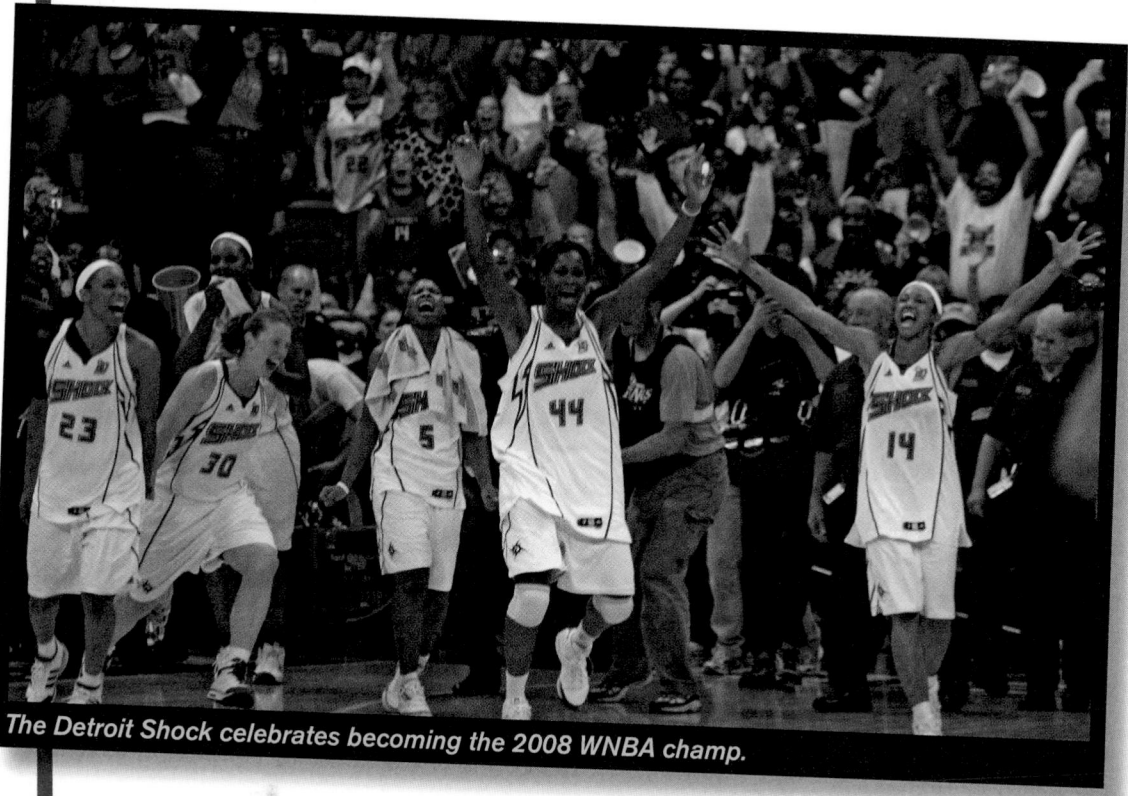

The Detroit Shock celebrates becoming the 2008 WNBA champ.

*TBA: To be announced. Actual dates of event not available at press time.

October 2009

7 MLB
Play-offs begin

8–11 Golf
The President's Cup, Harding Park, San Francisco, California

10 Track
Ironman Triathlon World Championship, Kona, Hawaii

12–18 Gymnastics
World Championships, London, England

14–18 Martial Arts
Taekwondo World Championships, Copenhagen, Denmark

15 MLB
League Championship Series begin

27 MLB
World Series begins

November 2009

1 Running
New York City Marathon

17–27 Weightlifting
World Championships, Goyang City, South Korea

22 NASCAR
Ford 400, Homestead, Florida
Final race of Chase for the Cup championship series

22 Soccer
MLS Cup, Seattle, Washington

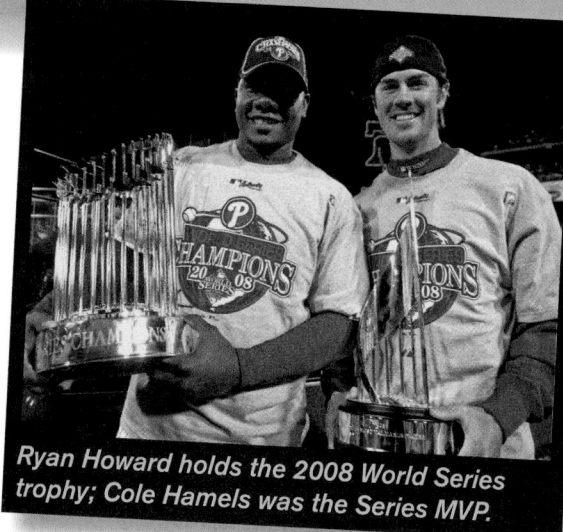

Ryan Howard holds the 2008 World Series trophy; Cole Hamels was the Series MVP.

December 2009

6 College Soccer
Women's championship game, College Station, Texas

5 College Football
ACC championship, Tampa, Florida
SEC championship, Atlanta, Georgia
Big 12 championship, Dallas, Texas

13 College Soccer
Men's championship game, Cary, North Carolina

January 2010

1 College Football
Rose Bowl, Pasadena, California
Allstate Sugar Bowl, New Orleans, Louisiana

4 College Football
Tostitos Fiesta Bowl, Tempe, Arizona

5 College Football
FedEx Orange Bowl, Miami, Florida

7 College Football
Bowl Championship Series national championship game, Pasadena, California

9–10 NFL
Wild-Card Play-off Weekend

14–24 Figure Skating
U.S. Figure Skating World Championships, Spokane, Washington

16–17 NFL
Divisional Play-off Weekend

18–31 Tennis
Australian Open, Melbourne

24 NFL
Conference Championship Games

28–31 Action Sports
Winter X Games, Aspen, Colorado

February 2010

7 NFL
Super Bowl XLIV, Land Shark Stadium, Miami, Florida

12–26 Winter Olympic Games
Vancouver, Canada

14 NBA
NBA All-Star Game, Dallas, Texas

14 NASCAR
Daytona 500, Daytona Beach, Florida

March 2010

7–20 Field Hockey
World Cup, New Delhi, India

22–28 Figure Skating
World Figure Skating Championships, Torino, Italy

April 2010

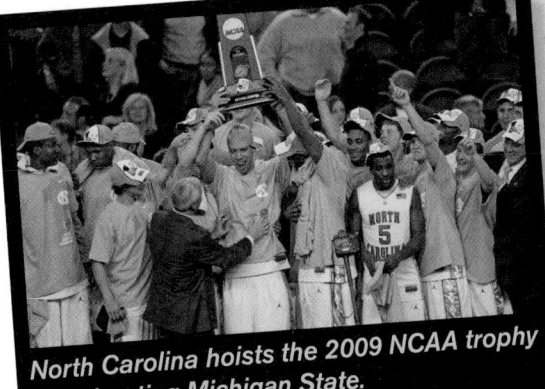

North Carolina hoists the 2009 NCAA trophy after beating Michigan State.

2–6 College Basketball
NCAA Men's and Women's Final Four, Indianapolis, Indiana

5–11 Golf
The Masters, Augusta, Georgia

May 2010

1 Horse Racing
Kentucky Derby, Churchill Downs, Louisville, Kentucky

15 Horse Racing
Preakness Stakes, Pimlico Race Course, Baltimore, Maryland

June 2010

5 Horse Racing
Belmont Stakes, Belmont Park, Elmont, New York

5–6 Tennis
French Open Championships, Paris, France

11 Soccer
World Cup begins in South Africa

TBA* Hockey
Stanley Cup championship series

TBA* NBA
NBA finals

17–20 Golf
U.S. Open Championship, Pebble Beach, California

19 College Baseball
College World Series, Omaha, Nebraska

21 Tennis
All-England Championships at Wimbledon begin

July 2010

1 Cycling
Tour de France begins, Rotterdam, Netherlands

8–11 Golf
U.S. Women's Open, Oakmont, Illinois

11 Soccer
World Cup championship game, Johannesburg, South Africa

13 MLB
All-Star Game, Anaheim, California

15–18 Golf
British Open Championship, St. Andrew's, Scotland

TBA* Action Sports
Summer X Games, site TBA

August 2010

TBA* Golf
LPGA Championship

TBA* Baseball
Little League World Series

12–15 Golf
PGA Championship, Kohler, Wisconsin

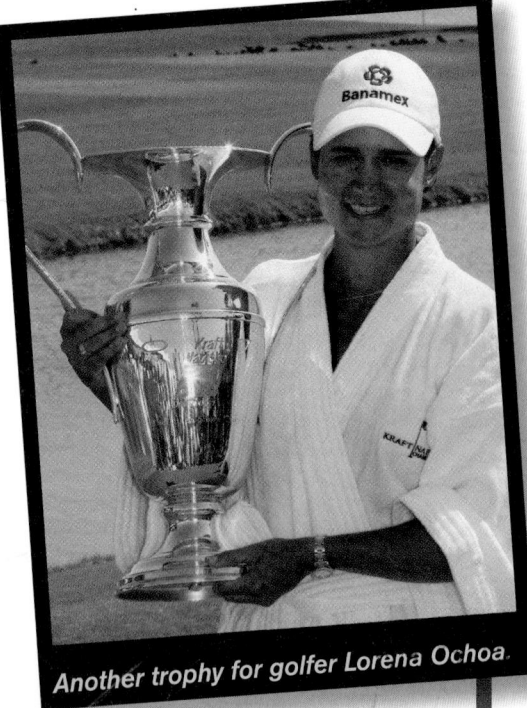

Another trophy for golfer Lorena Ochoa.

*TBA: To be announced. Actual dates of event not available at press time.

Produced by Shoreline Publishing Group LLC

Santa Barbara, California

www.shorelinepublishing.com

President/Editorial Director: James Buckley, Jr.

Designed by Tom Carling, www.carlingdesign.com

The *Year in Sports* text was written by

James Buckley, Jr., & Jim Gigliotti

plus **Craig Zeichner** (NHL), **Ted Keith** (College Basketball), and **John Walters** (College Football).

Thanks to Brenda Murray and her all-star pals at Scholastic for all their extra-inning and overtime help!

Photo research was done by the authors. Thanks to Steve Diamond and Dwayne Howard of Scholastic Picture Services for their assistance in obtaining the photos.

Photography Credits

Front cover, clockwise from top left: AP/Wide World (2); Tom DiPace/Getty Images; Jared Wickersham/Getty Images; Paul Spinelli/Getty Images. Back cover, from top to bottom: Doug Pensinger/Getty Images; Al Bello/Getty Images; AP/Wide World.

Interior: AP/Wide World: 5t, 8, 11, 13, 15, 16, 20, 22, 23, 25 (3), 26t, 31, 32, 33, 38, 39, 40t, 42, 43, 44, 45, 47, 48, 49, 52, 53, 58, 60 (2), 61, 63, 64, 65b, 66, 67t, 69, 72, 74, 76, 77b, 78, 79, 87, 89 (2), 90, 91, 93, 94b, 97, 100, 101, 102, 104, 105, 107, 114t, 115t, 116t, 117, 124, 125b, 126, 127, 129b, 135t, 139b, 144b, 146, 155b, 156, 157, 168, 169b, 171b, 175b, 177b, 179, 181t, 186, 187, 190; Corbis: Chris Williams/Icon SMI: 120; Getty Images (by photographer): AFP: 158, 169t, 172t; Greg Bartram/MLS: 142; Al Bello: 36; Doug Benc: 51, 180; Andrew D. Bernstein/NBA: 85; Lisa Blumenfeld: 30, 172b; Clive Brunskill: 5b, 160; Simon Bruty/SI: 147; David Cannon: 154t, 191; Robert Cianfione: 125t; Timothy A. Clary/AFP: 17, 175t; Collegiate Images: 56; Fabrice Coffrini: 167t; Chris Condon/PGA Tour: 14; Lucas Dawson: 176; Victor Decolongon: 144t; Adrian Dennis: 12; Carl De Souza: 159; Tom DiPace/SI: 151; Kevork Djansezian: 145b; Emmanuel Dunand/AFP: 4, 86; Stephen Dunn: 27l, 50; Craig Durling: 128; Elsa: 65t; D. Clarke Evans/NBA: 95; Express/Hulton Archive: 163; Marc Feldman: 153r, 155t; Jonathan Ferrey: 62; Getty Images: 134; Chris Graythen: 46, 123; Sam Greenwood: 114b, 114t, 115b; Jeff Gross: 28; John Gurzinski/AFP: 173b; Scott Halleran: 154b; John Harrelson: 111, 112b, 113; Jeff Haynes/AFP: 96; Harry How: 103, 139t, 166l; Jed Jacobsohn: 67b; Rusty Jarrett: 110, 122, 129t; Jeff Kardas: 131b; Robert Laberge: 10; Gavin Lawrence: 131t; Library of Congress: 170; D. Lippitt/Einstein/NBA: 92, 188; Andy Lyons: 77t, 170t, 171t; Jerry Markland: 112t; Ronald Martinez: 40, 84; Jim McIsaac: 73, 98; J. Meric: 9; Jonathan Moore: 132; Olivier Morin/AFP: 164; Joe Murphy: 70, 75; Joe Murphy/NBA: 82; Kiyoshi Ota: 167b; Doug Pensinger: 136, 137b, 137t, 140, 166r, 174; Rich Pilling/MLB: 29, 189; Alberto Pizzoli/AFP: 145t; Christian Pondella: 138, 141; Adam Pretty: 162; Mark Ralston/AFP: 173t; Andrew Redington: 152; Ron Rekomaa/AFP: 178; Bob Riha, Jr.: 130; Joe Robbins: 119, 181b; Jim Rogash: 21; Bob Rosato/SI: 59, 80; Kirstin Scholz/ASP: 135b; Gregory Shamus: 88; Ezra Shaw: 26b; Tim Sloan/AFP: 153l; Ron Vesely: 18; Ian Walton: 161; Todd Warshaw: 108; Dennis Wierzbicki: 24; Jonathan Willey/MLB: 27r; Alex Wong: 116b; Andrew Yates/AFP 177l.

PRESENTED BY 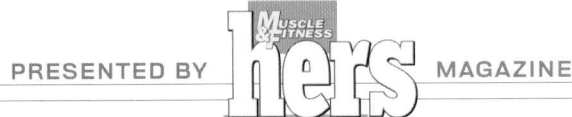 MAGAZINE

101 Fat-Burning
Workouts & Diet Strategies
For Women

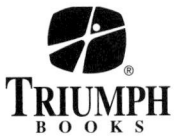

TRIUMPH
BOOKS

BY THE EDITORS OF *MUSCLE & FITNESS HERS*

Acknowledgments

This publication is based on articles written by Devin Alexander, Michelle Basta Boubion, NSCA-CPT, Ruth Carey, Mark Casselman, Mitzi Dulan, Tabatha Elliott, PhD, Kathleen Engel, Lara McGlashan, Robin Vitetta Miller, Jimmy Peña, Gretchen Roberts, Carey Rossi, Debra Wein and Joe Wuebben.

Cover photography by Ian Logan.

Photography by Art Brewer, Michael Darter, Miki Duisterhof, Mark Ferri/Envision, Naj Jamai, John Kelly, Carin Krasner, Marc Lecureuil, Ian Logan, Pornchai Mittongtare, Steven Needham/Envision, Joaquin Palting, Jim Purdum, Tom Rafalovich, Roni Ramos, Robert Reiff, Marc Royce, John Russo and Cory Sorensen.

Project editor is Carey Rossi.

Project managing editor is Vicki Baker.

Project copy editors are Erin Newman and James Riley.

Project design by Michael Touna and KiWon Ballman.

Photo assistant is Amina Cruz.

Editor in Chief/Group Editorial Director of MUSCLE & FITNESS HERS is Peter McGough.
Founding Chairman is Joe Weider. Chairman and CEO of American Media, Inc., is David Pecker.

ISBN: 978-1-60078-206-0

Printed in USA.

101 Fat-Burning Workouts & Diet Strategies
For Women

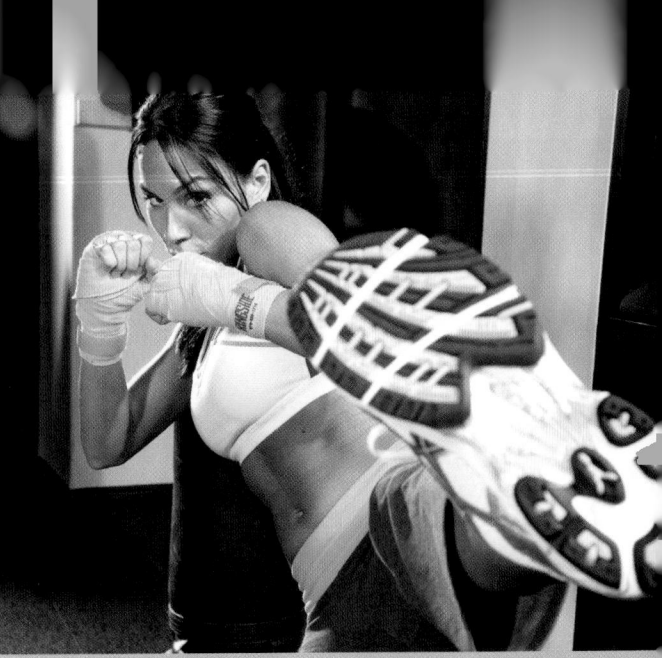

training

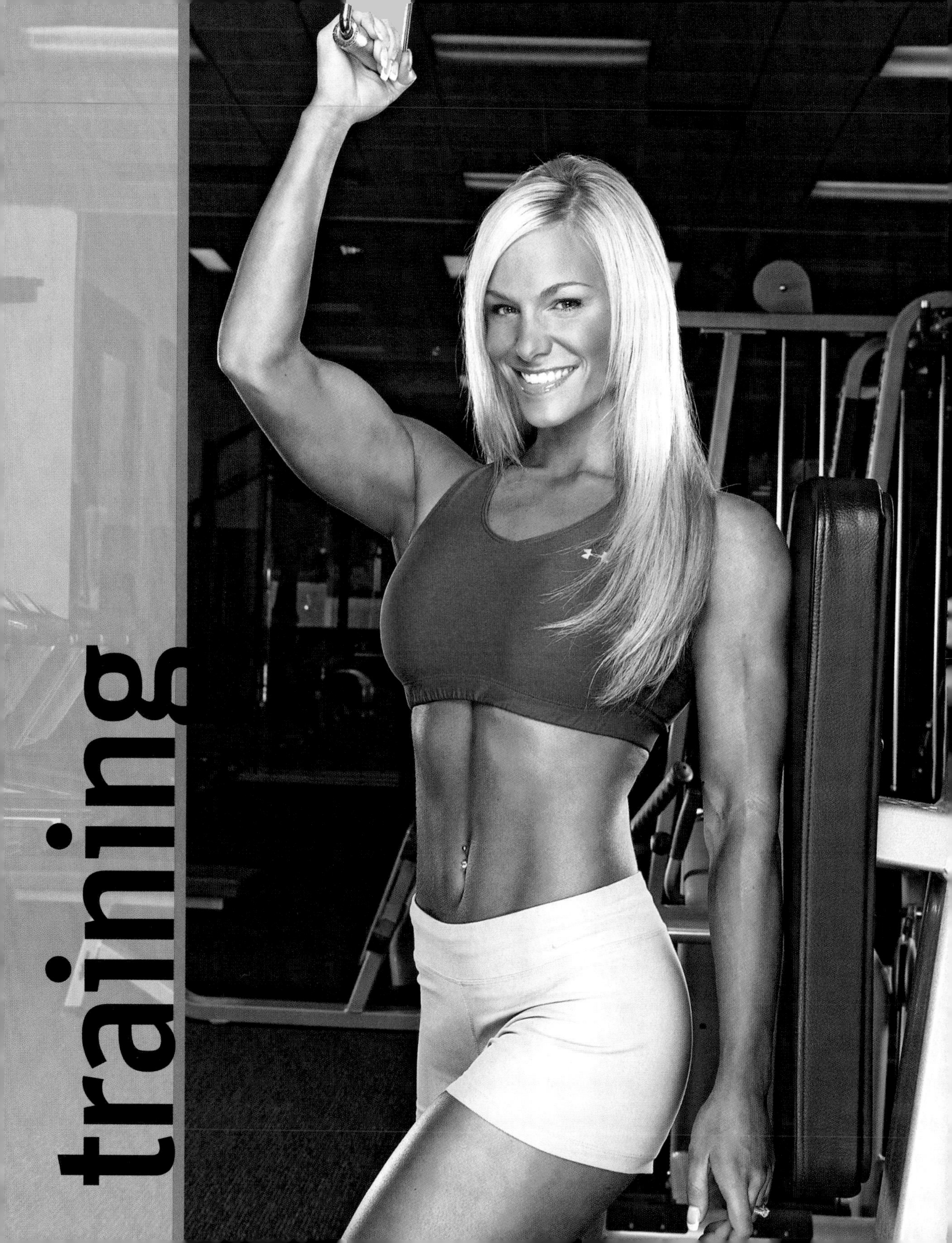

contents

The quest for your best body begins here. Over the next 60 pages you'll find an incredible array of effective exercise programs and routines that have been designed with one goal in mind: To help you lean out while also improve your fitness and strength at the same time. Turn the page to start sculpting the body of your dreams.

 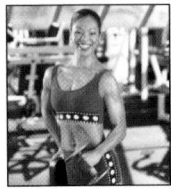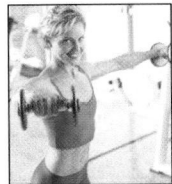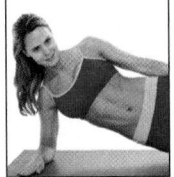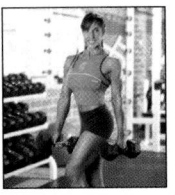

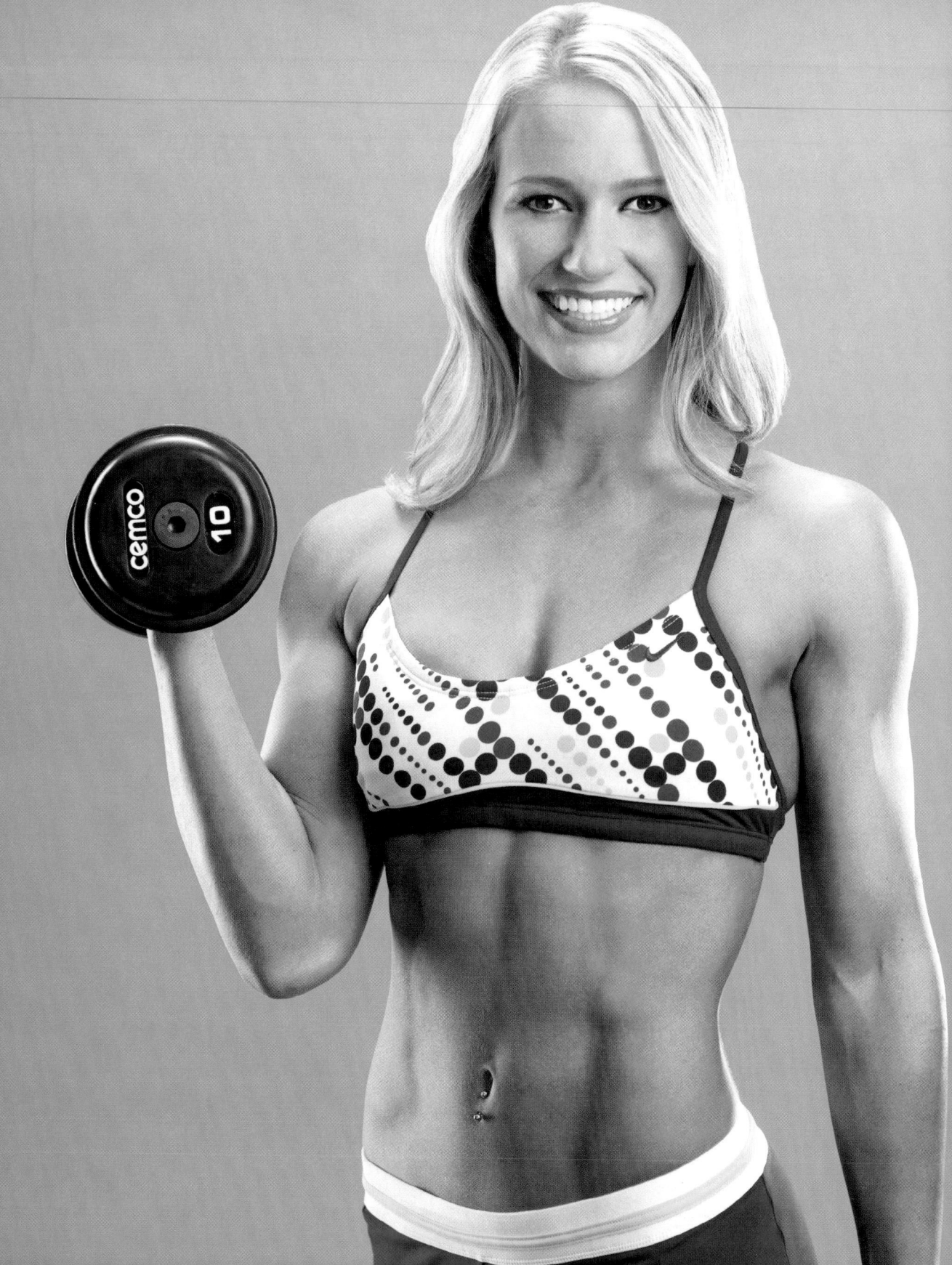

Chapter 1

Look Great In Eight

Burn fat and add sexy curves with this progressive eight-week body blast. Using a menu of exercises, basic training techniques and a calendar to put it all together, you will notice a difference in your physique in two months. The best part is that you get to choose the exercises to do. So forget about [insert your dreaded exercise here]. This program is about sculpting a lean physique and enjoying yourself.

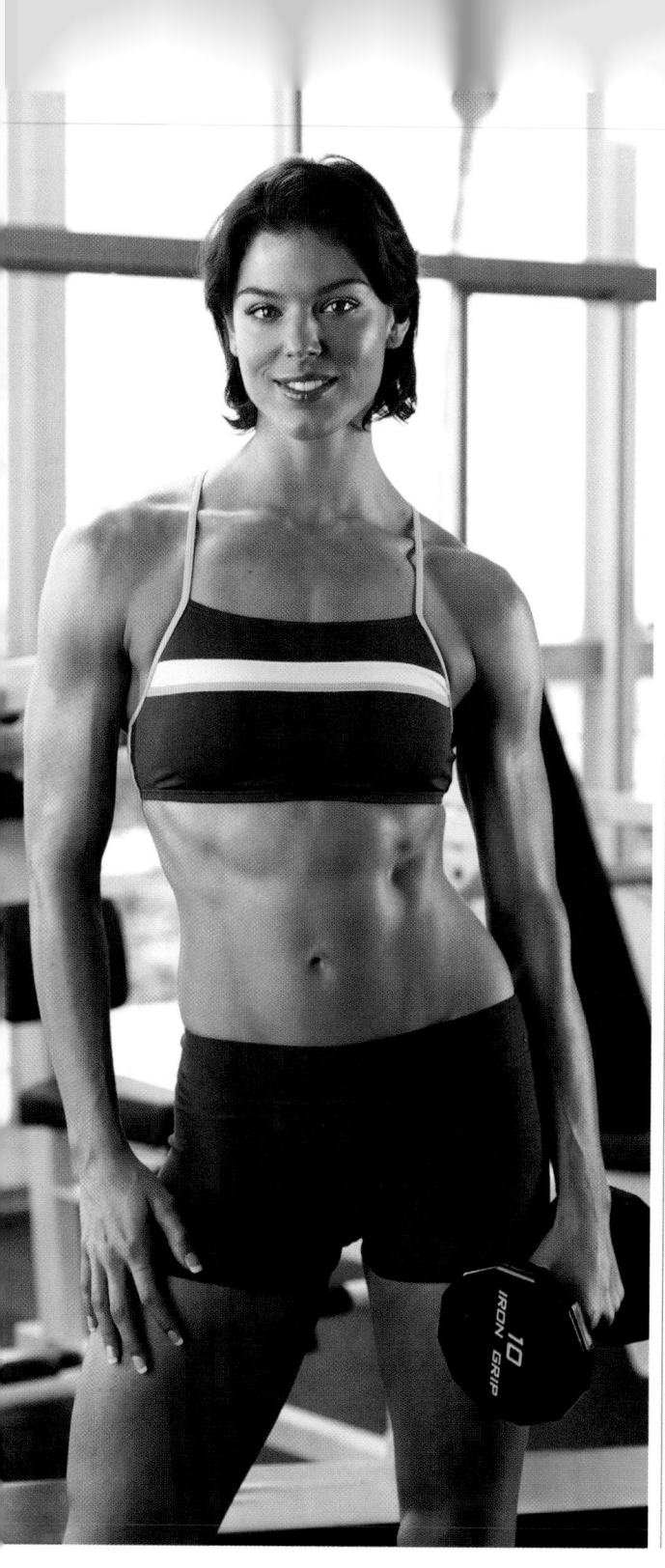

Hey you, the girl with the nice body and serious dedication to fitness. Yes, you! You work out all the time, you've been exercising for years, and even though you've noticed some great changes in your physique, you still want more, don't you? If it's true that the better shape you get in, the higher the bar rises for the shape you want to be in, then this is the workout for you.

Fast-paced and progressively challenging, this eight-week program focuses on increasing muscle tone and definition with an emphasis on wasting fat from your body. It's hardcore, serious and time-consuming. If you follow it — for the results it was intended to produce — be prepared to push your body beyond its comfort zone, further than you've ever taken it before. Be prepared to come out on the other side of eight weeks with a body that sets the standard rather than one that follows.

EIGHT THE HARD WAY

No doubt, this program will have you working hard, fast and often. It has to if it's going to be effective. Nothing good comes easy, but if you do it right, it may come a little quicker, and that's the premise of this workout. Eight weeks is a reasonable amount of time to commit to a serious exercise program without risking burnout, overload or boredom. It's time enough to see and feel your body transform, to reach new heights and realize more of your potential.

If you're looking for a way to lose 20 pounds or to build a fitness-competitor physique, we have to tell you, it's going to take longer than a mere eight weeks. It isn't going to happen in a couple of months, with this program or any other. But what you can expect is to have a stronger, leaner, shapelier body and to feel great about making the time and effort to achieve it.

Each week focuses on a different style of training, which helps to keep your body from becoming accustomed to a particular workout or set of exercises. You'll do circuit, heavy, high-rep and supersets training, repeating the cycle — with few changes — the last four weeks. The cardio portion of the program is progressive, geared to increase in not only frequency, but duration and intensity, as well. This is to kick your body into fat-burning mode, especially in the last few weeks when your metabolism is already burning hotter.

menu of exercises

BACK
Pull-Down
Seated Cable Row
Bent-Over Barbell Row
One-Arm Dumbbell Row
T-Bar Row
Machine Row

CHEST
Flat Bench Press
Push-Up
Dumbbell Flye
Incline Dumbbell Press
Pec-Deck Flye
Seated Machine Press

QUADS|GLUTES
Squat
Stationary Lunge
Walking Lunge
Step-Up
Leg Press
Leg Extension

HAMSTRINGS
Deadlift
Romanian Deadlift
Lying Leg Curl
Flat-Bench
  Dumbbell Leg Curl
Standing One-Leg Curl
Seated Machine
  Hamstring Curl

ABS
Crunch
Hip Thrust
Oblique Crunch
Cable Crunch
Swiss Ball Crunch
  with Feet on Wall
Vertical Bench Leg Raise

BICEPS
EZ-Bar Preacher Curl
Standing Barbell Curl
Cable Hammer Curl (with Rope)
Supinating Dumbbell Curl
Incline Dumbbell Curl
Machine Preacher Curl

TRICEPS
Dumbbell Kickback
Pressdown
Overhead Cable Extension
Lying Triceps Extension
Overhead Dumbbell Extension
Close-Grip Bench Press
Machine Dip

DELTS
Military Press
Arnold Press
Dumbbell Lateral Raise
Bent-Over Dumbbell
  Lateral Raise
Machine Press
Front Barbell Raise

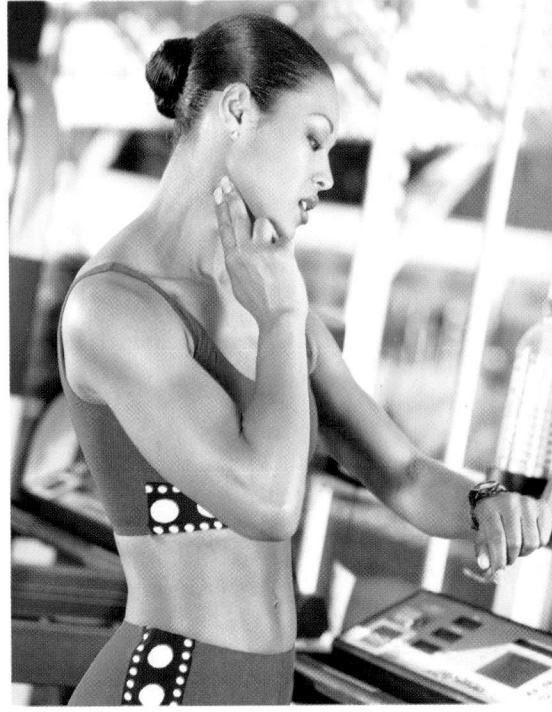

THE FINE PRINT

Don't neglect flexibility training. To help keep muscles supple, reduce the risk of injury and help maintain joint health, warm up for 5–10 minutes with a low-impact activity and then begin your stretch session. Two days of flexibility training are automatically built in. If you'd like to devote more time than that allotted to this part of your training, by all means, go right ahead.

You'll also notice three days during the eight weeks designated as rest days, where you have the day off completely. Don't train on these days — at all. Instead, take the time off to reflect on your level of dedication thus far and appreciate the downtime. Probably your most highly anticipated day will be the dietary cheat days, of which there are three. On these days, you have license to eat whatever you want, within reason. Bon appétit!

When doing the cardio intervals, follow the suggestions for the work-recovery ratios. For example, on a day where you do 30 minutes at 1:1, this means you warm up for five minutes, bump up the intensity for one minute (work), then bring it back down for one minute (recovery). During the work portion of the session, raise your heart rate to 80%–85% — or higher, depending on your level of fitness — then drop it back down to 60%–65% during the recovery phase. You can also extend the work-to-rest periods, as long as they're kept even. So if you'd rather, you can work at a high intensity for two minutes and then recover for two minutes. Or bring those numbers down if you prefer.

When doing resistance and cardio training on the same day, lift first. Hit the weights when your muscles are fresh to reduce the risk of injury. Follow the 90-minute rule: Keep your workouts under 90 minutes in length. As long as you spend your time wisely, you should be able to accomplish all the goals for each day within the time frame. And of course, we can't say it enough: Make sure that you take the time to stretch your muscles to reduce injury and soreness.

WEEK-BY-WEEK BREAKDOWN

#1 WEEK 1

RESISTANCE TRAINING FOCUS: CIRCUIT

Choose one exercise for each major muscle group. Go through the circuit, doing one set of each exercise and resting as little as possible. When finished, start at the beginning and repeat two more times. Choose weights that bring you to momentary muscle failure within 12 reps. This week, you'll work your entire body on three different days in a total-body workout. Rest between sets for only as long as it takes to set up your next exercise.

CARDIO: Do four days of cardio, focusing on long sessions — 40–60 minutes — in a lower heart-rate range. Do one day of higher-intensity intervals for a change of pace. On the recreational cardio day, this is your chance to break away from the routine and engage in whatever activity you enjoy most. You can go for a hike, a long walk, even go dancing; the important thing is to have fun and share the experience with someone.

#2 WEEK 2

RESISTANCE TRAINING FOCUS: HEAVY

Work on the bodyparts indicated for each day. Choose three exercises for each major muscle group being worked and do four sets of 8–10 reps. Lift heavy enough to reach muscle failure by the last couple of reps. Always use the first set of an exercise as a warm-up. This week you'll work each bodypart once in a split routine. Rest between sets will vary, depending on the bodypart being trained, but you'll probably need anywhere from 1–2 minutes to allow some muscle recovery.

CARDIO: This week, cardio sessions will remain at four; however, the emphasis is on higher-intensity training

flexibility training

An often-overlooked part of fitness, flexibility can enhance your workouts, your results and your life. On the designated days, dedicate 15–20 minutes to stretching all the muscle groups you train throughout the week. Below are some basic guidelines to follow, but you'll benefit much more by reading up on stretching and learning more than what we include here. (For explanations and pictures of most of the stretches included below, see the August/September 2001 issue of MUSCLE & FITNESS HERS.)

MUSCLE GROUP	USE THIS MOVE
Back	Upper back pull
Chest	Doorway chest stretch
Quads/Hip flexors	Standing quad pull
Glutes	Glute stretch
Hamstrings	Seated hamstring stretch
Biceps	Biceps pull
Triceps	Overhead triceps pull
Delts	Lateral pull
Low back	Trunk twist

cardio suggestions

The following activities are just a few of the many choices available to you when it comes to fulfilling your cardio requirement each week. Since the focus of this program is fat-burning — and the cardio workouts are progressive — you may need to get creative to avoid tedium. A word to the wise: Don't do the same thing more than twice a week. Keep your body guessing and keep moving toward that goal by varying your cardio activities.

MACHINES	FUN STUFF
Stair-stepper	Swimming laps
Treadmill	In-line skating
Stationary bike	Hiking
Elliptical trainer	Walking
FITNESS CLASSES	Dancing
Studio cycling	Outdoor cycling
Step	Running
Kickboxing	
Low impact	

— keeping your heart rate up for a relatively short amount of time. Three workouts will be 25–30 minutes long at 80%–85% of your max heart rate, with one long, lower-intensity day thrown in for variety.

#3 WEEK 3
RESISTANCE TRAINING FOCUS: HIGH REPS
Work on the bodyparts indicated for each day. Choose three exercises for each major muscle group being worked and do three sets of 15–20 reps. Choose weights heavy enough to fatigue your muscles within the suggested rep range. This week you'll work each bodypart twice in a split routine. Rest between sets should last 60–90 seconds.
CARDIO: Bumped up to five times this week, you'll train for 30–40 minutes at 70%–75% of your max heart rate during four of the sessions. You'll also do one session of higher-intensity intervals for 30 minutes.

#4 WEEK 4
RESISTANCE TRAINING FOCUS: SUPERSETS
This is where you work two muscle groups back to back with no rest. For example, when you train biceps and triceps, you'll do a set of dumbbell curls, then without rest, go straight into an overhead dumbbell extension. Work on the two bodyparts indicated for each day. Choose three exercises for each major muscle group being worked and do three sets. Choose weights heavy enough to reach muscle failure in 12 reps. Move quickly between exercises, resting as little as possible. This week, you'll train each bodypart only once. Take no downtime between sets here: Move right from one exercise to the other.
CARDIO: Staying at five sessions this week, most cardio sessions will last 25–30 minutes and you'll train at 75%–80% of your max heart rate. Of course, one workout will consist of training at a lower intensity for a longer period.

WEEK 5
RESISTANCE TRAINING FOCUS: CIRCUIT
Follow guidelines for Week 1.
CARDIO: Sessions are similar. The only change is an extra day of cardio.

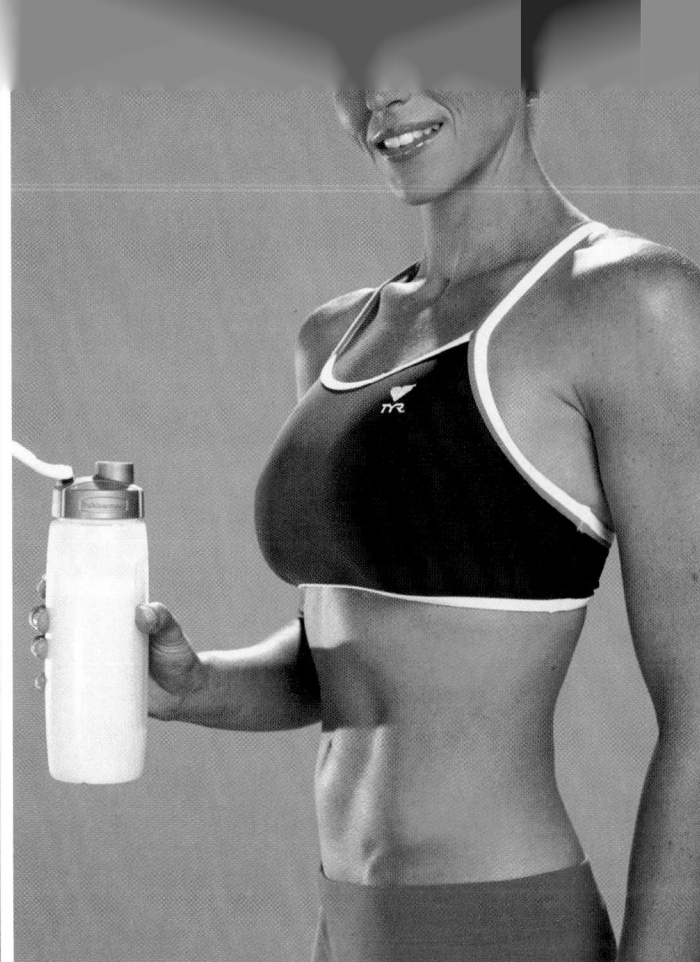

WEEK 6
RESISTANCE TRAINING FOCUS: HEAVY
Follow guidelines for Week 2.
CARDIO: Sessions are similar. The only change is an extra day of cardio.

WEEK 7
RESISTANCE TRAINING FOCUS: HIGH REPS
Follow guidelines for Week 3. Bodyparts trained together will differ from Week 3.
CARDIO: Sessions are similar. The only change is an extra day of cardio.

WEEK 8
RESISTANCE TRAINING FOCUS: SUPERSETS
Follow guidelines for Week 4. Bodyparts trained together will differ from Week 4.
CARDIO: Sessions are similar. The only change is an extra day of cardio.

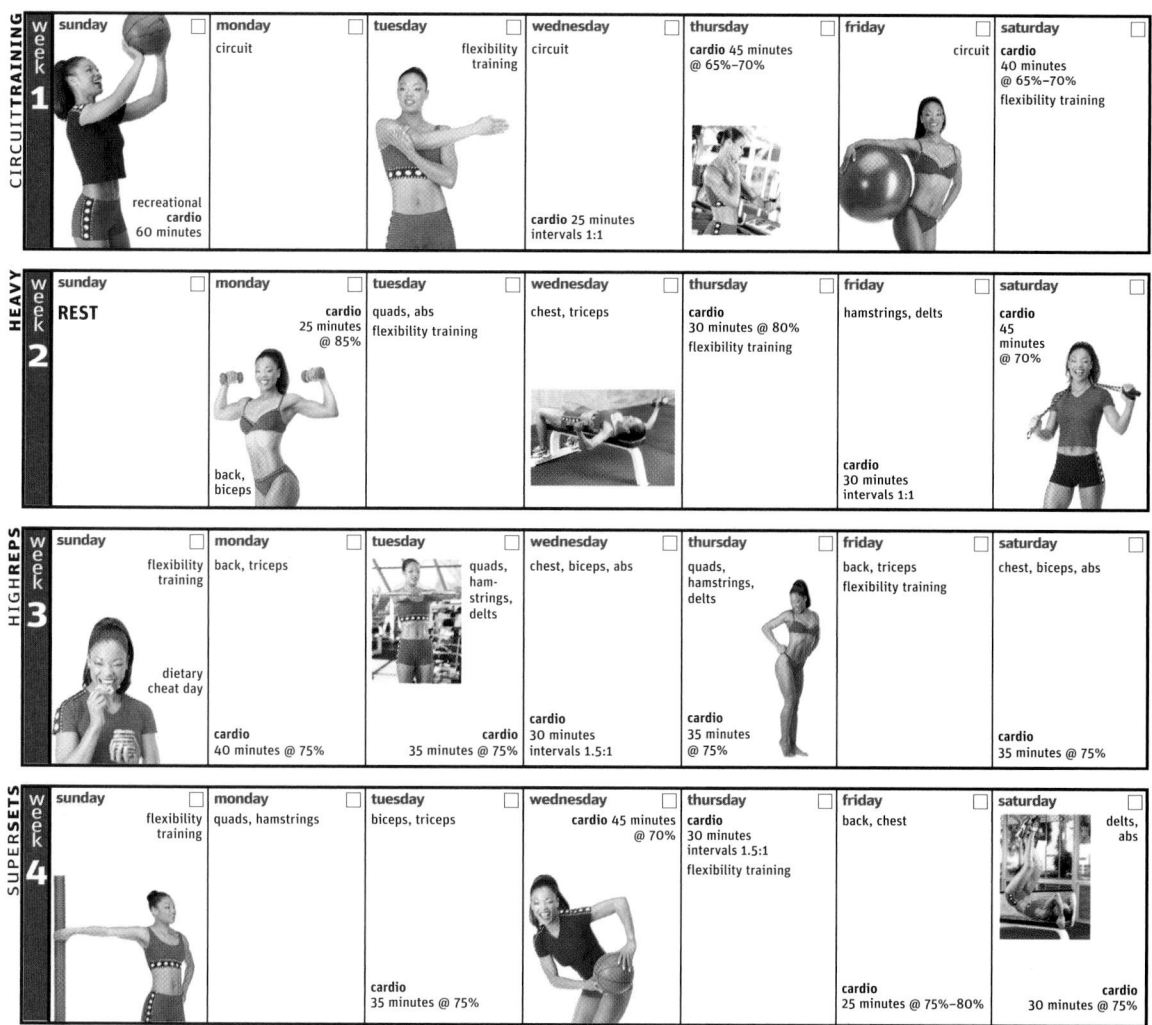

CIRCUIT TRAINING — week 1

	sunday	monday	tuesday	wednesday	thursday	friday	saturday
	recreational **cardio** 60 minutes	circuit	flexibility training	circuit / **cardio** 25 minutes intervals 1:1	**cardio** 45 minutes @ 65%–70%	circuit	**cardio** 40 minutes @ 65%–70% / flexibility training

HEAVY — week 2

	sunday	monday	tuesday	wednesday	thursday	friday	saturday
	REST	**cardio** 25 minutes @ 85% / back, biceps	quads, abs / flexibility training	chest, triceps	**cardio** 30 minutes @ 80% / flexibility training	hamstrings, delts / **cardio** 30 minutes intervals 1:1	**cardio** 45 minutes @ 70%

HIGH REPS — week 3

	sunday	monday	tuesday	wednesday	thursday	friday	saturday
	flexibility training / dietary cheat day / **cardio** 40 minutes @ 75%	back, triceps / **cardio** 35 minutes @ 75%	quads, hamstrings, delts	chest, biceps, abs / **cardio** 30 minutes intervals 1.5:1	quads, hamstrings, delts / **cardio** 35 minutes @ 75%	back, triceps / flexibility training	chest, biceps, abs / **cardio** 35 minutes @ 75%

SUPERSETS — week 4

	sunday	monday	tuesday	wednesday	thursday	friday	saturday
	flexibility training	quads, hamstrings	biceps, triceps / **cardio** 35 minutes @ 75%	**cardio** 45 minutes @ 70%	**cardio** 30 minutes intervals 1.5:1 / flexibility training	back, chest / **cardio** 25 minutes @ 75%–80%	delts, abs / **cardio** 30 minutes @ 75%

week-by-week breakdown

week 1 CIRCUIT**TRAINING**

Train your entire body three times this week. Choose one exercise for each major muscle group listed and go through the circuit three times. Do 12 reps with a weight that brings you to momentary muscle failure within 12 reps and rest as little as possible. Rest between sets for only as long as it takes to set up your next exercise. Do three days of cardio — 40–60 minutes each — in a lower heart-rate range. Do one day of higher-intensity intervals for a change of pace. On the recreational cardio day, choose something fun that you enjoy.

week 2 HEAVY

Train each bodypart once, choosing three exercises for each major muscle group. Do four sets of 8–10 reps. Lift heavy enough to reach muscle failure by the last couple of reps. Always use the first set of an exercise for a new bodypart as a warm-up. Rest roughly 1–2 minutes between sets. Do four cardio sessions with an emphasis on higher-intensity training — keeping your heart rate up for a relatively short amount of time. Three workouts will be 25–30 minutes long at 80%–85% of your max heart rate, with one long, lower-intensity day.

week 3 HIGH**REPS**

Train each bodypart twice, choosing three exercises for each major muscle group being worked. Do three sets of 15–20 reps with weights heavy enough to fatigue your muscles within the suggested rep range. Rest 60–90 seconds between sets. Do five cardio sessions this week, 30–40 minutes at 70%–75% of your max heart rate during four of the sessions. Do one session of higher-intensity intervals for 30 minutes.

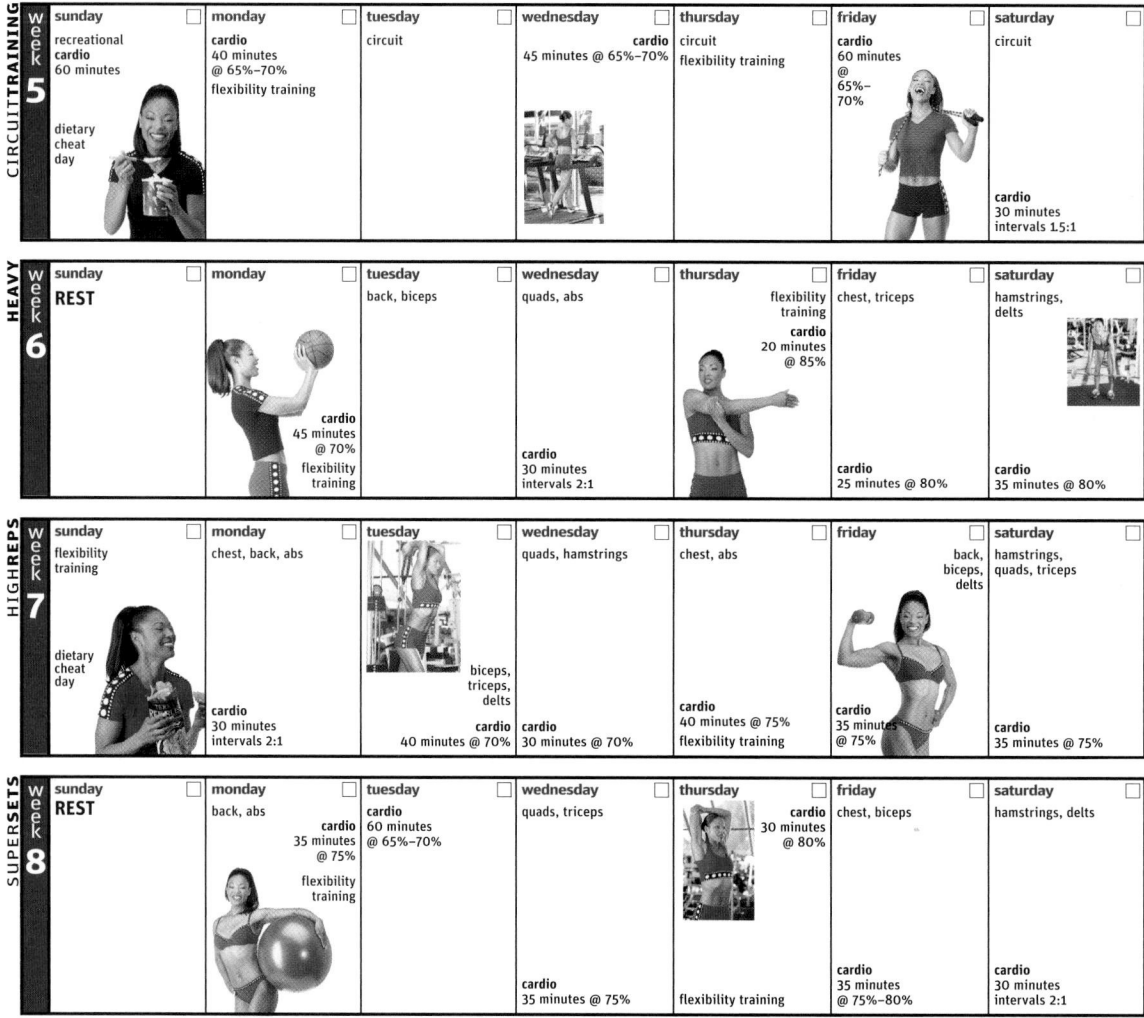

Week 5 — CIRCUIT TRAINING

sunday	monday	tuesday	wednesday	thursday	friday	saturday
recreational **cardio** 60 minutes	**cardio** 40 minutes @ 65%–70% flexibility training	circuit	**cardio** 45 minutes @ 65%–70%	circuit flexibility training	**cardio** 60 minutes @ 65%–70%	circuit
dietary cheat day						**cardio** 30 minutes intervals 1.5:1

Week 6 — HEAVY

sunday	monday	tuesday	wednesday	thursday	friday	saturday
REST		back, biceps	quads, abs	flexibility training **cardio** 20 minutes @ 85%	chest, triceps	hamstrings, delts
	cardio 45 minutes @ 70% flexibility training		**cardio** 30 minutes intervals 2:1		**cardio** 25 minutes @ 80%	**cardio** 35 minutes @ 80%

Week 7 — HIGH REPS

sunday	monday	tuesday	wednesday	thursday	friday	saturday
flexibility training	chest, back, abs	biceps, triceps, delts	quads, hamstrings	chest, abs	back, biceps, delts	hamstrings, quads, triceps
dietary cheat day **cardio** 30 minutes intervals 2:1		**cardio** 40 minutes @ 70%	**cardio** 30 minutes @ 70%	**cardio** 40 minutes @ 75% flexibility training	**cardio** 35 minutes @ 75%	**cardio** 35 minutes @ 75%

Week 8 — SUPERSETS

sunday	monday	tuesday	wednesday	thursday	friday	saturday
REST	back, abs **cardio** 35 minutes @ 75% flexibility training	**cardio** 60 minutes @ 65%–70%	quads, triceps	**cardio** 30 minutes @ 80%	chest, biceps	hamstrings, delts
			cardio 35 minutes @ 75%	flexibility training	**cardio** 35 minutes @ 75%–80%	**cardio** 30 minutes intervals 2:1

week-by-week breakdown

week 4 SUPERSETS
Train each bodypart only once, working two muscle groups back to back with no rest in between. Choose three exercises, doing three sets of 12 reps. Choose weights heavy enough to reach muscle failure in 12 reps. Move quickly between exercises, resting as little as possible. Do five cardio sessions this week, most of which will last 25–30 minutes at 75%–80% of your max heart rate. Do one workout at a lower intensity for a longer period and one interval workout.

week 5 CIRCUIT TRAINING
Follow guidelines given for Week 1. Cardio sessions are similar. The only change is the extra day of cardio.

week 6 HEAVY
Follow guidelines given for Week 2. Cardio sessions are similar. The only change is the extra day of cardio.

week 7 HIGH REPS
Follow guidelines for Week 3. Bodyparts trained together will differ from Week 3. Cardio sessions are similar. The only change is the extra day of cardio.

week 8 SUPERSETS
Follow guidelines for Week 4. Bodyparts trained together will differ from Week 4. Cardio sessions are similar. The only change is the extra day of cardio.
Congratulations, you've made it!

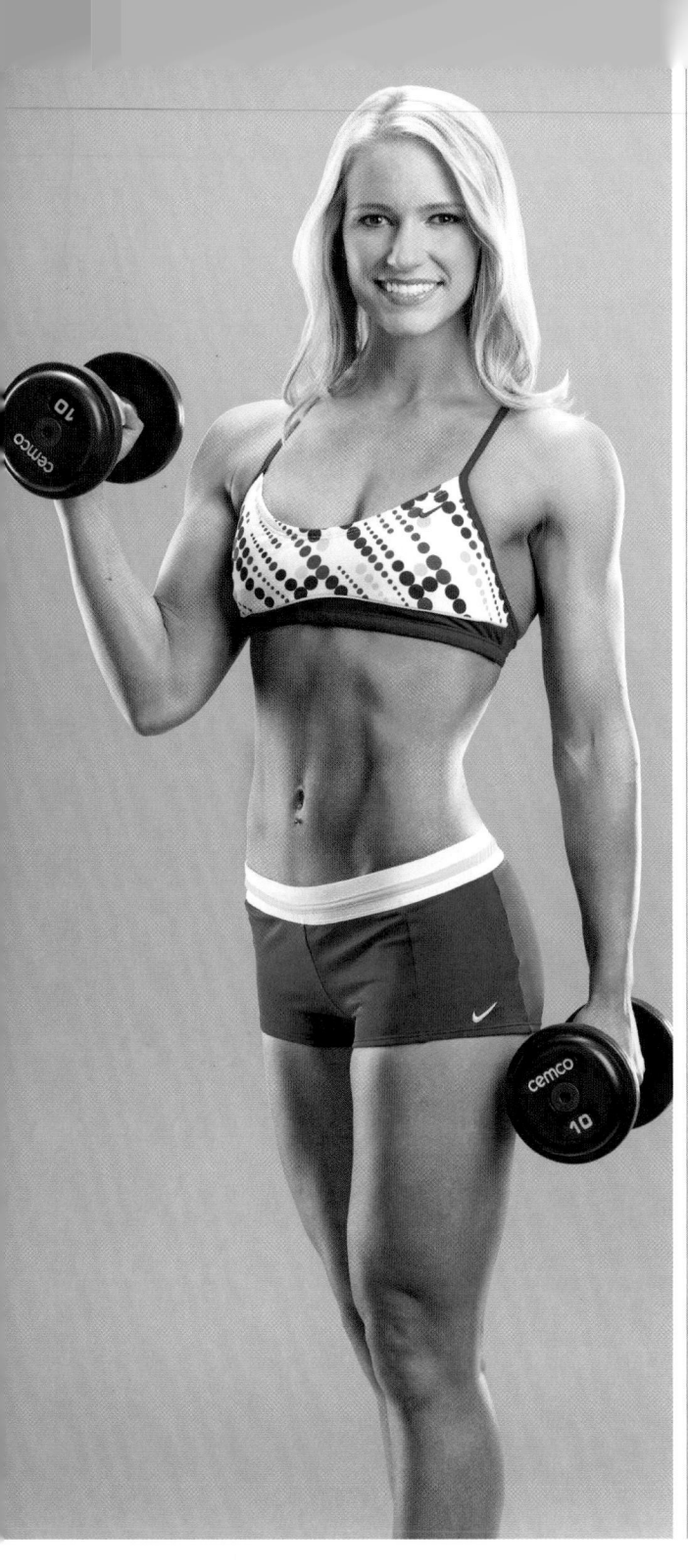

STICKING WITH IT

If after the eight weeks you like what you've accomplished and want to keep going, it's simple to do. Since the program already has variations built in, you can repeat the eight weeks over again, making small changes such as introducing new exercises into the mix and matching up different bodyparts to train together the second time around. You can also try breaking up the workouts into a.m. and p.m. splits: Do cardio in the morning and weight training in the evening. If you really want to blast whatever fat you might still want to lose, try doing cardio twice a day a couple of days a week (also in the a.m. and p.m.). Just remember to keep the intensity low and go long. (You could also follow "The Next Level" program in Chapter 2.) Finally, to keep the fire burning, schedule in a week of rest every once in a while. This gives both your mind and your body a much-needed break, helping you to return to the gym renewed, refreshed and ready to go!

IF YOU'RE A BEGINNER ...

Don't be discouraged by the hardcore nature of this program. With a few modifications, you can follow along and expect an even more dramatic change in your mind and body than those who've been doing this a long time. Instead of following the calendar as it's given, make these changes and then proceed (after getting your doctor's approval, of course).*

• Weeks 1–4: Follow the circuit format of resistance training. Choose one exercise per bodypart and do two rounds of each, keeping reps at 12–15. Do not go to muscle failure. Cut all cardio sessions down to 20 minutes and delete the interval days.

• Weeks 5–8: Follow the high-rep suggestions of weeks 3 and 7. Choose two exercises for each bodypart and do two sets of 15–20 reps for each. Again, don't go to muscle failure; there's plenty of time for that later. Do four days of cardio, two days at 20 minutes and two days at 25 minutes, if possible. Keep your heart rate steady at 65%–70% of your max.

* Consult your physician before starting a workout program if you're inactive, have a health condition or if you plan to increase the frequency, duration and intensity.

abs

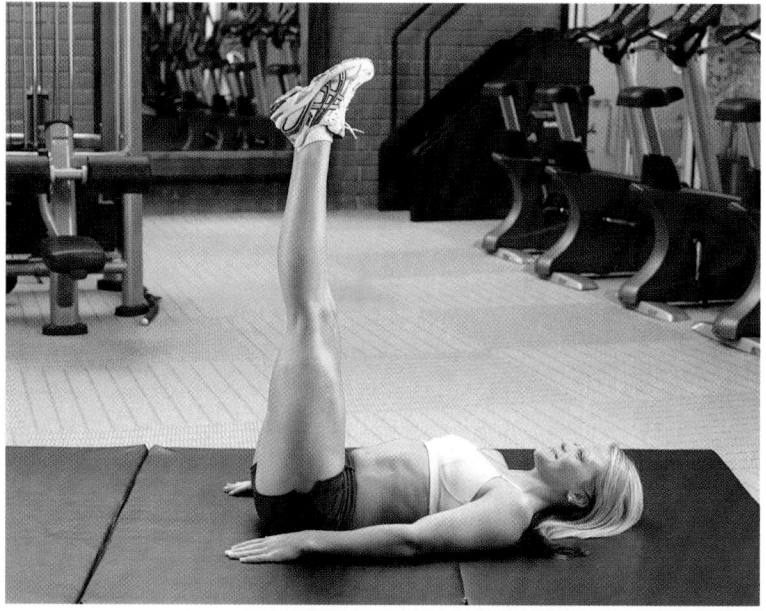

Hip Thrust

Lie face-up on the floor with your hands extended at your sides. Lift your feet up so your legs are roughly perpendicular to the floor. Contract your abs to raise your hips and glutes straight up off the ground, pushig your feet toward the ceiling. Hold this position for a count before lowering your glutes back to the floor. Repeat for reps.

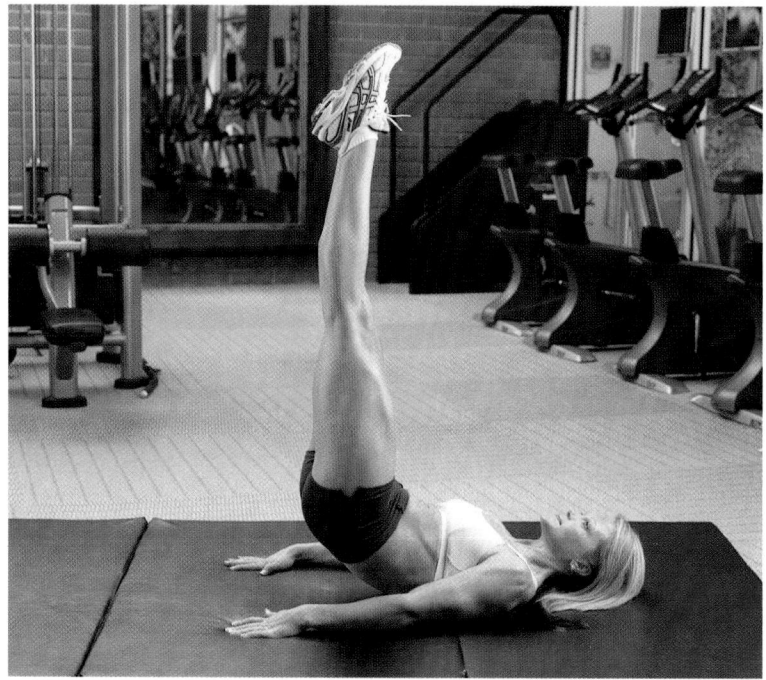

delts

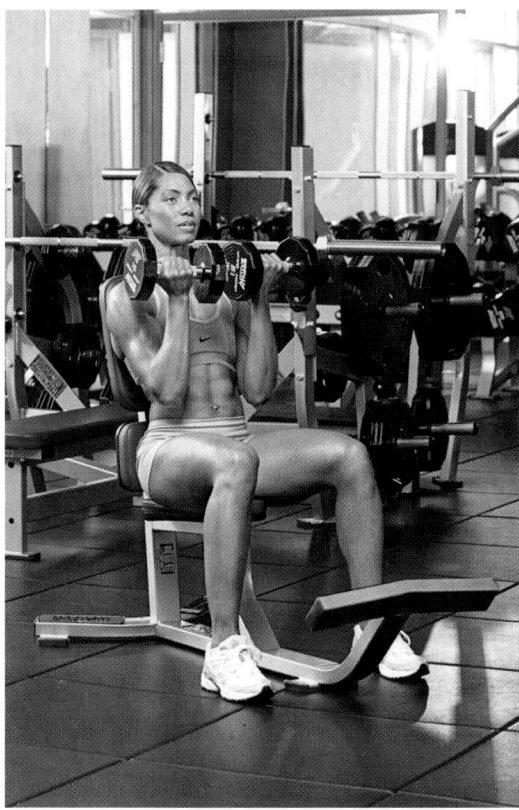

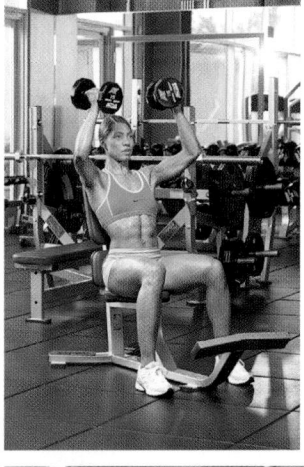

Arnold Press

Sit in a low-back bench and hold a dumbbell in each hand above shoulder level with a pronated grip (palms facing forward), your head straight and eyes focused forward. Keeping your shoulders back, press the dumbbells overhead in an arc, but don't let the weights touch at the top. Slowly reverse the motion to return to the start position.

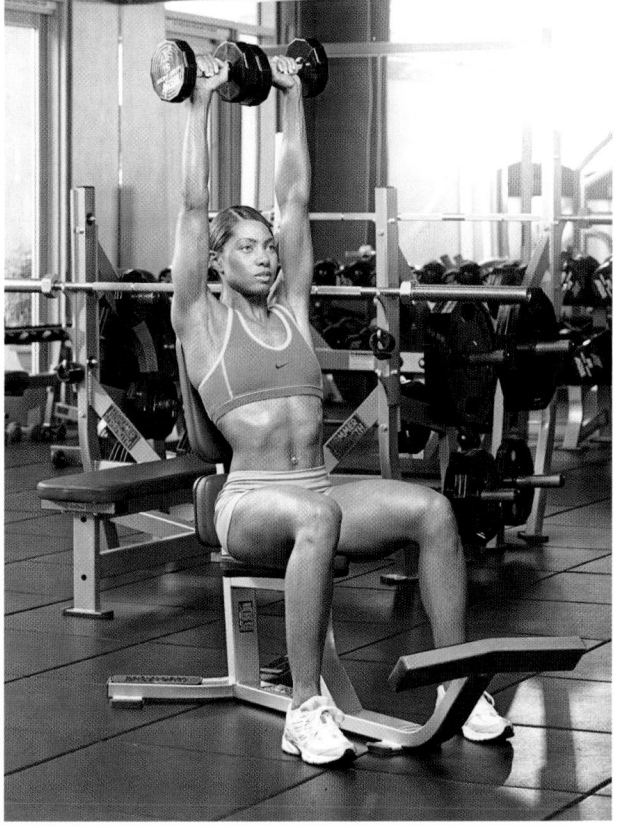

quads

Leg Press

Sit squarely in the leg press machine and place your feet on the sled, shoulder-width apart. Keeping your chest up and lower back pressed into the back support, carefully unlock the weight from the safeties. Bend your knees to lower the weight, stopping before your glutes lift off the pad. Hold for a brief count, then extend your legs to press the weight up, stopping just short of locking out your knees. Squeeze your legs hard at the top, then repeat for reps.

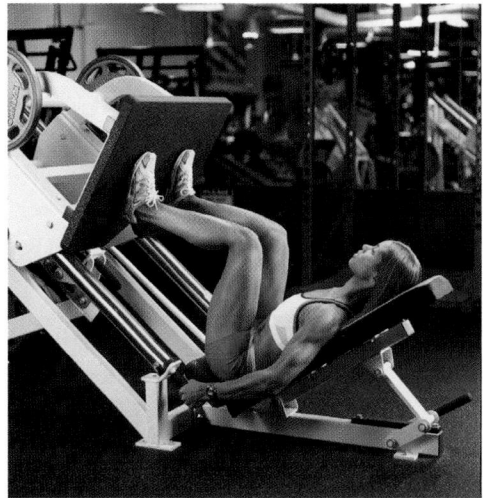

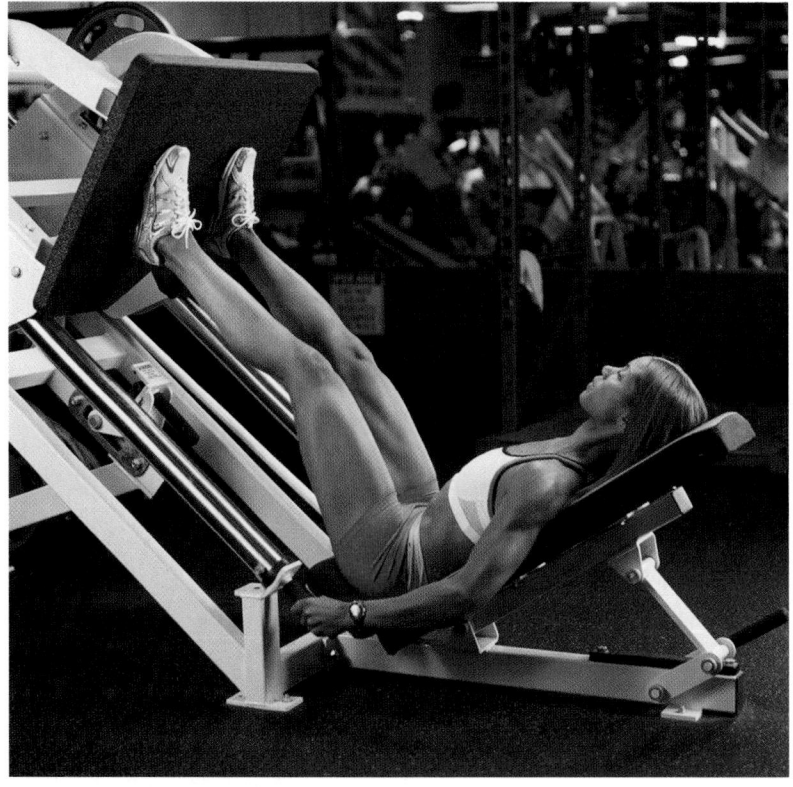

back

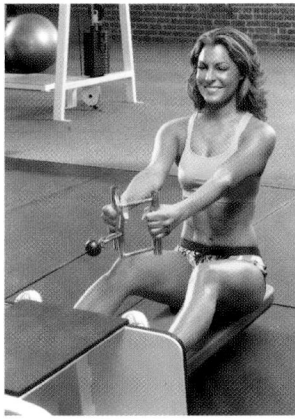

Seated Cable Row

Attach a close-grip handle to a row apparatus and sit upright on the bench facing the weight stack. Place your feet on the platform, legs slightly bent. Reach forward to grasp the handles; keep your back flat and chest up. With your torso erect, arms fully extended, pull the handles toward your midsection. Keep your elbows in, your torso erect and your head in a neutral position. Squeeze your back muscles. Hold for 1-2 seconds before slowly reversing the motion to return to the start position.

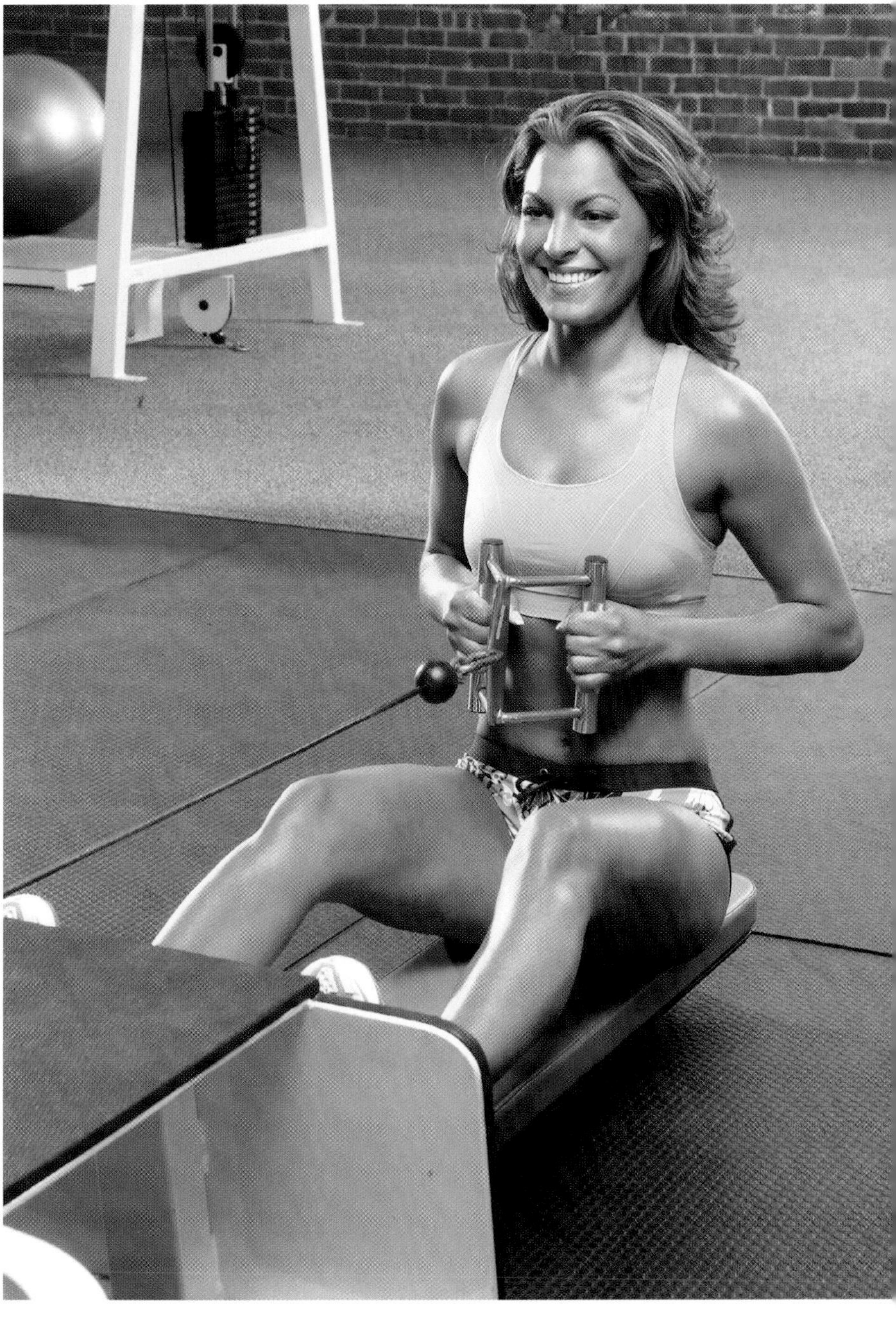

hams

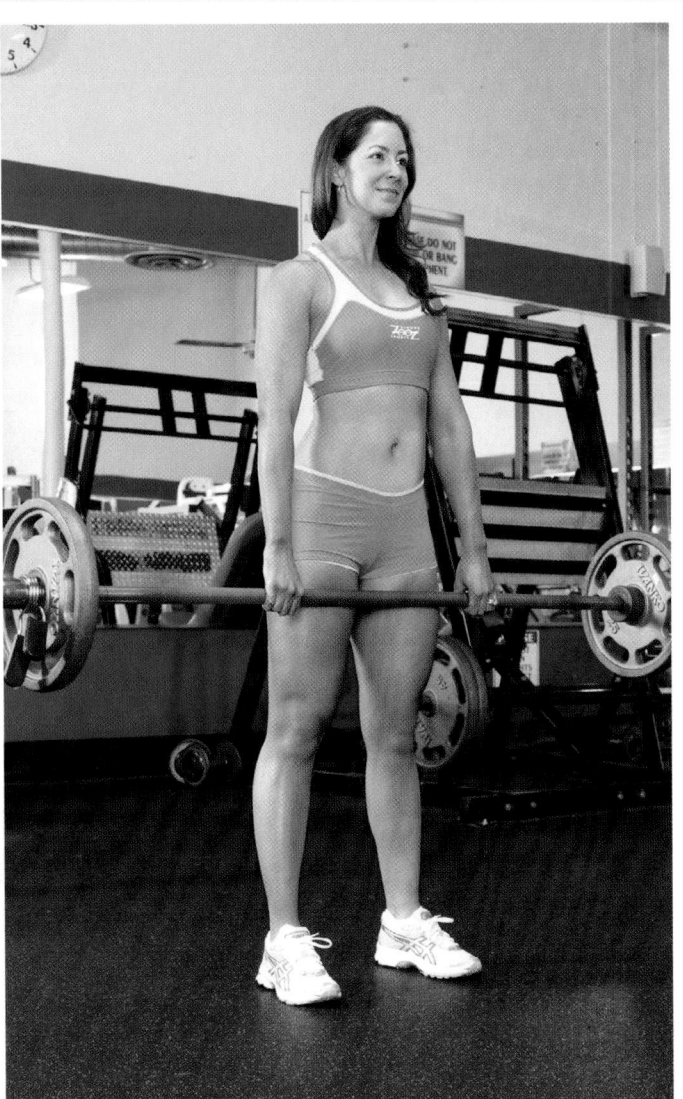

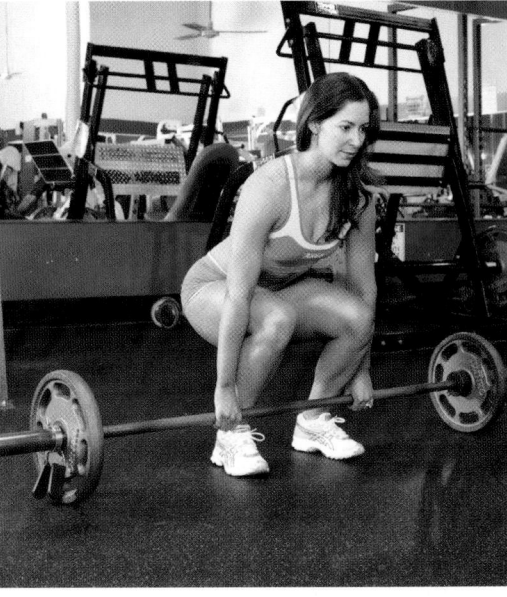

Deadlift

Feet flat under a bar, squat down and take a slightly wider than shoulder-width grip. Allow the bar to rest against your shins. With your chest up and back flat, lift the bar by extending your hips and knees fully. Keep your arms straight throughout the movement, as you drag the bar up your legs till you are in a standing position. Squeeze your back, legs and glutes, then lower the bar along the same path until it touches the floor. Allow the bar to settle before beginning the next rep.

hams

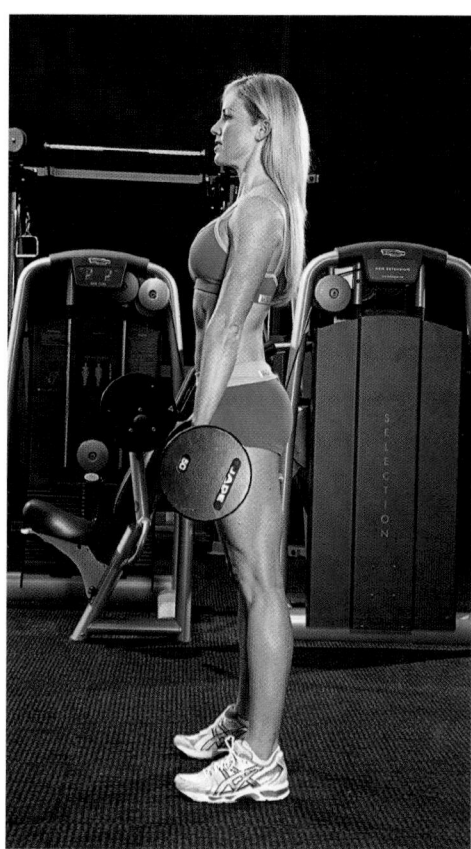
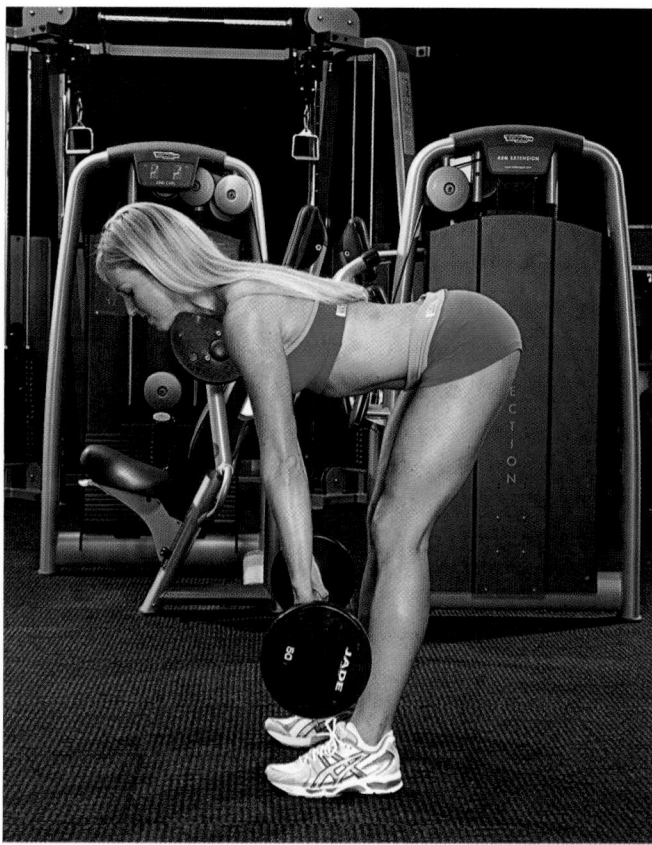

Romanian Deadlift

Stand upright holding a barbell in front of your upper thighs with a pronanted (overhand) grip. Keep your feet shoulder-width apart and a slight bend in your knees. Keeping your chest up, abs tight and the natural arch in your low back, lean forward from your hips, pushing them rearward until your torso is roughly parallel to the floor. As you lean forward, keep your arms straight and slide the bar down your thighs toward the floor until it reaches your shins. At the bottom, keep your back flat, head neutral and the bar very close to your legs. Flex your hamstrings and glutes and lift your torso while pushing your hips forward until you bring the bar back to the start position.

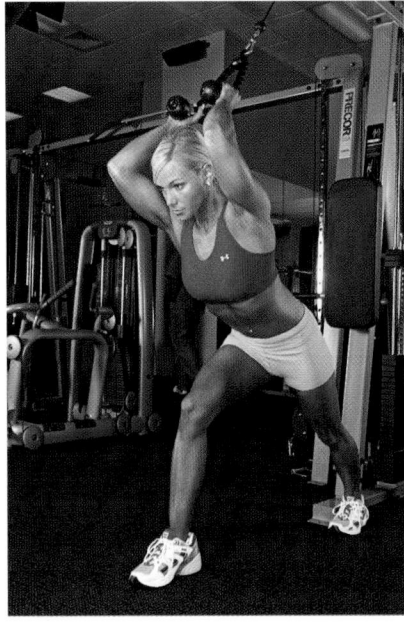

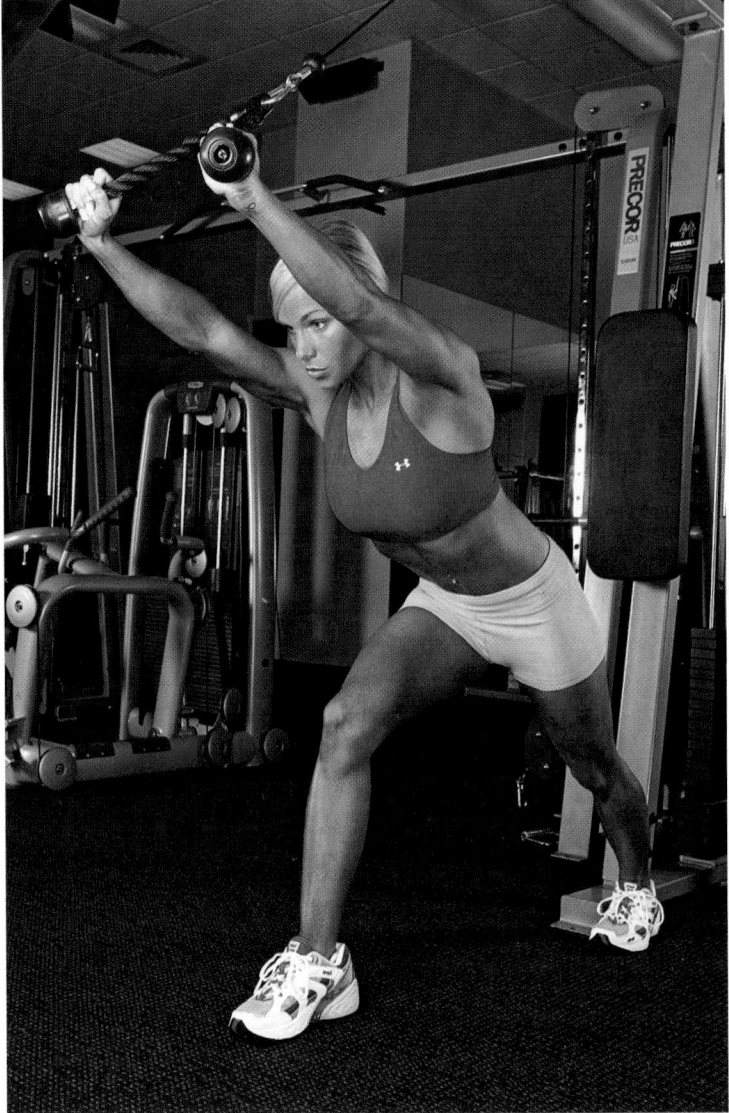

Overhead Cable Extension

Sit or stand facing away from a high cable pulley. Grasp a straight bar or rope (shown) attachment with your arms bent at 90 degrees. Squeeze your triceps as you straighten your arms to full extension. Hold for 1-2 seconds then reverse the motion to return to the start position. Repeat for reps.

biceps

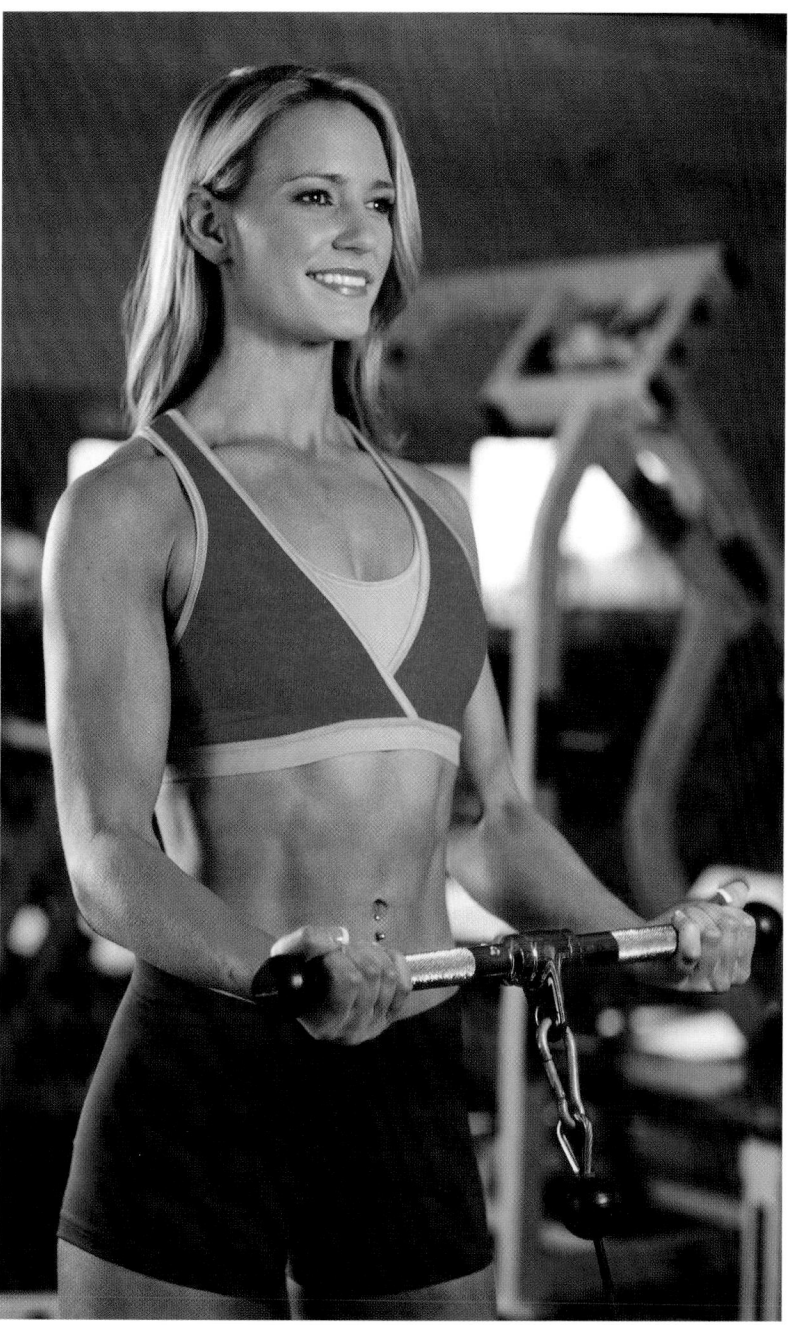

Cable Curl

Stand facing a cable weight stack. Attach a curl bar to the low pulley cable. Take an underhand, shoulder-width grip on the bar. With abs tight, chest up and head straight, contract your biceps to curl the bar toward your chest, keeping your elbows at your sides. Hold and squeeze at the top, then slowly return the bar along the same path. Repeat for reps.

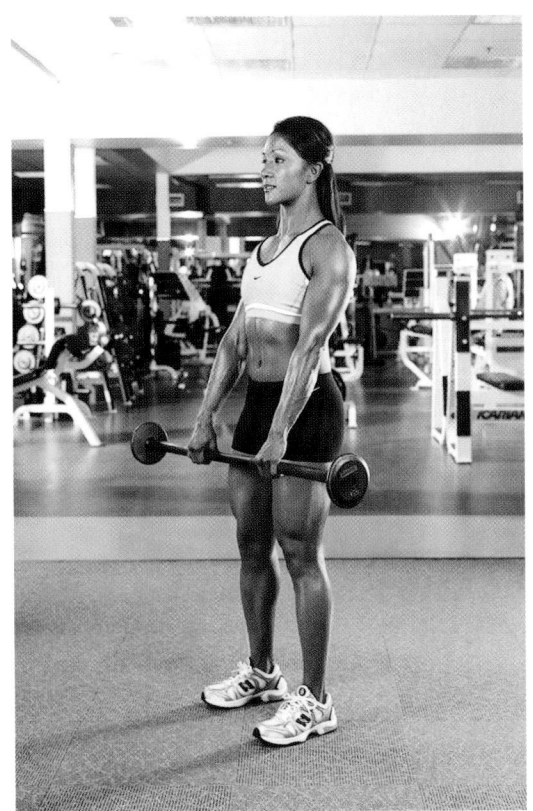
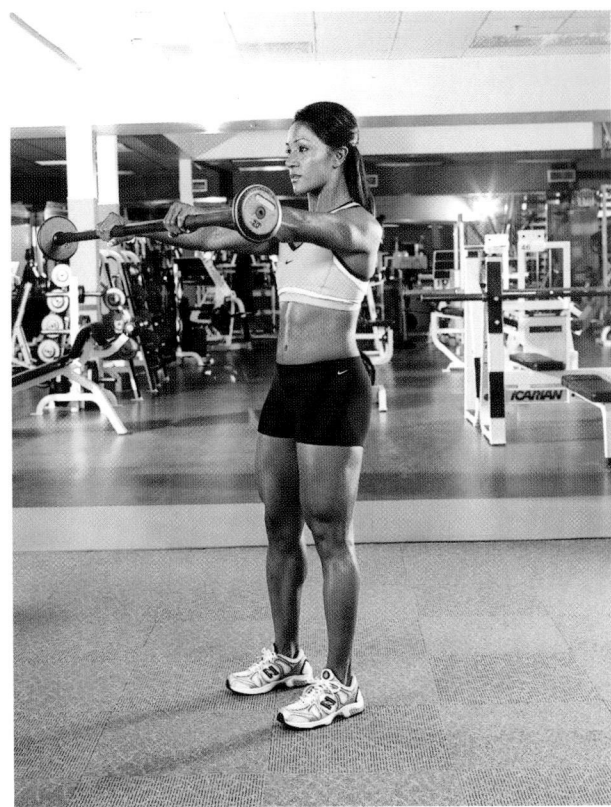

Front Barbell Raise

Stand holding a loaded barbell directly in front of your thighs, your abs tight and chest up. Keeping your arms straight, raise the barbell in front of you just above parallel to the floor. Pause, then lower to the start position and repeat for reps.

chest

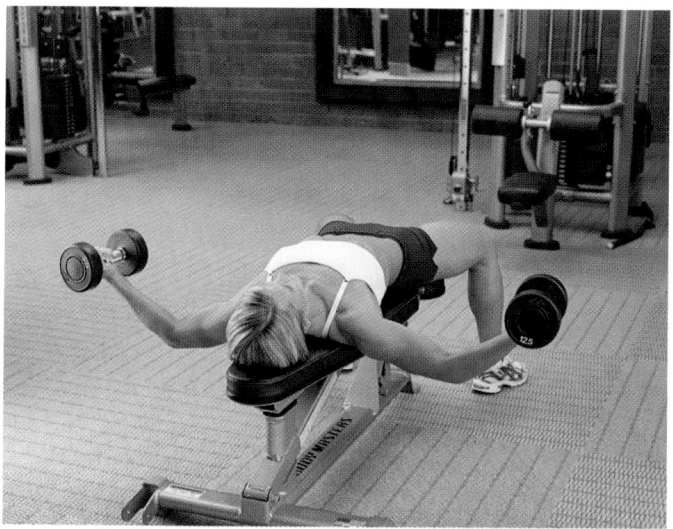

Dumbbell Flye

Lie face-up on the bench with your feet flat on the floor. Hold a dumbbell in each hand with a neutral grip and extend your arms above your chest. Bend your elbows slightly. Slowly lower the dumbbells in a wide arc down to your sides. Keep your elbows locked in the slightly bent position throughout the movement. Stop when your elbows reach shoulder level before reversing the motion.

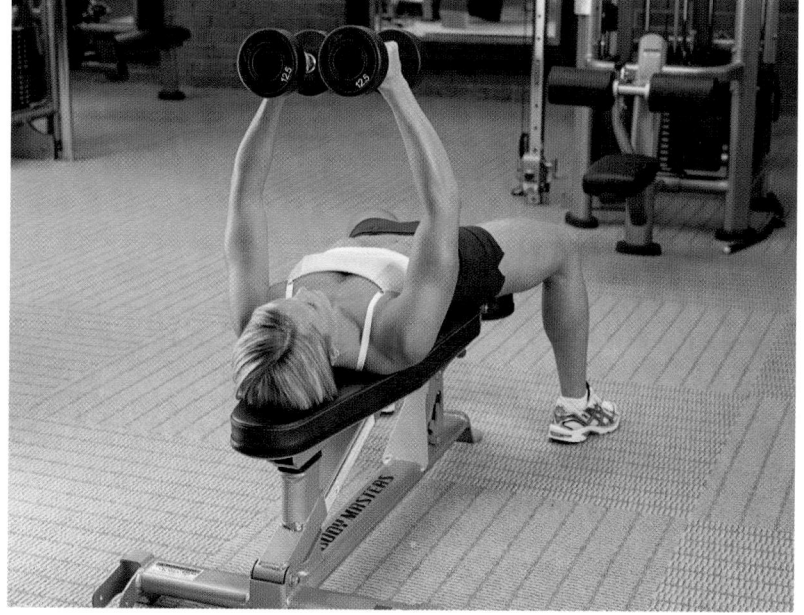

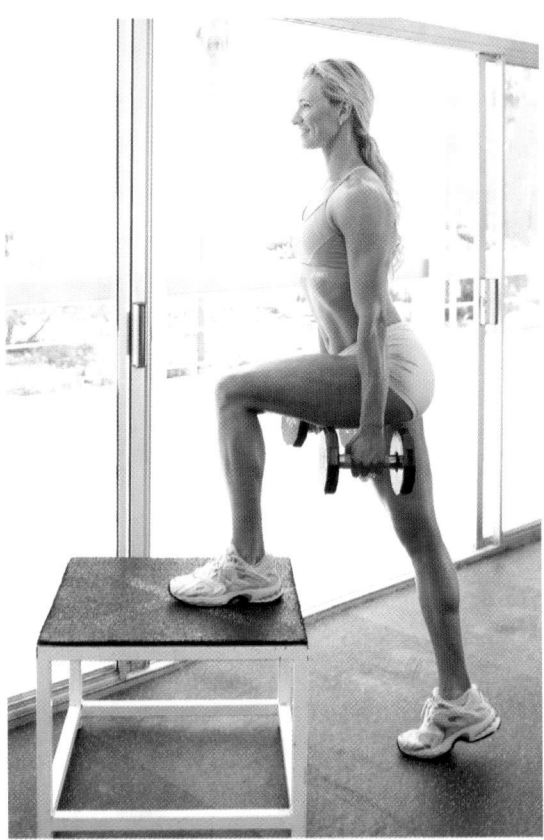

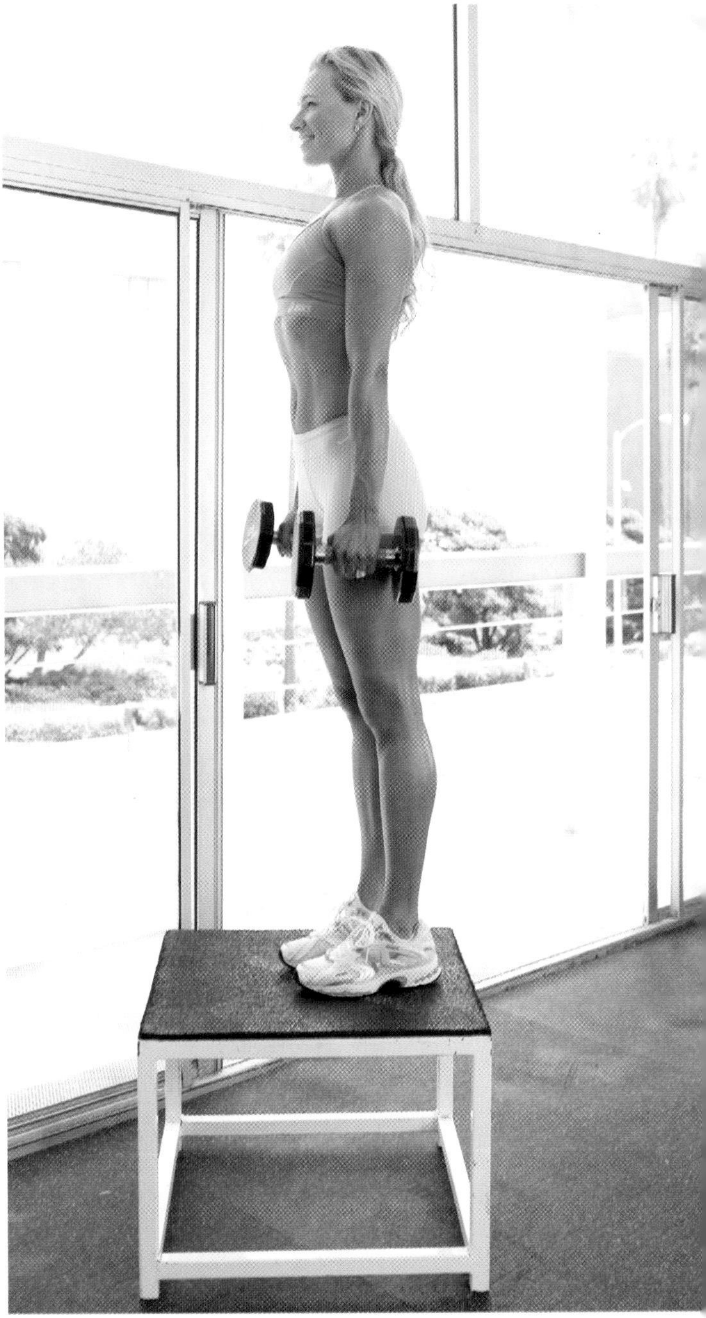

Step-Up

Stand erect with your feet close together facing a bench. Step up onto the bench with your left leg, pushing through your left heel as you rise. Bring your right foot up onto the bench, then step down with your left foot followed by your right. Repeat, leading with the right. Alternate the leading foot for reps.

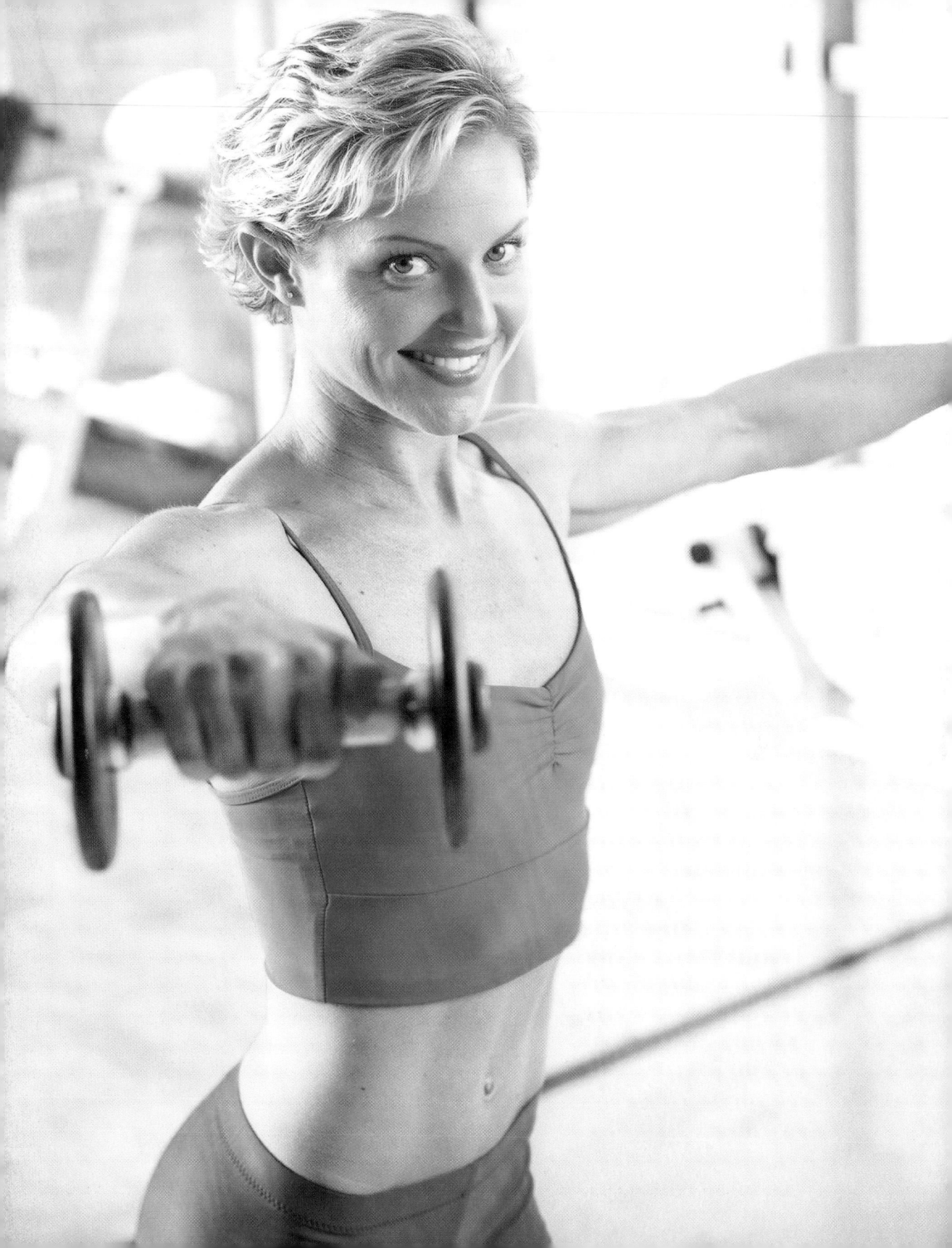

Chapter 2

The Next Level

If you've got at least six months of consistent training under your belt and want to take your body to the next level, check out this fast-paced, fast-acting workout program. We'll guide you through, step by step, on how to transform your body from adequate to astonishing — but it'll take a good six-week effort on your part!

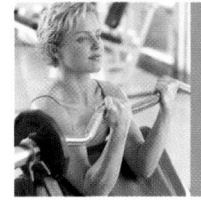

upper body

After doing the "Look Great in Eight" program, consider this the second phase in your journey to a leaner and more balanced-looking physique. But to see results, you need to be ready to kick up the intensity. We have a few tricks up our sleeves.

Using a combination of advanced training techniques — employed in an aggressive workout schedule — paired with a solid cardio routine and your kick-ass attitude to keep the intensity where it needs to be, you will be able to transform your physique yet again. Think about it: If you want it bad enough, you'll do it. Now what are you waiting for? Shouldn't you be at the gym?

THE PROGRAM

This program is somewhat unconventional in its design, although many components may be familiar to you. It's made up of compound (multijoint) and isolation (single-joint) exercises, and the set and rep ranges vary, calling for low reps for compound exercises and relatively high reps for the isolation movements. "This program is for show and go," says Kelly Williams, PhD, CSCS, who devised the routine. This means the multijoint exercises — the ones that increase size and strength — serve as a base for the single-joint moves, which help improve muscle shape. With workouts broken down into upper- and lower-body splits, you'll lift four days during each week and do cardio 3–4 days each week.

Every set of compound exercises for upper body calls for three sets of 10 reps

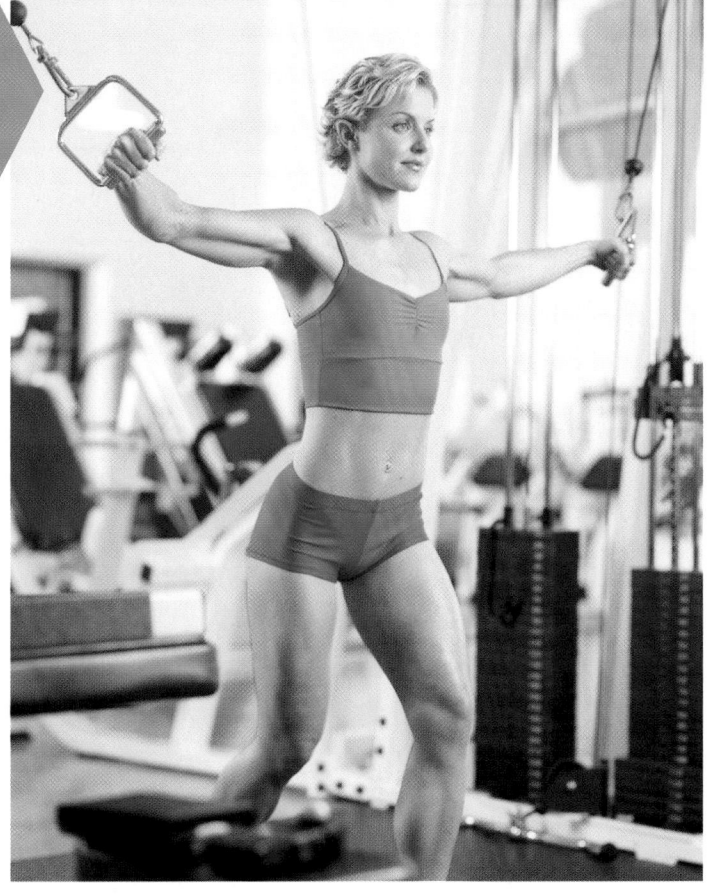

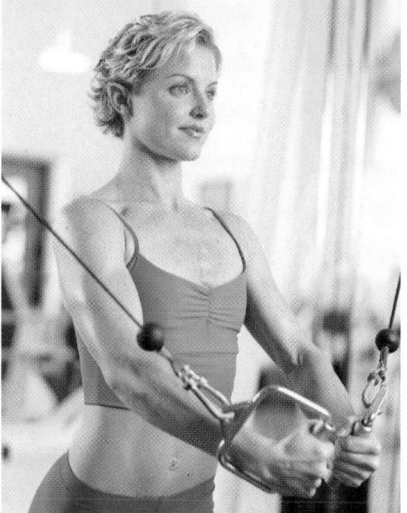

CABLE CROSSOVER

Execution Tips: Stand erect with a slight forward lean, head up and elbows slightly bent. Without changing the angle in your elbows, squeeze your pecs to bring the handles down in an arc to meet in front of your midsection.

How to Make It Tougher: Save this exercise for last and do drop sets until even the weight of the pin seems too heavy.

upper-body blitz

Train upper body on days 2 and 5. Start with the compound exercise and complete the sets and reps listed for each week. Follow that with the isolation movement for each body part. Incorporate the advanced training techniques only on the final sets of the week.

For Week 1, start by training chest first; Week 2, train back first; Week 3, train biceps first; Week 4, train triceps first; Week 5, train shoulders first; and Week 6, train your weakest body part first.

CHEST

Bench Press	Compound
Dumbbell Flye or Cable Crossover	Isolation

BACK

Front Pull-Down	Compound
Seated Cable Row	Compound

BICEPS

EZ-Bar Curl	Isolation
Preacher Curl	Isolation

TRICEPS

Dumbbell Kickback	Isolation
Lying Triceps Extension	Isolation

SHOULDERS

Upright Row	Compound
Lateral Raise or Bent-Over Lateral Raise	Isolation

Week	Day	Intensity	Sets x Reps (compound)	Sets x Reps (isolation)	Advanced Techniques
1	2	medium	3x10	3x12-15	
	5	hard	3x10	3x12-15	Stripping
2	2	light	3x10	3x12-15	
	5	hard	3x10	3x12-15	Stripping
3	2	medium	3x8	3x12-15	
	5	hard	3x8	3x12-15	Partials
4	2	light	3x8	3x12-15	
	5	hard	3x8	3x12-15	Partials
5	2	medium	3x6	3x12-15	
	5	hard	3x6	3x12-15	Supersets
6	2	light	3x6	3x12-15	
	5	hard	3x6	3x12-15	Supersets

INTENSITY KEY: Hard = push to failure; Medium = stop a couple of reps short of failure; and Light = stop several reps short of failure.

during the first two weeks, eight reps the second two weeks and six reps the final two weeks. "For the isolation lifts, you'll stay with 12–15 repetitions throughout the six weeks," explains Williams, an associate professor at Missouri Western State College in St. Joseph.

Likewise, for lower-body compound movements, you'll do four sets of 15 reps (4x15) the first two weeks, 4x12 the next two and 4x10 the last two weeks; however, you'll stick with three sets of 15 for all isolation exercises the entire six weeks. "I have some real fun ways to make it less than routine," Williams warns. Alternating between low-, medium- and high-intensity workouts, as well as lifting progressively more weight and doing fewer reps, will keep your muscles from adapting to the workload. Which brings us to the subject of intensity.

Since intensity plays such a vital role in any workout designed to initiate positive change, it has been built into this program. You'll notice that the six weeks are broken down into segments that indicate particular intensity levels: low, medium and high. As a reminder, to make progress, muscles need to be pushed beyond what they're used to doing. This breaks down the muscles, which then need to be repaired to come back stronger the next time you work out.

A little-understood fact is that you actually experience more gains when you cycle the intensity of your workouts. Going hard and heavy 24/7 is a prescription for overtraining and limited progress. Working at varying levels — not always hard and heavy — reduces the risk of injury and burnout and helps keep you motivated. Therefore, cycling the intensity of your workouts will help you maximize success.

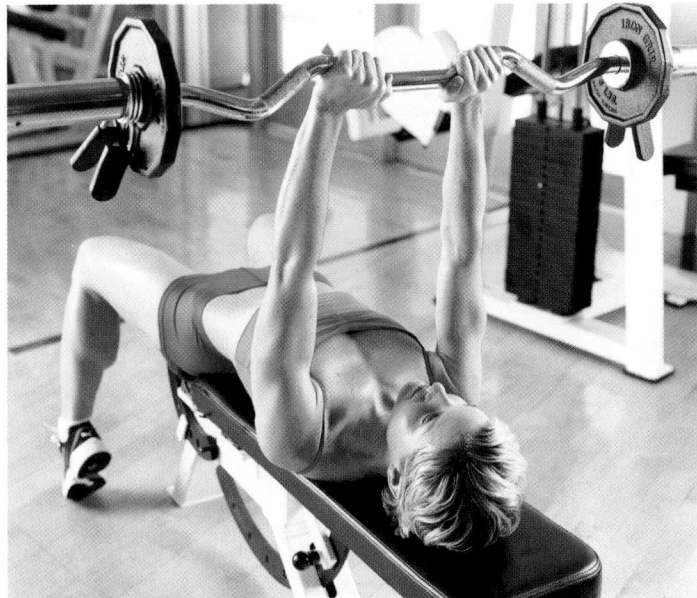

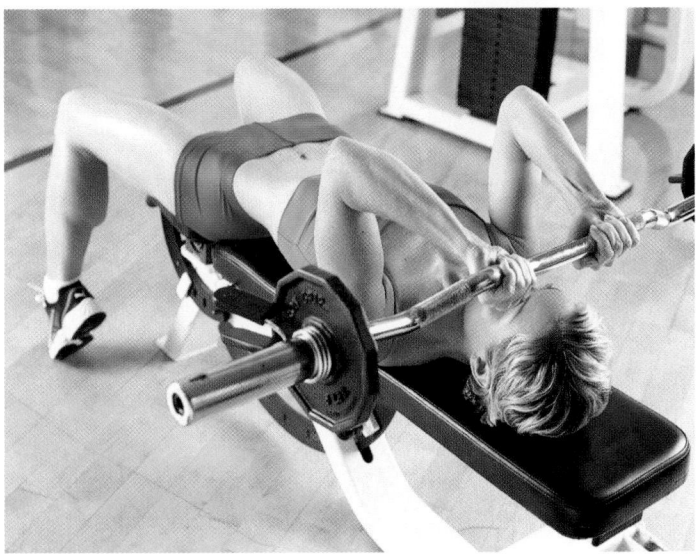

LYING TRICEPS EXTENSION

Execution Tips: Hinge only at the elbows — your shoulder joints should not move at all — to lower the weight toward your forehead. Press the bar back up, again making sure you move only at the elbows.

How to Make It Tougher: After each set, go right into a set of 10 close-grip bench presses, keeping your elbows from flaring out.

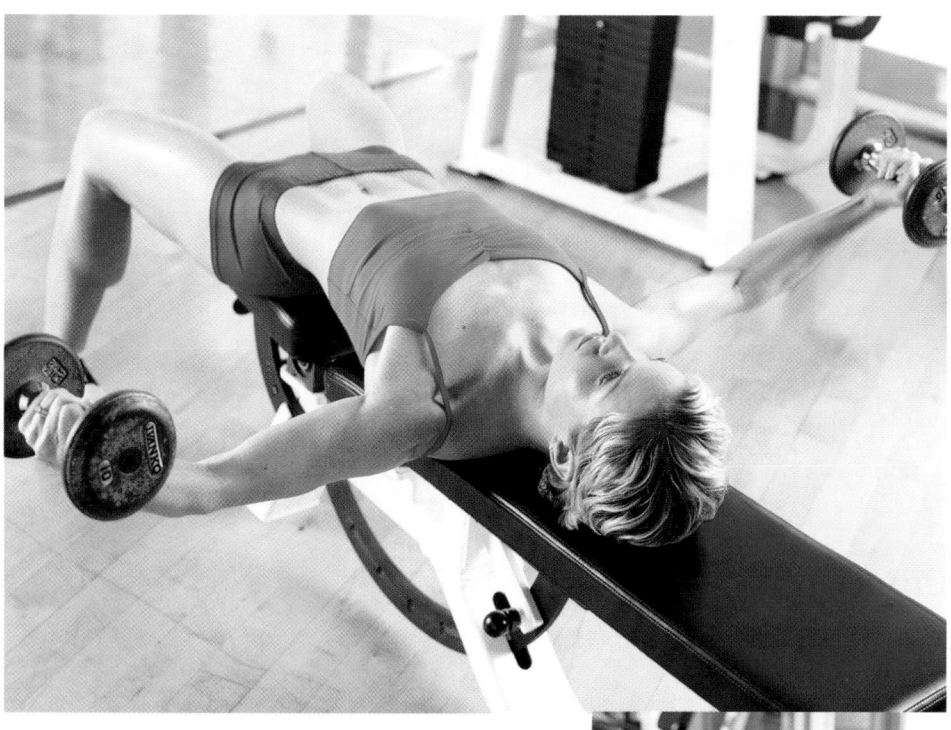

DUMBBELL FLYE

Execution Tips: Keeping a slight angle locked in your elbows, lower the weights directly out to your sides, stopping when your upper arms are just short of parallel to the floor. Squeeze your chest muscles to raise the dumbbells back up.

How to Make It Tougher: When you finish your set of flyes, do a quick set of 10 flat-bench presses for chest with the weights, having your spotter ready.

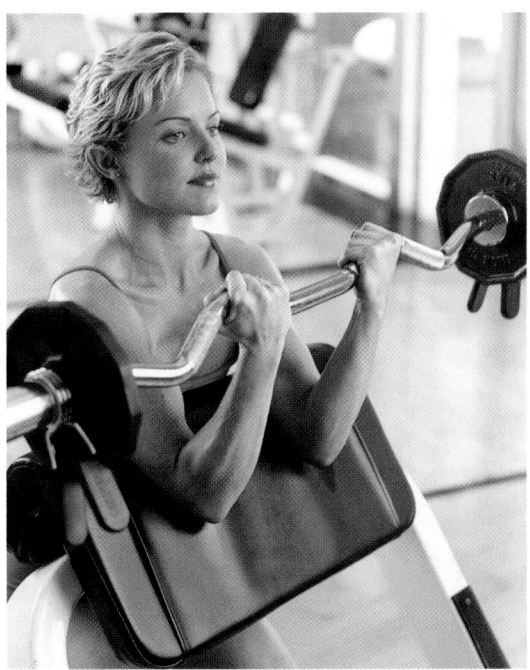

PREACHER CURL

Execution Tips: Keep your triceps firmly against the pad and ensure that your shoulders, elbows and wrists line up in the same plane. Really squeeze the biceps at the top. Keep those wrists strong.

How to Make It Tougher: Do partial reps, going down halfway and coming almost all the way back up.

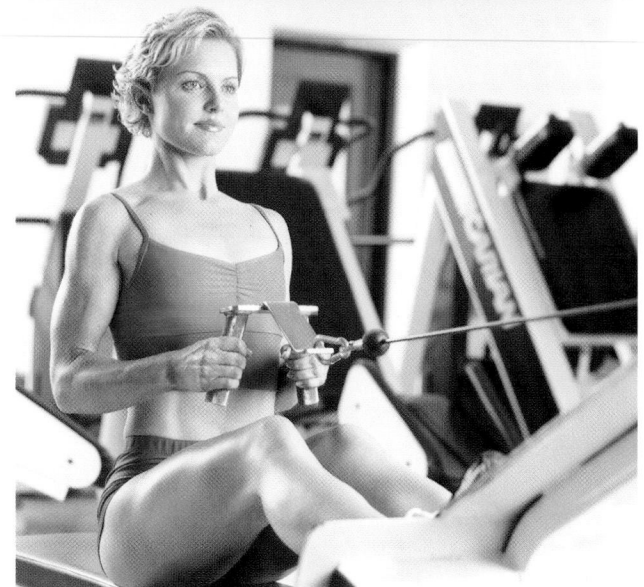

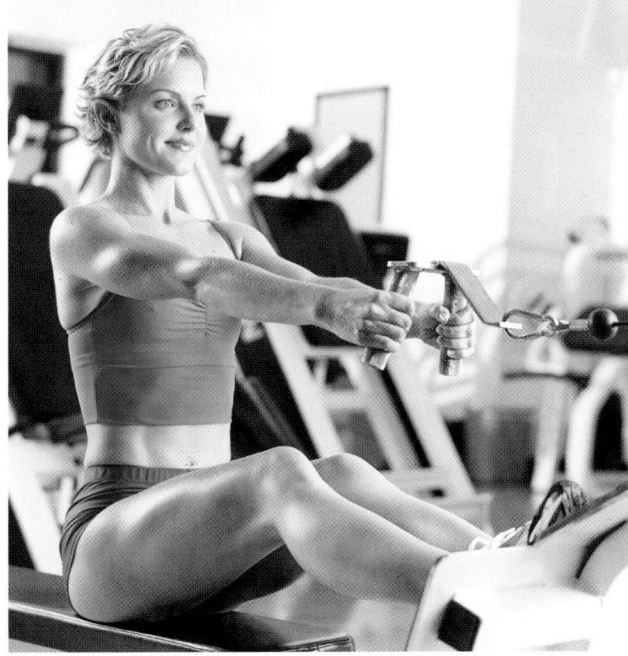

SEATED CABLE ROW

Execution Tips: Keep your knees slightly bent, abs tight and chest high. Don't round your back when lowering the weight stack or lean forward too far. Be sure to squeeze those shoulder blades together and open your chest when pulling the handle into your midsection.

How to Make It Tougher: When you pull the handle toward you and squeeze your shoulder blades together, hold for a two-count, then slowly return the weight for a four-count.

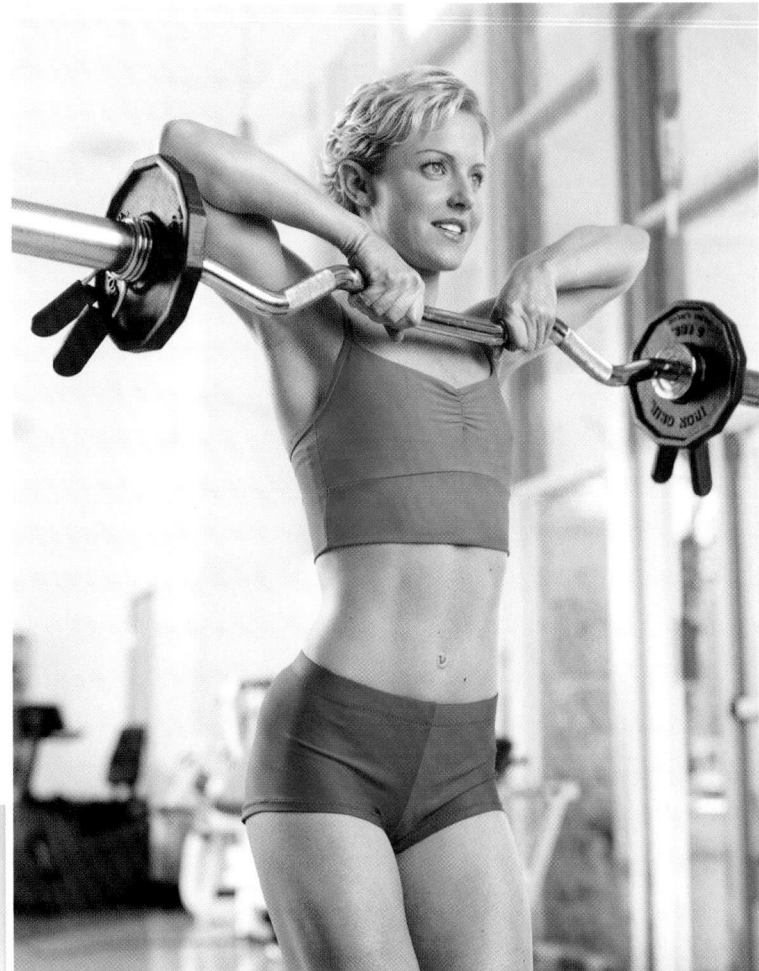

UPRIGHT ROW

Execution Tips: With a medium-width grip, relax your shoulders and raise the bar or dumbbells to your upper chest. Keep your elbows higher than your hands throughout the movement.
How to Make It Tougher: Pair this exercise with an overhead press to really work your shoulders.

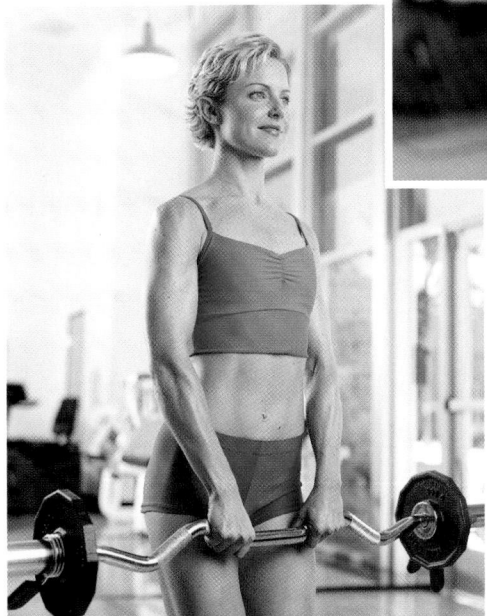

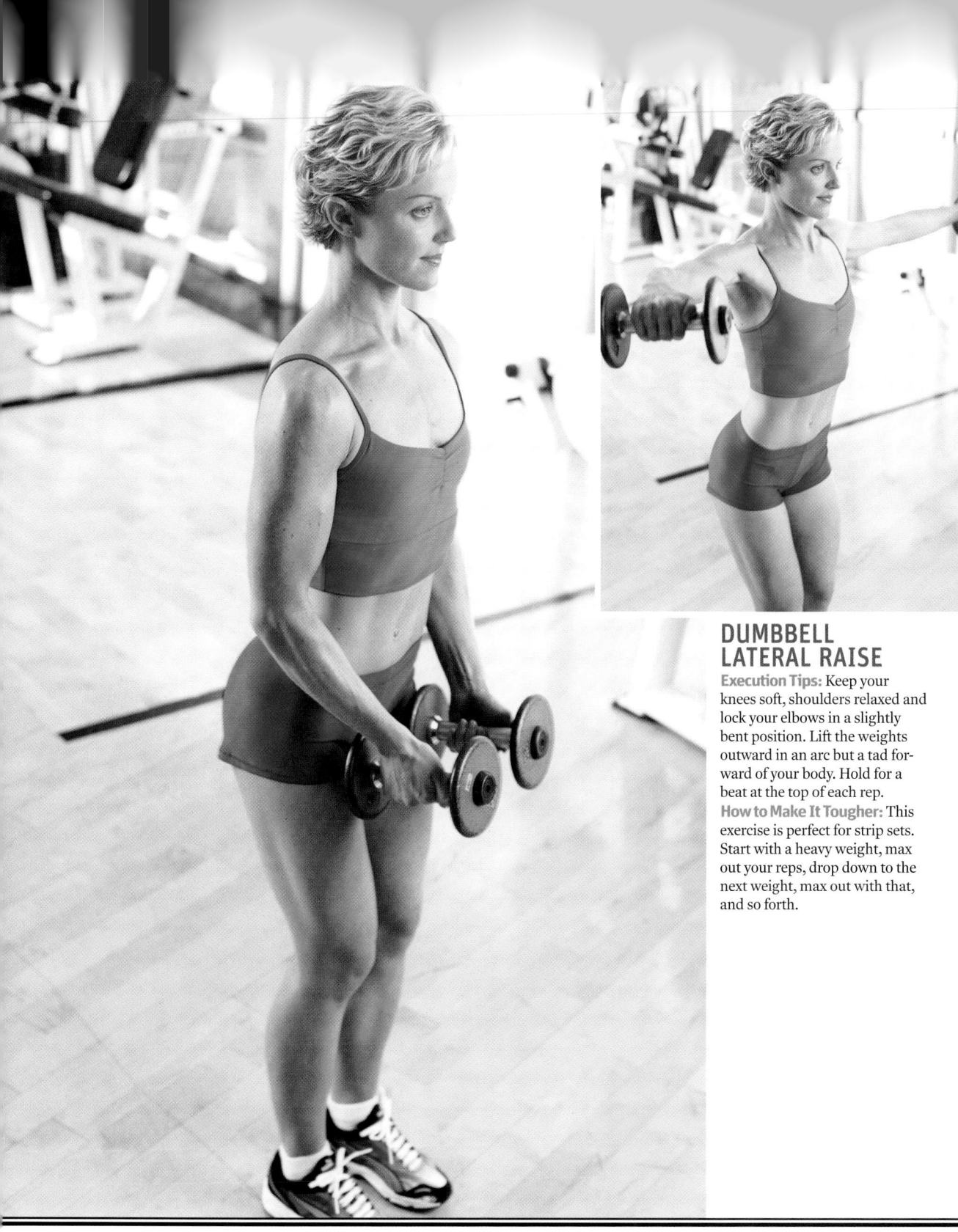

DUMBBELL LATERAL RAISE

Execution Tips: Keep your knees soft, shoulders relaxed and lock your elbows in a slightly bent position. Lift the weights outward in an arc but a tad forward of your body. Hold for a beat at the top of each rep.

How to Make It Tougher: This exercise is perfect for strip sets. Start with a heavy weight, max out your reps, drop down to the next weight, max out with that, and so forth.

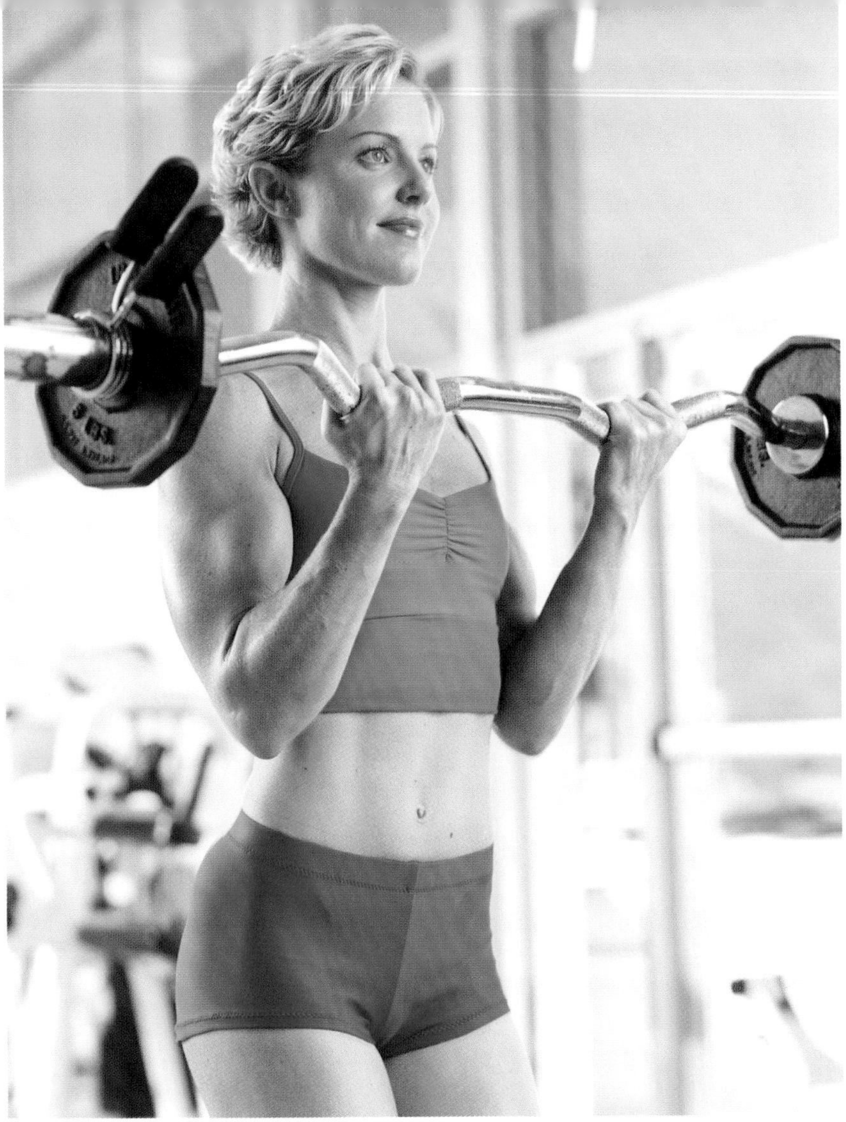

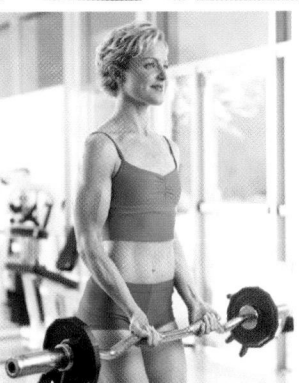

BENCH PRESS

Execution Tips: Grip the bar just a little wider than your shoulders. Keep your wrists straight and lower the bar to the middle of your upper chest, but don't let it touch.

How to Make It Tougher: With a spotter there to assist you, end each set with 8–10 partial reps.

FRONT PULLDOWN

Execution Tips: Tighten your abs, lift your chest, squeeze your shoulder blades together and arch your back slightly, then pull the bar down to your upper chest. Let the bar rise as high as possible to stretch your lats before repeating.

How to Make It Tougher: Take a wide grip on the bar and don't use momentum.

DUMBBELL KICKBACK

Execution Tips: Keep your back flat, abs contracted and your upper arm parallel to the floor, locking your elbow at your side. Fully extend your arm to get a full range of motion.

How to Make It Tougher: Do a compound set of this exercise and dips off the side of a flat bench.

BENT-OVER LATERAL RAISE

Execution Tips: Choose a weight light enough to move through a full range of motion. Pause at the top of the motion and don't rest at the bottom. Watch out for body swing.

How to Make It Tougher: Do this exercise after training your back, when your rear delts are already well on their way to being fatigued.

EZ-BAR CURL

Execution Tips: Relax your shoulders, keep your knees soft and your wrists straight. Contract your biceps hard at the top of the movement, and don't lose that tension as you lower the bar.

How to Make It Tougher: With the assistance of a training partner — and after a warm-up set — do negatives. Add some weight to the bar and have your partner help you raise the weight, then slowly lower it by yourself.

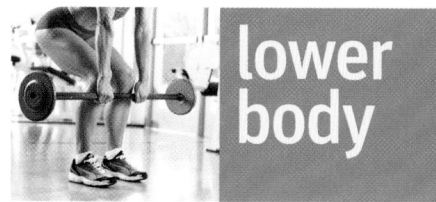

lower body

THE BONUSES

Take a deep breath, because you are about to dance to that intensity tune one more time. "On high-intensity days — and you'll probably come to call them 'killer' days — you'll use advanced training techniques," states Williams. Here's a warning, er, we mean an explanation of the methods he suggests.

Stripping: "No, it doesn't involve G-strings or Chippendales' dancers. On your last set of one exercise — after you've hit the failure point — quickly reduce the weight and keep going, doing as many reps as you can with the lightened load. When you hit failure again, remove — or strip — more weight, continuing on and resting only long enough to lighten your load, until all that's left is the bar." Optimally, your strip set should include 5–6 reps at three different weights (that is, two strips).

Partials: "This will make you very sore and is performed more effectively if you have a reliable and strong training partner. Do this on your last set of an exercise. Start the set and lift to near failure. After the last rep — when you're having trouble raising the weight — have your partner lift the weight for you. Very slowly, and under your own power, carefully lower the weight. Repeat this process several times until you're reduced to a quivering pile of jelly." If you don't have a training partner, you may opt to do partial reps. On the last set of the last exercise, do half-reps, where you lower the weight halfway and raise it all the way up for peak contraction.

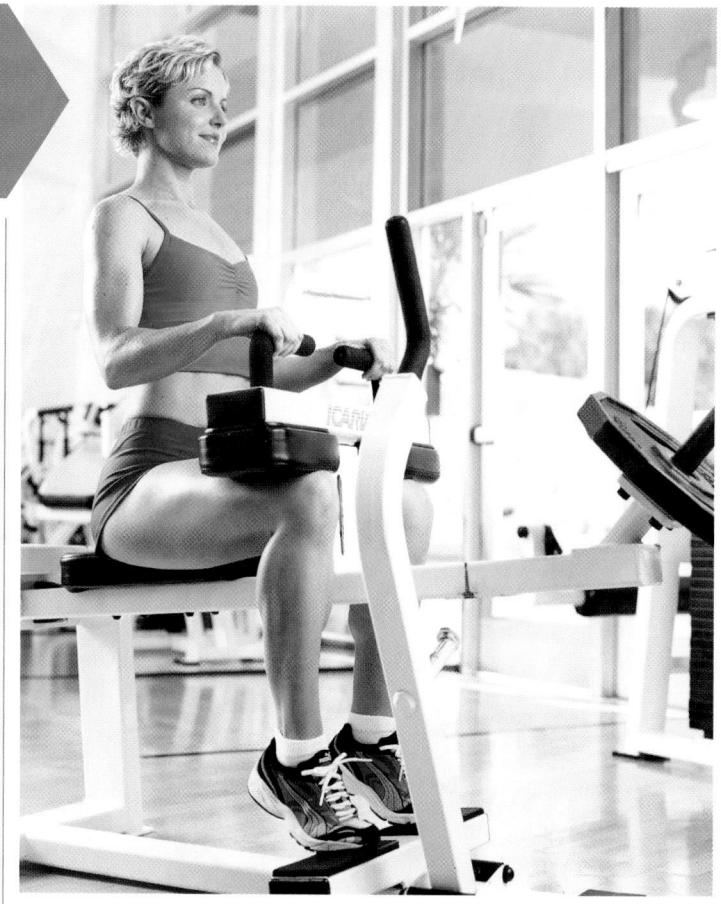

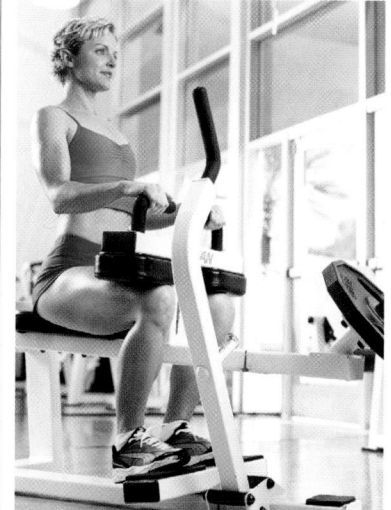

SEATED CALF RAISE

Execution Tips: Place the balls of your feet on the platform, toes in a neutral position. Place your hands on the handles or at your sides, and avoid swinging back when you lift the weight.

How to Make It Tougher: Change your foot placement within each set. Start with your toes outward for 10 reps, followed by toes straight ahead for 10, ending with toes out for 10. Can you say burn?

lower-body blast

Train upper body on days 1 and 4. Start with the compound exercise and complete the sets and reps listed for each week. Follow that with the isolation movement for each body part — except when supersetting. In this case, superset quads with hamstrings, doing the remaining quad exercise by itself. Then do the rest of the exercises in the order in which they are listed. Incorporate the advanced training techniques only on the final sets of the week.

For Week 1, start with squats; Week 2, lunges; Week 3, single-leg squats; Week 4, deadlifts; Week 5, squats; and Week 6, train abdominals first.

QUADS/GLUTES
Squat	Compound
Stationary Lunge	Compound
Single-Leg Squat	Compound

HAMSTRINGS
Romanian Deadlift	Compound
Lying Leg Curl	Isolation

CALVES
Standing Calf Raise	Isolation
Seated Calf Raise	Isolation

LOW BACK
Back Extension	Isolation

ABDOMINALS
Crunch	Isolation
Decline Crunch	Isolation
Reverse Crunch	Isolation
Exercise-Ball Crunch	Isolation

Week	Day	Intensity	Sets x Reps (compound)	Sets x Reps (isolation)	Advanced Techniques
1	1	medium	4x15	3x15	
	4	hard	4x15	3x15	Stripping
2	1	light	4x15	3x15	
	4	hard	4x15	3x15	Stripping
3	1	medium	4x12	3x15	
	4	hard	4x12	3x15	Partials
4	1	light	4x12	3x15	
	4	hard	4x12	3x15	Partials
5	1	medium	4x10	3x15	
	4	hard	4x10	3x15	Supersets
6	1	light	4x10	3x15	
	4	hard	4x10	3x15	Supersets

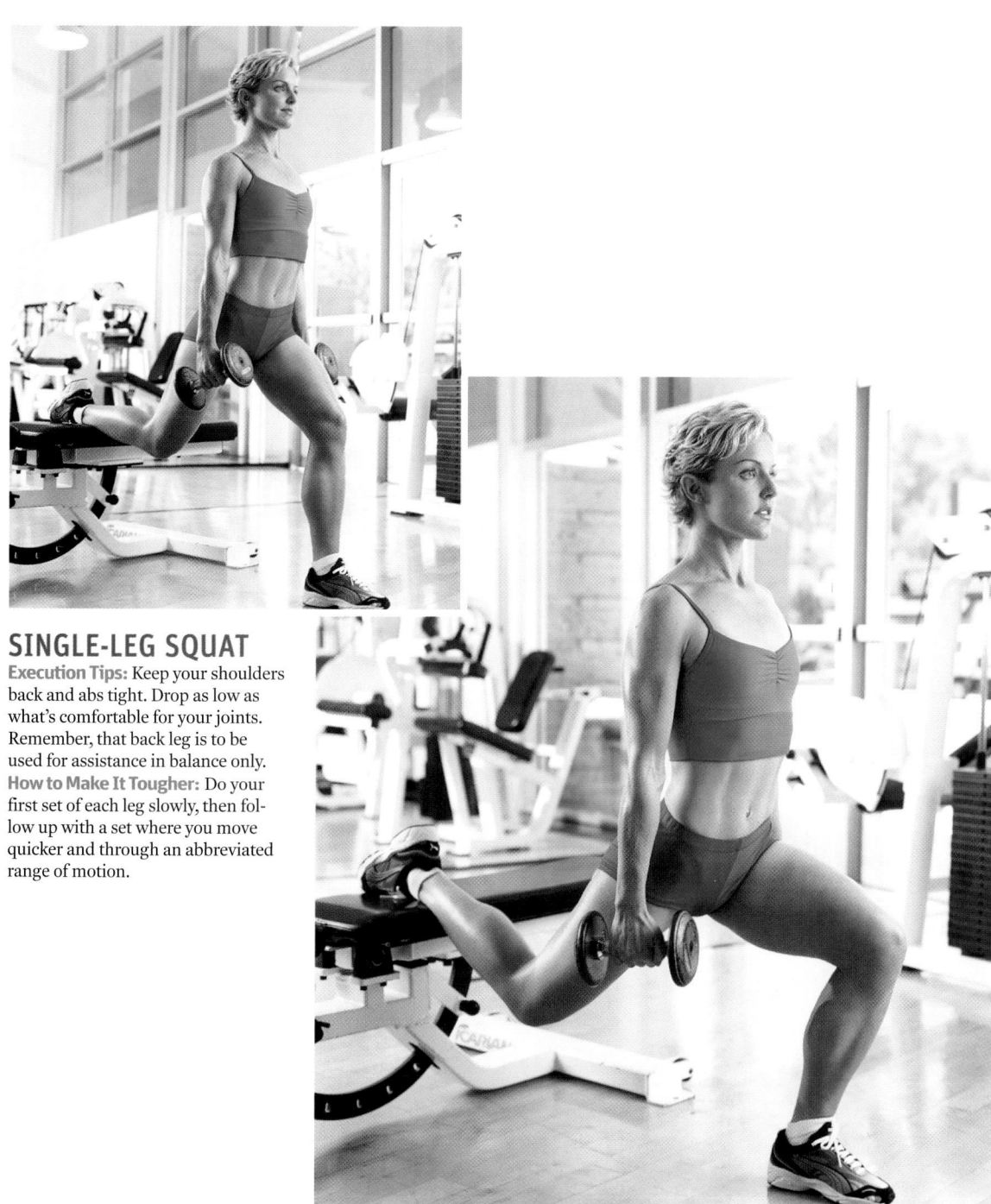

SINGLE-LEG SQUAT

Execution Tips: Keep your shoulders back and abs tight. Drop as low as what's comfortable for your joints. Remember, that back leg is to be used for assistance in balance only.
How to Make It Tougher: Do your first set of each leg slowly, then follow up with a set where you move quicker and through an abbreviated range of motion.

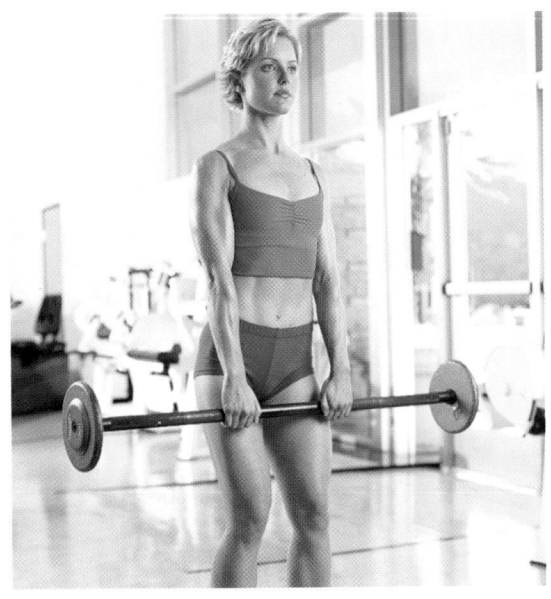
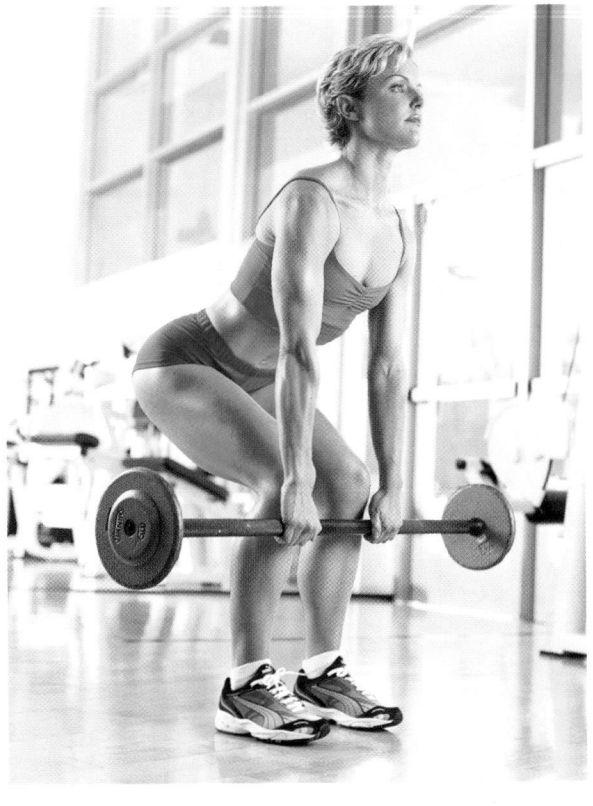

ROMANIAN DEADLIFT

Execution Tips: Keep your back slightly arched and head up; by the time you get to the bent-over position, your back is flat instead of rounded. Go down only as far as your flexibility allows. Squeeze through your hamstrings and glutes as you pull your hips forward to rise.

How to Make It Tougher: Superset these with walking lunges.

#7

cardio combustion

Train within the suggested heart-rate zones. To estimate percentages of your maximum heart rate (MHR), subtract your age from 220, then multiply by 0.60 for 60%, 0.65 for 65%, 0.75 for 75%, and so on. These numbers are guidelines only. Another way to gauge intensity is by rate of perceived exertion. On a scale of 1-10, with 10 representing maximum intensity, you should work between 6 and 8. (Six correlates to about 60% of your MHR and 8 is about 80%.)

Week	Frequency	Duration	Intensity
1	4 times per week	30 minutes	75%-80% of MHR
2	3 times per week	40 minutes	65%-75% of MHR
3	3 times per week	50 minutes	60%-65% of MHR
4	3 times per week	60 minutes	60% of MHR
5	4 times per week	30 minutes	75%-80% of MHR
6	3 times per week	60 minutes	60%-65% of MHR

Supersets: "This is a great one to use when you're pressed for time, since you put two exercises for opposing muscle groups together. Perform a lift, followed immediately by an exercise for the antagonistic muscle. For example, do a set of dumbbell curls for biceps followed by triceps extensions."

THE CARDIO EQUATION

The cardio portion of the program will follow along the same lines as your weight training, with low-, medium- and high-intensity days, varying in length and difficulty. "I'm a bit of a purist," admits Williams. "I don't particularly like to mix cardio and weight training in the same session, but that doesn't mean it can't be done." If you can, do your cardio in the morning and weights in the evening. If that's not possible, just do your cardio after weights. "Any lactic acid formed during the workout will be metabolized during aerobic exercise," Williams notes.

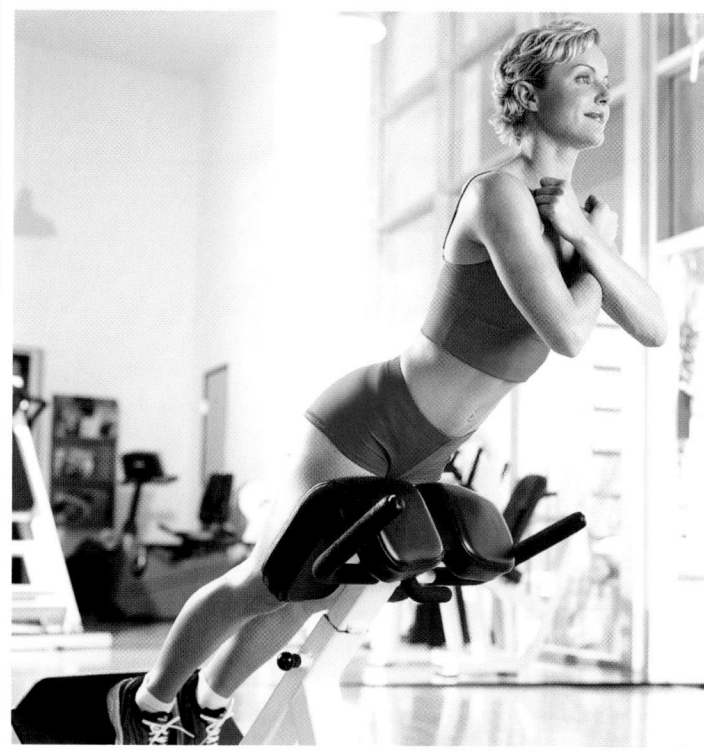

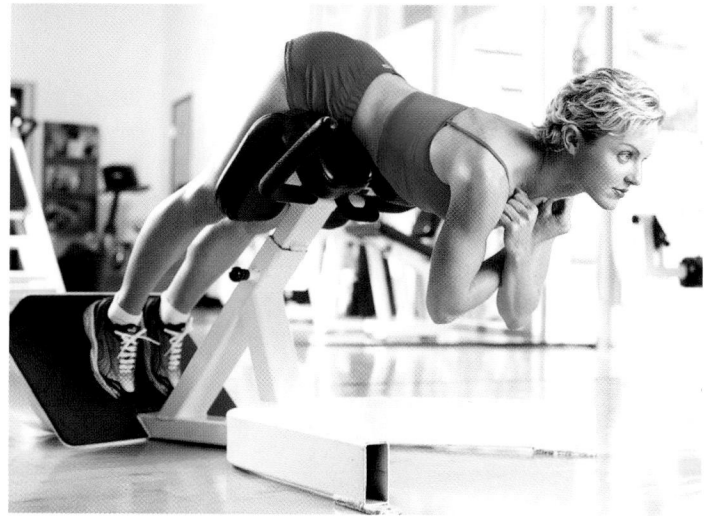

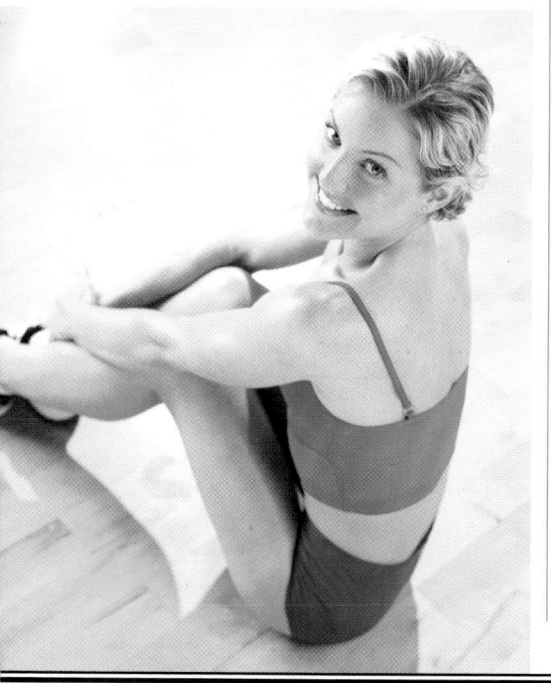

BACK EXTENSION

Execution Tips: Come up only as far as your natural body position, avoiding hyperextension of the back. Squeeze your glutes at the top.
How to Make It Tougher: Add a little weight to this exercise by holding a small plate tightly against your chest.

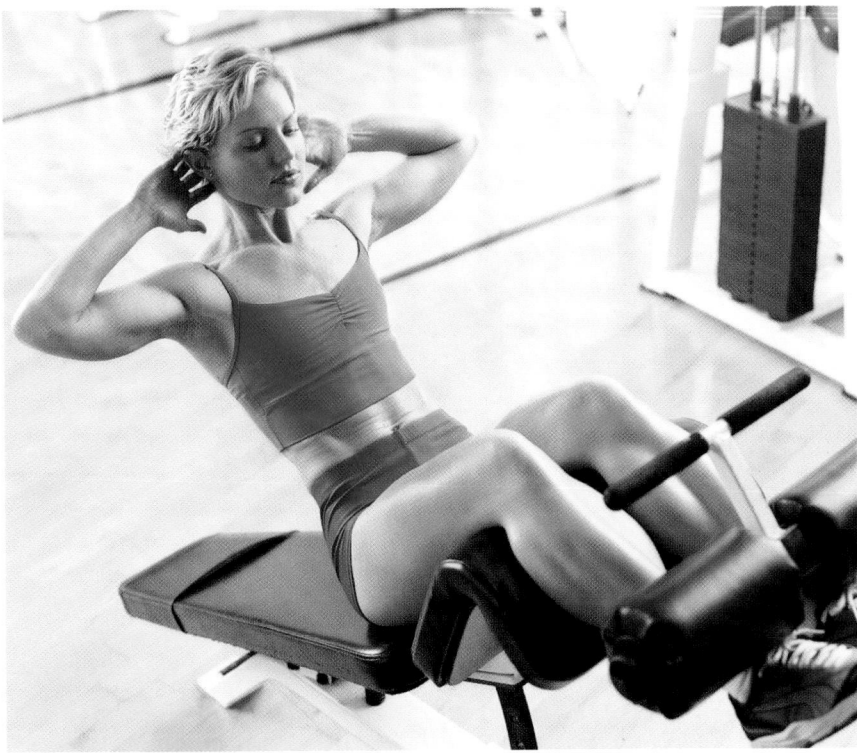

DECLINE CRUNCH

Execution Tips: Tuck your legs under the support pad of the decline bench. Range of motion is very small here, so don't try to come all the way up.

How to Make It Tougher: Start with sets of slow-count reps followed by faster-paced ones as your muscles begin to burn.

STANDING CALF RAISE

Execution Tips: Do one leg at a time. Make sure you go as high and as low as you can, working through a full range of motion.

How to Make It Tougher: To feel this one from your heels all the way up your glutes, try this: Lift up halfway on your working leg, hold for a second then lift higher and hold for two seconds before lowering your heel.

SQUAT

Execution Tips: Begin the movement by pushing your hips back, ensuring that your knees stay behind your toes as you descend into a deep knee bend. Go down until your thighs are parallel to the floor and push through your heels when you rise.

How to Make It Tougher: Move slowly through a full range of motion, taking two seconds to squat down and four to rise.

LYING LEG CURL

Execution Tips: Keep your hips pressed down and into the pad of the machine. Squeeze your glutes and hamstrings at the top of each rep. Your feet, knees and hips should remain in line.

How to Make It Tougher: Begin this as a unilateral exercise, doing three sets for each leg. Then really wear them out by doing 1–2 more sets using both legs.

CRUNCH

Execution Tips: Lightly cup the back of your head with your hands; don't pull on it. Curl forward, raising your shoulder blades up off the floor and slowly lower.

How to Make It Tougher: Extend your arms above your head and clasp your hands together, resting your head on your upper arms.

REVERSE CRUNCH

Execution Tips: Keep your upper body tight and stable, and use your abdominals — not momentum — to curl your hips off the floor toward your chest.

How to Make It Tougher: Lift your hips and hold for a two-count.

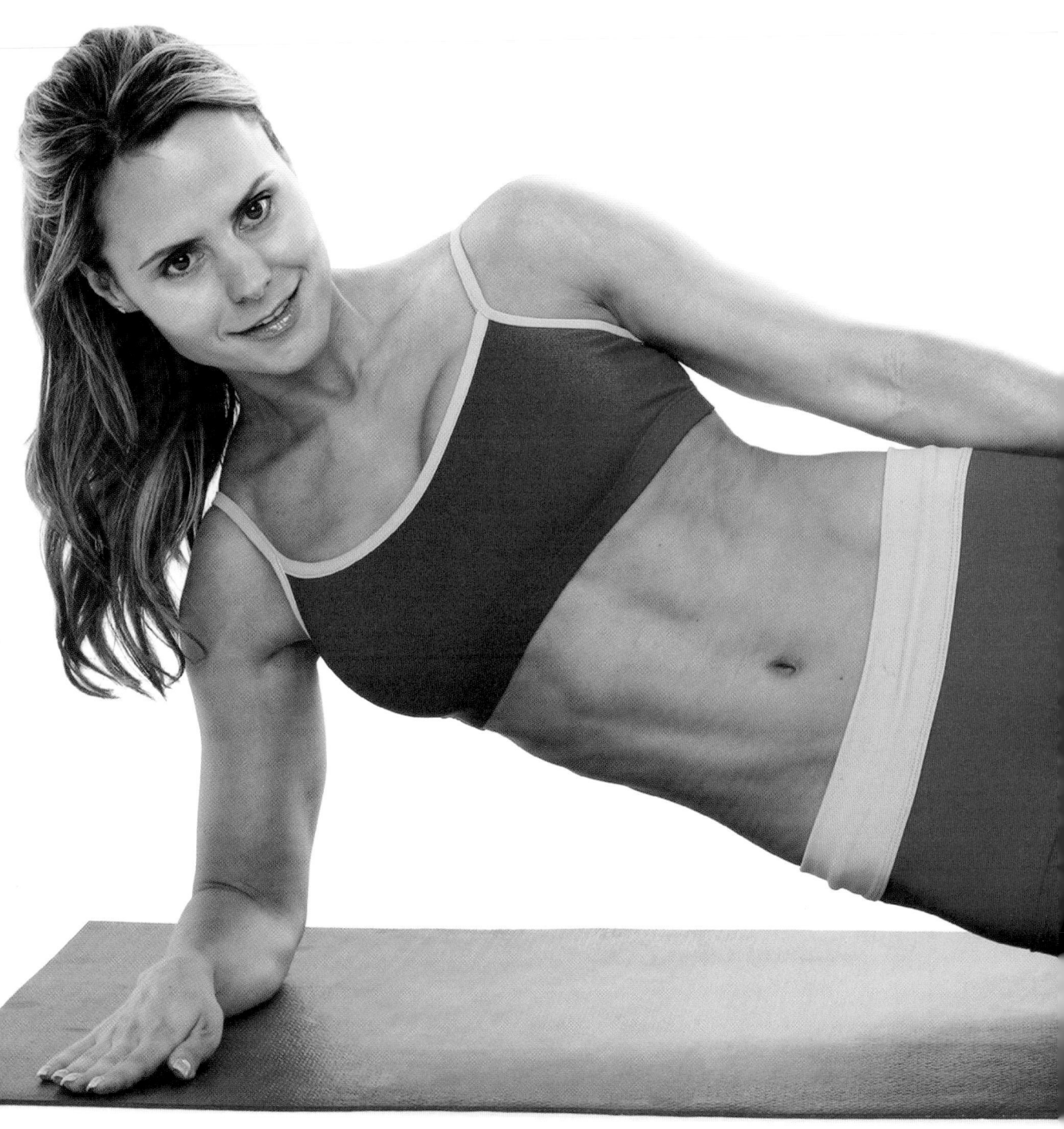

Chapter 3

Abs In 12 Weeks, Flat!

Doing hundreds of crunches won't give you the abs you want, but a well-thought-out workout program performed over a sustained period combined with a diet structured with fat loss in mind will. To attain the holy grail of a lean, tight midsection, you must progressively make your abs stronger, burn the flab hiding them and dial in your diet. This program will help you do that.

The training regimen is broken down into three four-week phases. In Phase One, you create the basic foundation that lets you proceed to more advanced routines in Phases Two and Three. As you progressively work your abs harder, you'll refine your diet each week to prepare for the unveiling of those fabulous abs. The guidelines listed here help you ease into and fine-tune your existing diet, but to really rev up the fat-burning furnace, use this routine in tandem with "The Ultimate No-Brainer Diet" beginning on page 99. This program is designed to fit into your regular training and cardio routines as prescribed and swap out your usual ab work for these routines three days a week, resting at least 48 hours between workouts.

»Phase One...

Weeks 1—4:
CREATING THE FOUNDATION

This month is about adapting to the exercises that form the foundation of this program. Perform your regular weight-training routine while using the workout below to train your abs three times a week, resting at least 48 hours between sessions. Do cardio at a moderate to high intensity 4–5 days a week for 30 minutes.

EXERCISE BALL CRUNCH

TARGETS: Upper abs
START: Lie face-up on a large exercise ball with your lower and middle back supported, knees bent and feet flat on the floor. Cross your arms over your chest. (For increased difficulty, place your hands lightly behind your neck as shown or, to make it even harder, extend your arms overhead.)
MOVEMENT: Raise only your head and shoulders as you contract your abs to move your upper body toward your pelvis. Slowly return to the starting position.

#8

EXERCISE	SETS	REPS
Exercise Ball Crunch	2–3	10–15
V-Twist	2–3	10–15 (to each side)
Reverse Crunch	2–3	10–15
Straight-Leg Raise	2–3	10–15
Plank	3	25–30 sec.

V-TWIST

TARGETS: All regions, with emphasis on the obliques and core

START: Sit on the floor with your knees slightly bent and hold your arms at 90-degree angles with your hands out in front of you. Lift your feet about 6 inches off the floor. Cross your ankles and lean back about 45 degrees while balancing on your glutes.

MOVEMENT: Pull your belly button toward your lower back, then rotate your torso to the left so your right shoulder points toward your knees. Twist to the right and repeat; continue twisting until you've done 10 reps to each side, or 20 total.

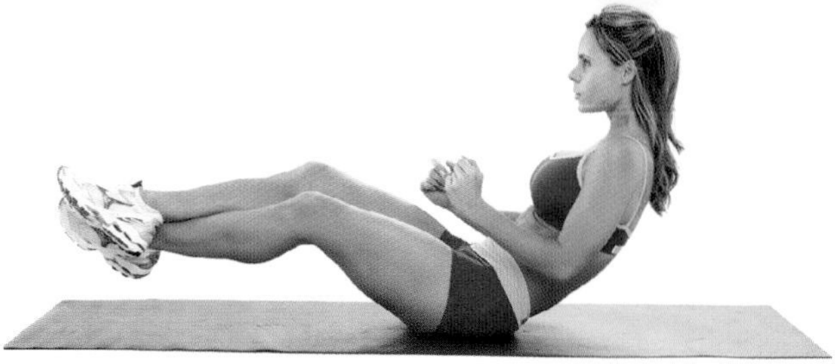

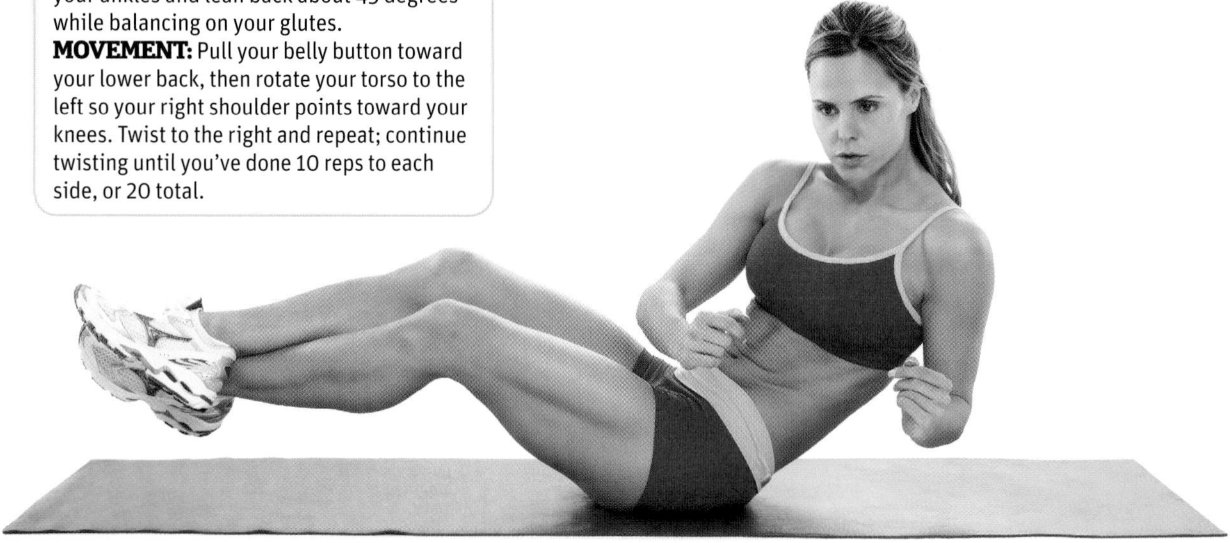

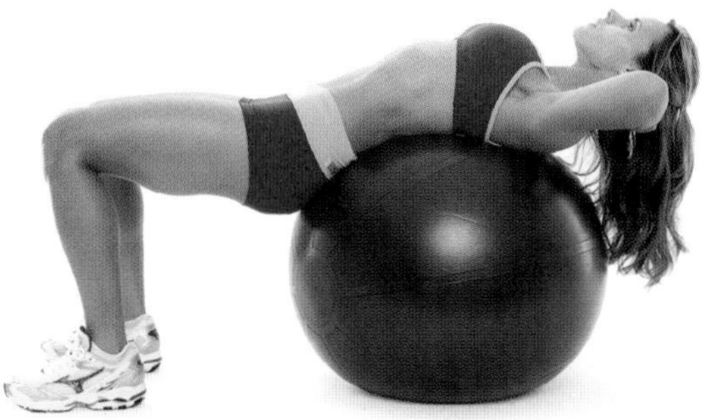

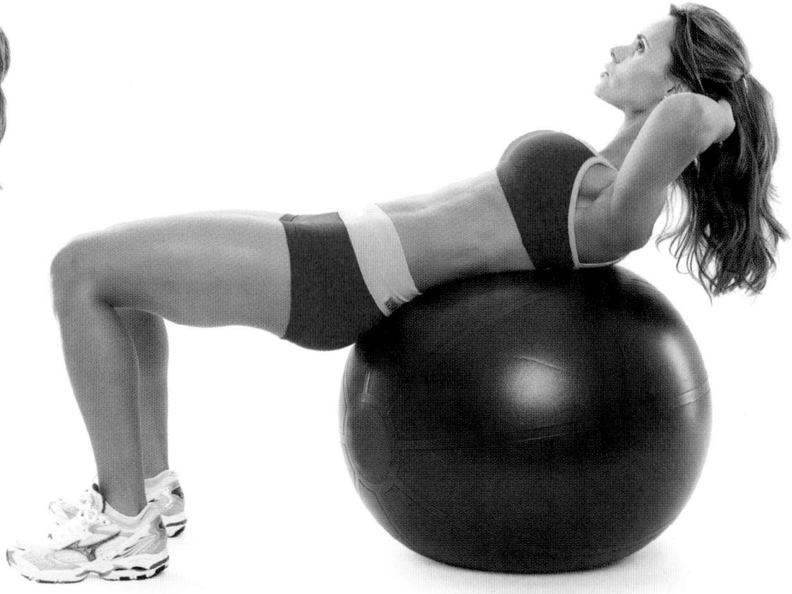

Make sure the movement originates from your abs, contracting them to raise your shoulders and head.

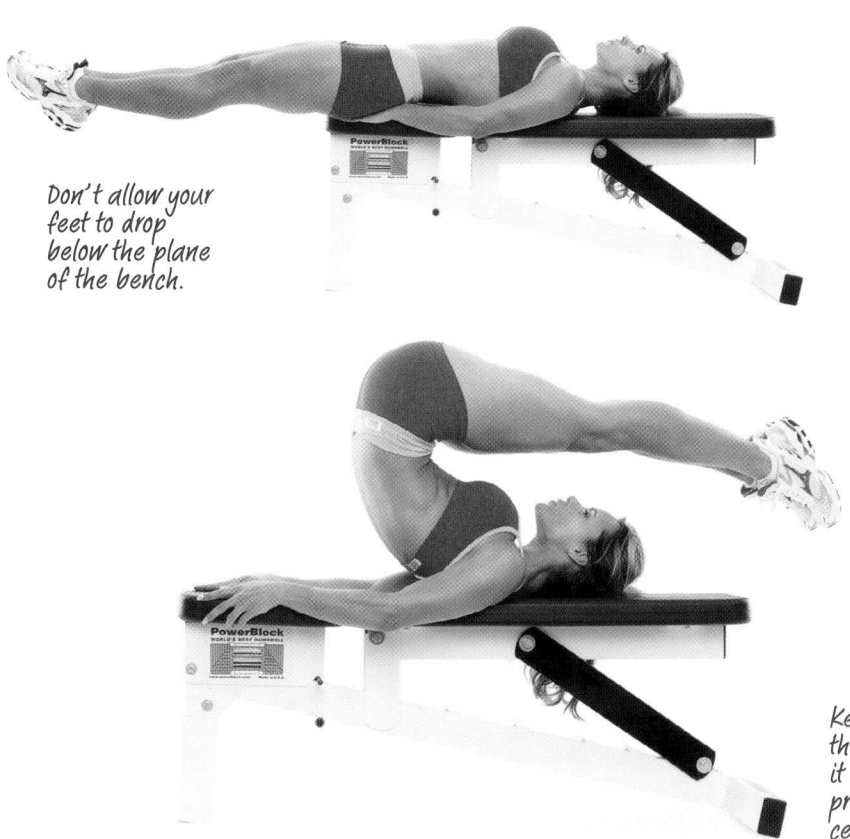

Don't allow your feet to drop below the plane of the bench.

STRAIGHT-LEG RAISE

TARGETS: Lower abs
START: Lie face-up on a bench with your glutes at its edge. Extend your legs, keeping them parallel to the floor. Place your hands next to your head and grasp the sides of the bench, or near your hips as shown.
MOVEMENT: Keeping your legs as straight as possible, raise them slowly until you're in a jackknife position. Your head and shoulders shouldn't move — make sure your abs do all the work. Unfold your body slowly and under control, lowering your legs back to the start position.

Keep your head on the bench; raising it can put undue pressure on your cervical spine.

PLANK

TARGETS: Core
START: Lie face-down on the floor and prop yourself up on your forearms with your elbows bent 90 degrees. Extend your legs and flex your feet so your toes touch the floor.
MOVEMENT: Keeping your abs pulled in tight and your back flat, lift your hips so your bodyweight is supported by your forearms and toes. Hold this position for up to 30 seconds. Maintain a tight low back and squeeze your glutes to prevent your body from sagging in the middle.

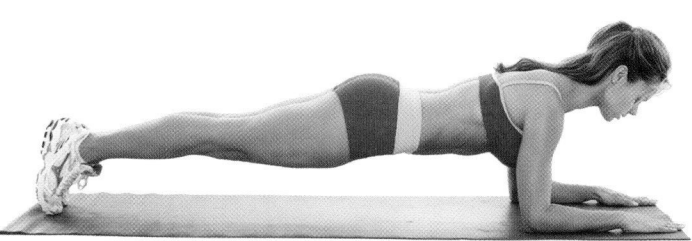

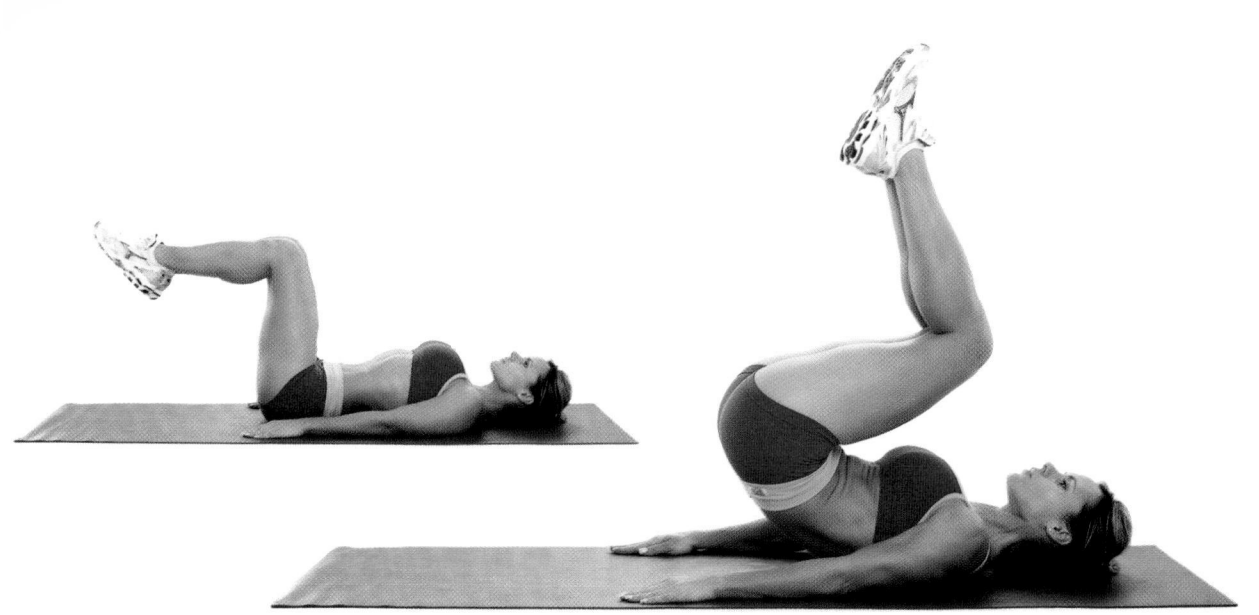

REVERSE CRUNCH

TARGETS: Lower abs
START: Lie face-up on the floor, feet up and thighs perpendicular to the floor. Place your arms down by your sides, palms on the floor.
MOVEMENT: Using your lower abs, bring your knees to your chest. Return slowly to the starting position and repeat.

WEEKLY NUTRITION GOALS

Week 1: Write It Down
Research shows that people who keep a food journal are more successful at losing and maintaining weight. It simply makes you more accountable: When you write down every morsel you put in your mouth and note how certain foods make you feel or affect your performance mentally and physically, you can easily make adjustments. Continue doing this throughout the program.

Week 2: Carry Water
Regular water keeps digestion, nutrient absorption, temperature regulation and waste elimination running smoothly. Plus, a 2003 study found that drinking a half-liter of cold water increased metabolic rate by 30% for more than an hour after drinking.

To calculate your water-intake goals, take your bodyweight in pounds and divide that number by two. That gives you the minimum number of ounces of water you should drink daily.

Week 3: Eat Protein at Every Meal
Eating protein makes you feel satisfied, therefore decreasing hunger sensations. If you eat only carbs, you'll crave more; more carbs can turn into a vicious cycle leading to poor energy and weight gain because of increased calorie intake. Aim to consume 20–30 grams of protein at every meal.

Week 4: Make One New Recipe Per Week
Doing this accomplishes a few things: Cooking at home eliminates eating out (where you can't control portions or ingredients), it introduces a variety of foods into your diet, and did we mention portion control?

≫Phase Two...

Weeks 5-8:
MAKING PROGRESS

Time to build some muscle. This month, add weight to the exercises from Phase One. Just like last month, do the program below in the order listed, three days a week, resting at least 48 hours between workouts. In addition, perform your regular weight-training routine and increase your cardio to 45 minutes per session 4–5 days a week.

#9

EXERCISE	SETS	REPS
Exercise Ball Crunch with Medicine Ball	3	12
Weighted V-Twist	2	10 (to each side)
Hip Thrust with Medicine Ball	3	10
Weighted Plank	3	25–30 sec.

WEIGHTED V-TWIST

TARGETS: All regions, with emphasis on the obliques and core
START: Sit on the floor with your legs extended but slightly bent. Hold a medicine ball with both hands in front of your abdominals and bend your arms slightly. Cross your ankles and lean your upper body back about 45 degrees. Elevate your feet about 6 inches off the floor.
MOVEMENT: Twist your torso to one side until the ball touches the floor. Smoothly return to center, then repeat the motion to the other side. Keep your abs tight throughout the exercise. Do 10 reps to each side.

You can also do this with a weight plate.

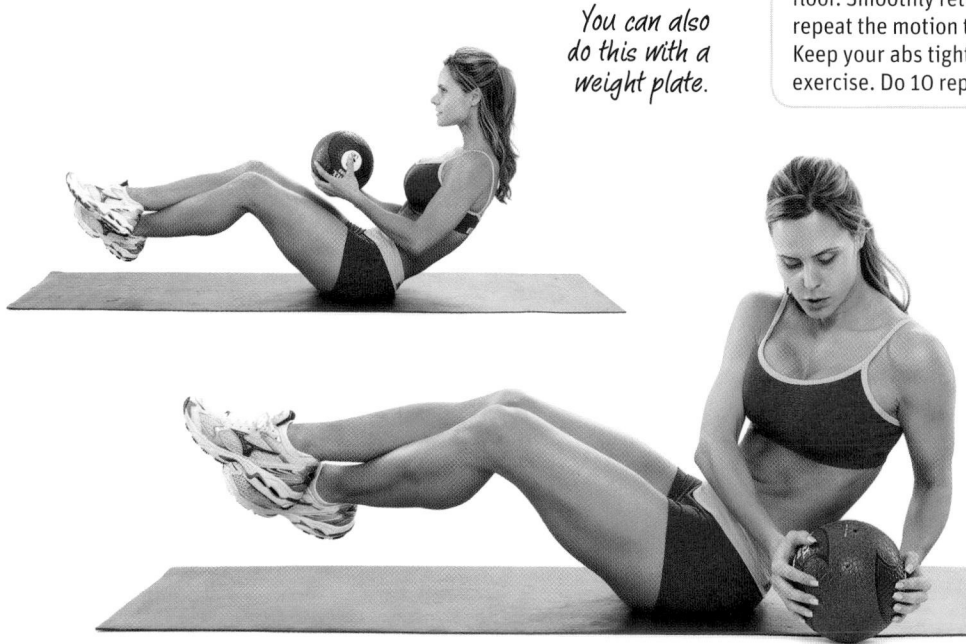

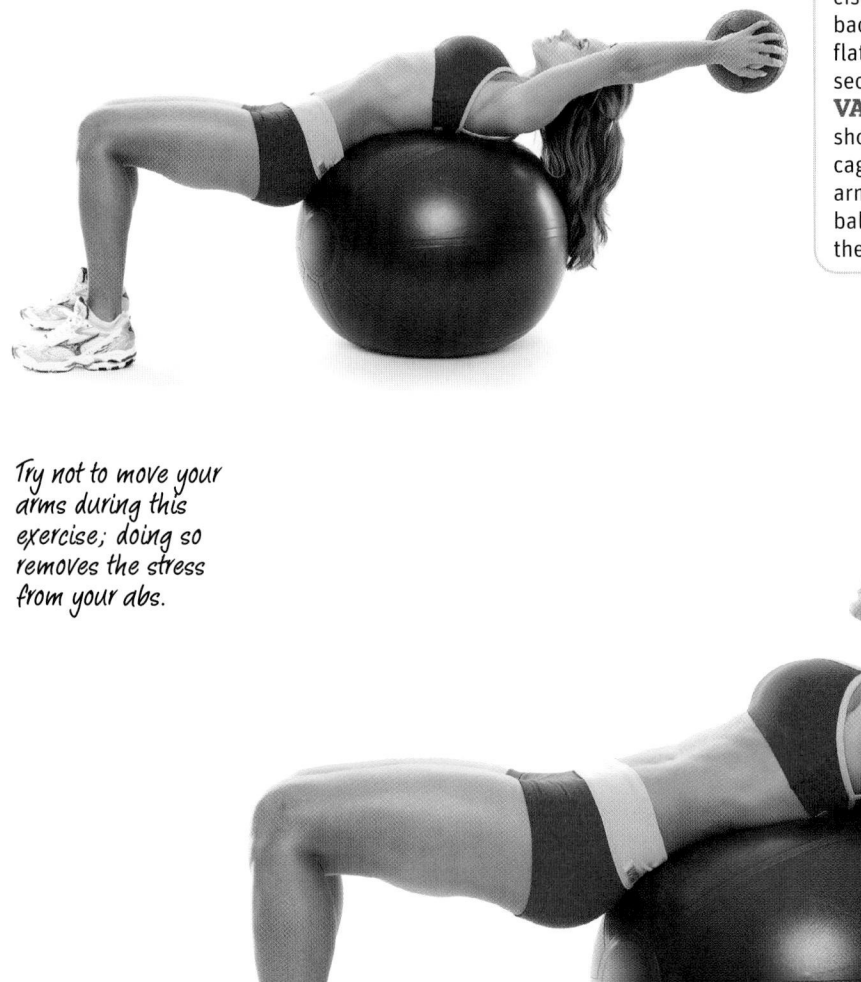

EXERCISE-BALL CRUNCH WITH MEDICINE BALL

TARGETS: Upper abs

START: Lie face-up on a large exercise ball with your lower and middle back supported, knees bent and feet flat on the floor. Hold a medicine ball securely overhead at arm's length.

VARIATION: Raise your head and shoulders as you crunch your rib cage toward your pelvis. Keep your arms straight so that the medicine ball is overhead. Contract your abs at the top of the motion for a one-count.

Try not to move your arms during this exercise; doing so removes the stress from your abs.

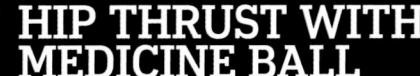

HIP THRUST WITH MEDICINE BALL

TARGETS: Lower abs
START: Lie face-up on the floor with your arms at your sides, palms down. Lift your legs until your thighs are perpendicular to the floor. Hold a medicine ball securely between your knees.
MOVEMENT: Use your abs to lift your hips. At first this will be only a few inches off the floor; the stronger you get, the higher you'll be able to lift.

Begin with a light medicine ball to get the form down; you can also start using just an ordinary ball.

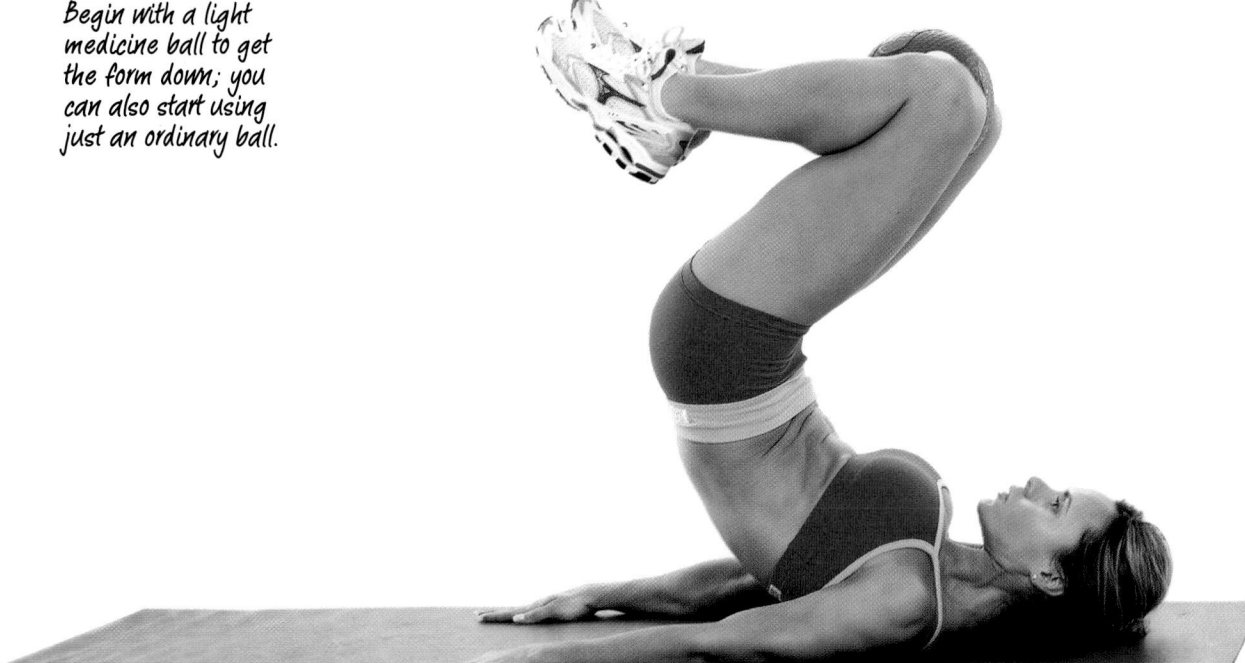

You may need to enlist someone to place the plate on your back.

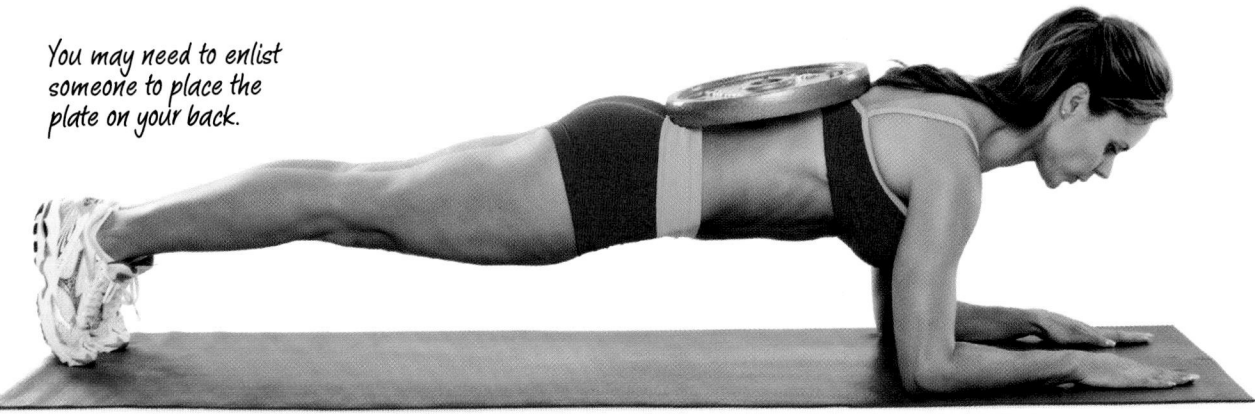

WEIGHTED PLANK

TARGETS: Core
START: Lie face-down on the floor with a weight plate balanced on your lower back. Prop yourself up onto your forearms with your elbows bent 90 degrees. Extend your legs and flex your feet so your toes touch the floor.

MOVEMENT: Keeping your abs pulled in tight and your back flat, lift your hips so your forearms and toes support your bodyweight. Hold this position for up to 30 seconds. Maintain a tight low back and squeeze your glutes to prevent your body from sagging in the middle.

WEEKLY NUTRITION GOALS

Week 5: Load Up on Fruits and Vegetables
Consider the colors of your fruits and vegetables as your map to beneficial phytochemicals and antioxidants. Each color represents different phytochemicals that work in different parts of your body's cells. Consuming a rainbow of foods during the day helps fight off the cell damage that intense exercise can provoke.

Week 6: Forget Late-Night Munchies
Avoid eating three hours before bed. However, if you must, eat protein like low-fat cottage cheese, a part-skim mozzarella cheese stick or a boiled egg. Do not eat carbs during this three-hour period since any food intake is more easily stored as fat when you're asleep.

Week 7: Avoid Drinking Your Calories
Consider this: Drinking a 10-ounce glass of fruit juice each day can add 51,100 calories in a year, or nearly 15 pounds. Tired of water? Drink green tea or coffee; both benefit your health and training without calories. Green tea contains antioxidants and can help burn fat. Coffee has been shown to improve performance in the gym when consumed before training.

Week 8: Eat Whole Grains
Whole grains are higher in fiber, protein and other important nutrients, and they make you feel satisfied and full longer. Research also shows that women who eat whole grains weigh less than those who don't. Choose 100% whole-wheat bread, brown rice and whole-wheat pastas. This step will help you avoid sugar and refined wheat, preparing you for next week's goal.

Weeks 9-12: THE FINAL STRETCH

Welcome to the last four weeks of your fab ab journey. This month's goal is to build muscle endurance. Perform the program below three days per week, resting at least 48 hours between workouts. Do your regular weight-training routine and increase your cardio to 4–5 days a week, 45–60 minutes per session.

#10

EXERCISE	SETS	REPS
Side Plank	2	25–30 sec.
Boat Sit	2	25–30 sec.
Weighted Plank on BOSU	2	25–30 sec.
Weighted Single Leg Plank	2	25–30 sec.

This small movement will test your oblique strength.

SIDE PLANK

TARGETS: Core
START: Lie on your left side with your legs extended. Prop yourself up on your left elbow, which should be directly below your shoulder.
MOVEMENT: Keeping your left elbow and left foot in contact with the floor, raise your hips as high as possible without rolling forward or back. Keep your body in a straight line and your abs tight. Hold this position as long as you can, working up to 20 seconds. Slowly lower your hips to return to the starting position, and repeat for reps. Switch sides and repeat.

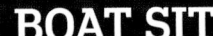

BOAT SIT

TARGETS: Core

START: Sit on the floor with your legs extended, abs tight and back straight. Extend your arms in front of you so they're parallel to the floor.

MOVEMENT: Lean back 45 degrees, then lift your feet off the floor about 6 inches. Hold for as long as possible while maintaining good form; work up to 30 seconds.

Concentrate on using only your ab power during this exercise.

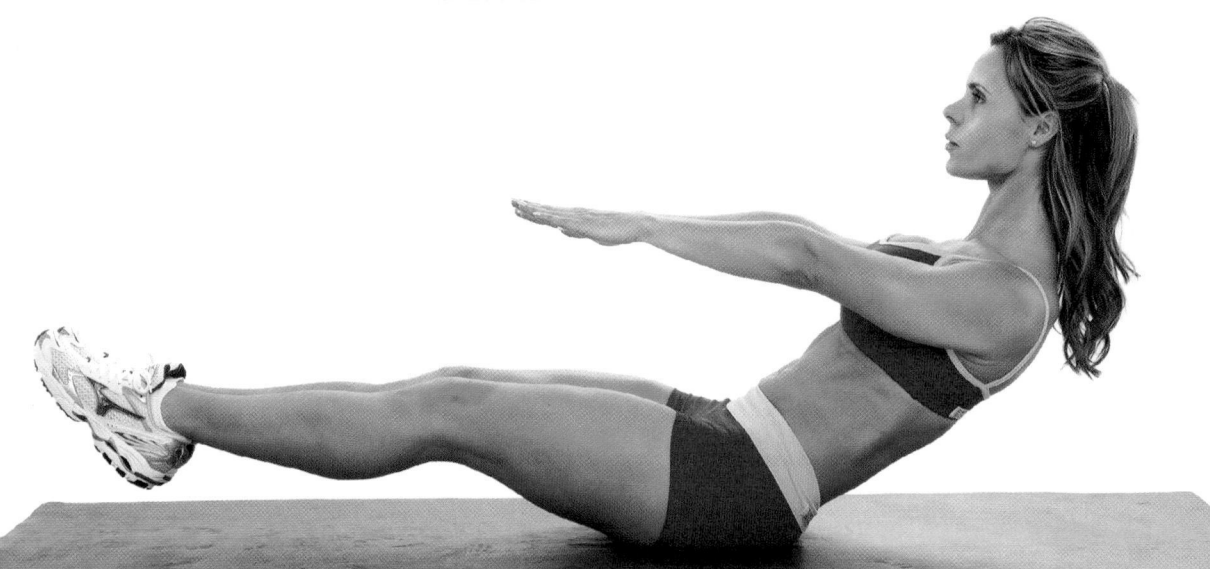

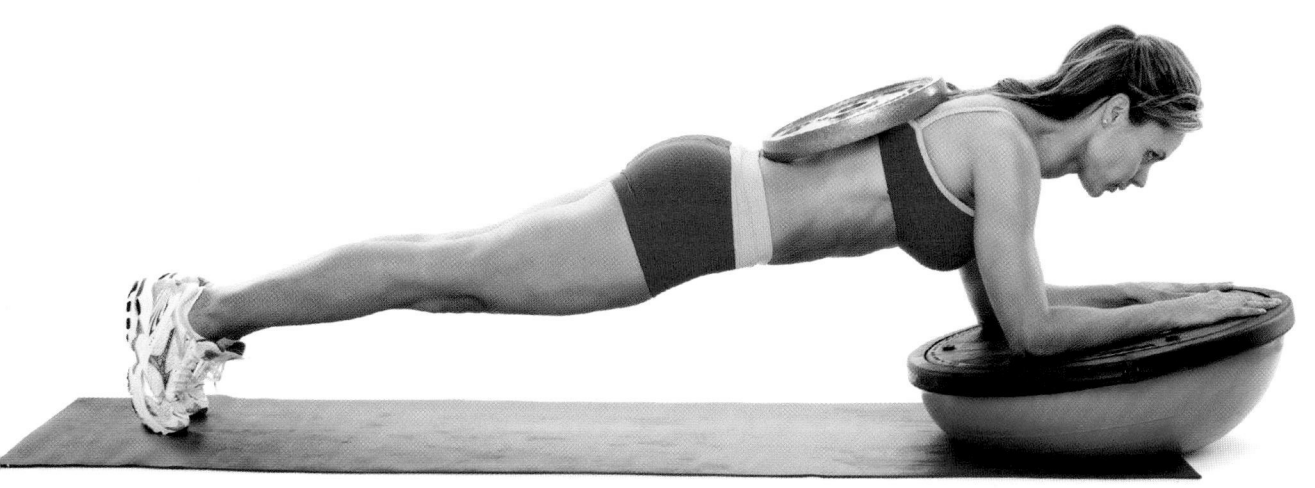

WEIGHTED PLANK ON BOSU

TARGETS: Core
START: Kneel on all fours with your arms on the flat side of a BOSU and a weight plate balanced on your back. Position your elbows under your shoulders and extend your forearms and hands forward. Extend your legs and flex your feet so your toes touch the floor. You may need a training partner to place the plate.
MOVEMENT: Keeping your abs pulled in tight and your back flat, lift your hips so your forearms and toes support your bodyweight. Hold this position for up to 30 seconds. Maintain a tight low back and squeeze your glutes to prevent your body from sagging in the middle.

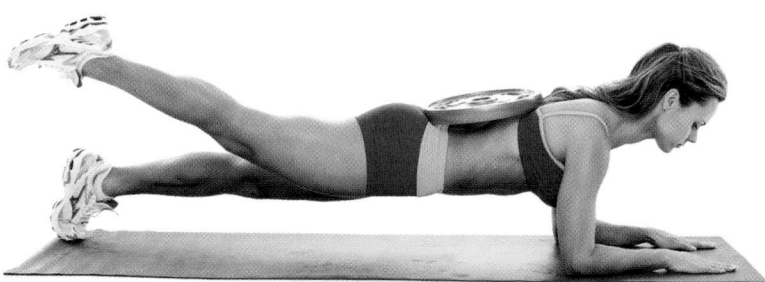

WEIGHTED SINGLE-LEG PLANK

TARGETS: Core
START: Lie face-down on the floor with a weight plate balanced on your lower back. Prop yourself up onto your forearms with your elbows bent 90 degrees. Extend your legs and flex your feet so your toes touch the floor.
VARIATION: Keeping your abdominals pulled in tight and your back flat, lift your hips so that your forearms and toes support your bodyweight. Maintain a tight low back and squeeze your glutes to prevent your body from sagging in the middle. Lift one foot off the ground about 6 inches, or as high as you can, while keeping your back flat. Hold this position as long as you can. Lower and repeat with the other foot. Work your way up to holding the position for 30 seconds.

WEEKLY NUTRITION GOALS

Week 9: Eat "Clean"

Start eating clean, which means you need to eat more fresh fruits and vegetables, whole grains, low-fat dairy, nuts, seeds, and lean meats and fish. Minimize the intake of foods with preservatives, artificial ingredients, chemically altered fats and high sodium.

Week 10: Subtract Added Sugar

Consider that the average American consumes 20 teaspoons of added sugar daily — in the forms of corn syrup, glucose and table sugar added into processed foods — and that adds about 320 calories per day. Cutting these unwanted calories can help you lose the fat that seems to be holding onto your midsection.

Week 11: Revisit Your Journal

Two weeks to your goal, how's your diet? Look over your food journal entries. Have you been eating enough protein? How's your vegetable intake? Can you crank each up a notch? Identify the areas in which you might have been a bit lax and renew your commitment.

Week 12: Eliminate Salt

At this point, you have only seven days until it's time to reveal your abs at the pool, beach, park or gym. So if you've been using frozen meals for portion control, canned vegetables to get your five-a-day or deli meat for your protein fix, say no to them this week because they contain higher levels of sodium than fresh foods. Too much of this mineral can promote water retention and bloating — two things that can hide your hard-earned ab definition. Look at your journal to identify the sneaky ways salt gets in your diet and cut back. It may mean breaking up with your saltshaker.

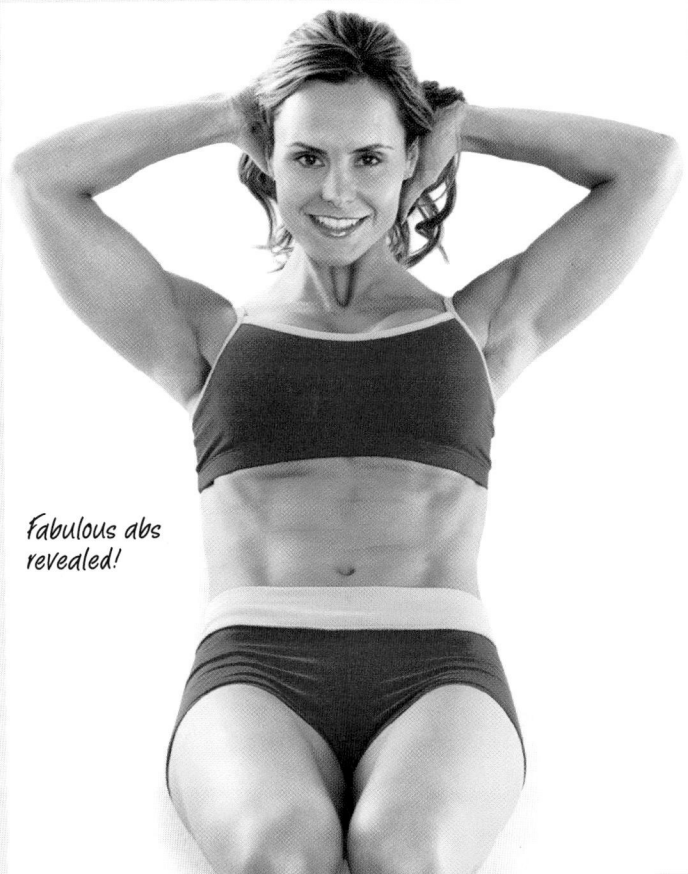

Fabulous abs revealed!

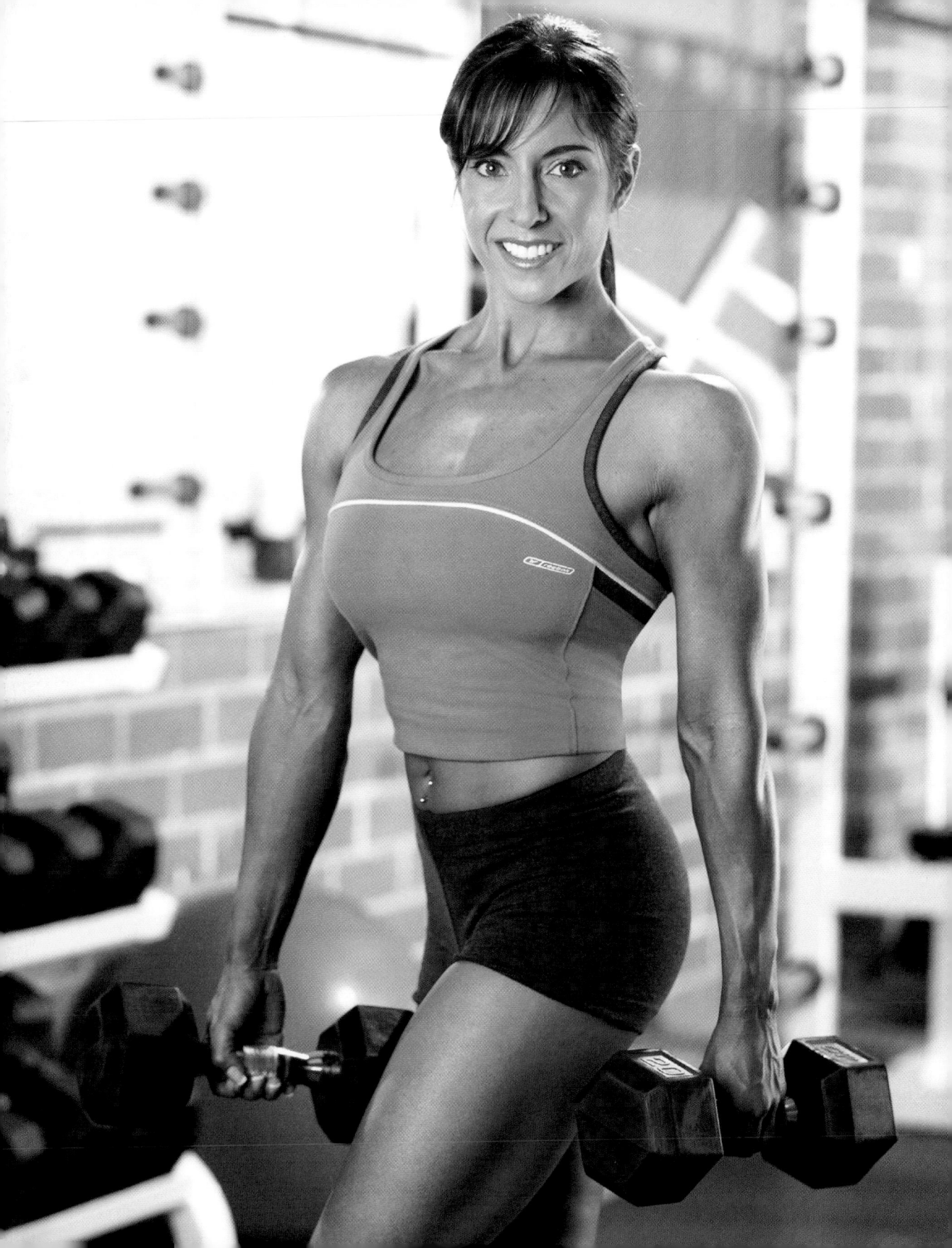

Chapter 4

Empowering Exercises

Have you ever watched a professional sporting event on TV and marveled at the physiques of the participants while silently cursing your genetic code for providing you with a less-than-magnificent body? While pro athletes are often blessed with superior physical traits that help them reach the top of their games, they also train hard, utilizing techniques and exercises that you don't.

This is especially true of athletes who play sports that involve explosive movements. Olympic sprinters, WNBA players, pro tennis players and beach volleyball divas all sprint, lunge, jump, serve, block and shoot with power. To be the best they can, these athletes overload their fast-twitch muscle fibers with power exercises and sprints, and this steady diet of explosive training is what provides the stimulus necessary for developing a world-class physique.

Remember this next time you're about to spend an hour moving at a sluggish pace on the stair-stepper or pumping out rep after rep on a weight machine. If you really want to make some serious changes to your physique, it's time to change your style of training. Incorporate these seven power exercises into your workout routine, and you'll look like a pro — in and out of the gym!

TRAIN LIKE A PRO

IFBB fitness pro Carla Sanchez was introduced to power training as a college basketball player. Today, she uses this style of training to improve her physique and make her a better athlete, capable of performing the exciting routines required in her sport. She employs a combination of speed-strength training, powerlifting (squats, deadlifts, bench presses), Olympic lifts (high pulls, snatches, cleans), and plyometrics to create a show-stopping body capable of executing powerful gymnastics movements.

Sanchez admits her program is unlike that of many of her fellow fitness competitors, but she credits this style of training with helping her develop a sexy, lean and athletic look. "Power training utilizes high levels of energy stores, burns fat and feels like a real workout," she says. "When you leave the gym, you'll definitely feel as

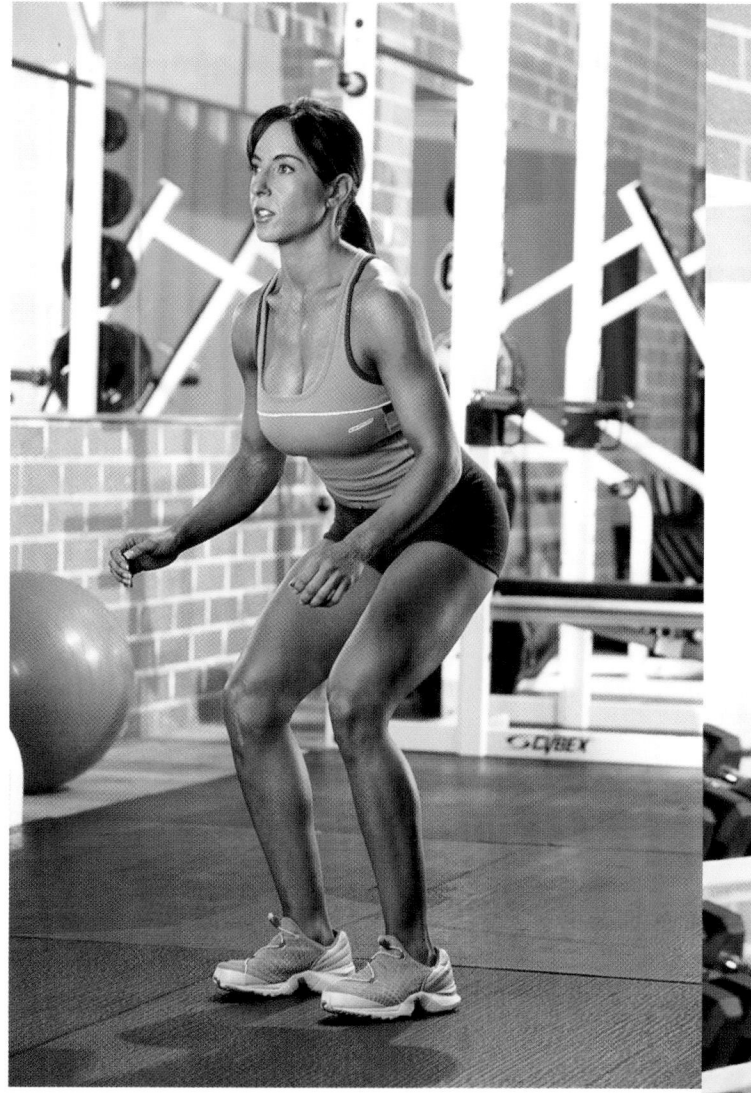

Tuck Jump

Muscle groups worked: abs, glutes, hamstrings, quads, calves. Execution: Take an athletic stance with your feet about shoulder-width apart. Hold your hands at about waist height, palms facing the ground to give your knees a target as you jump. Once you master the technique of pulling your knees as high as possible on each jump, you can drop your arms and swing them to gain maximum jumping height. To initiate each jump, quickly bend your knees (to about half-squat position), then instantly explode up into the air. Once airborne, use your hip flexors and abdominals to pull your knees as high as possible up to your chest so that they touch your hands. Upon landing, quickly change directions and explode into the air again. Picture yourself jumping on hot coals to reduce the amount of time you spend on the ground between reps.

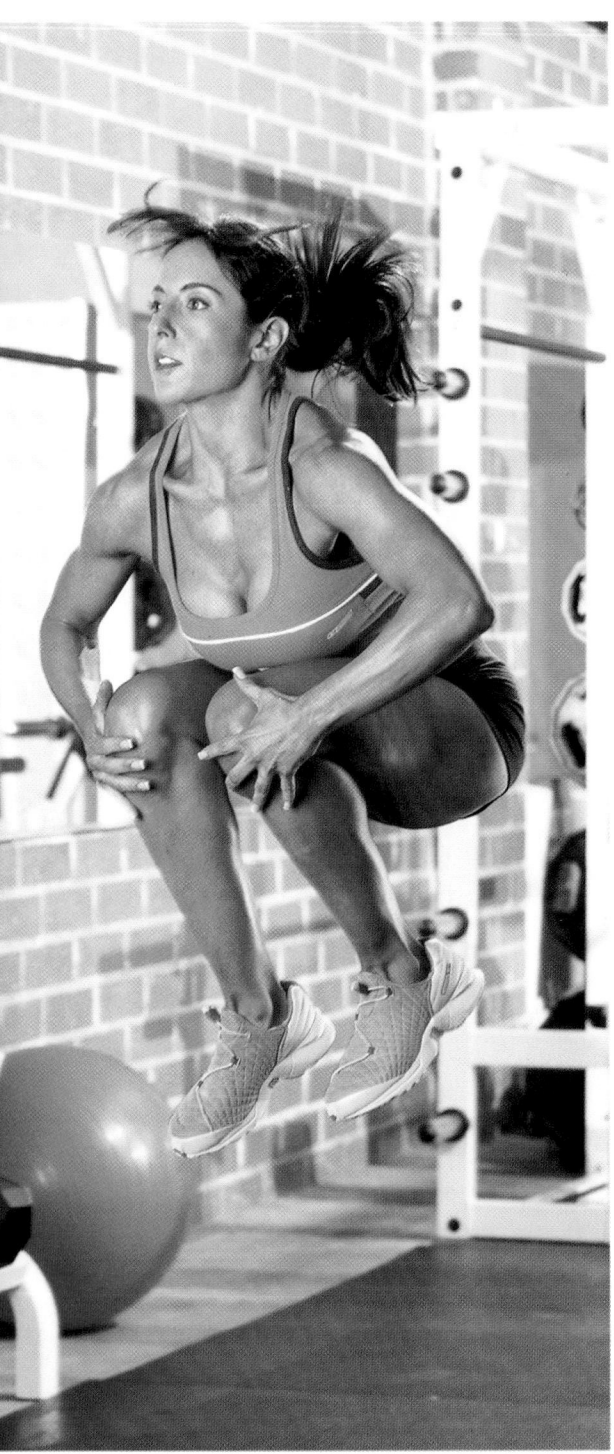

though you've put your body to the test."

Unlike the traditional body-sculpting workout that focuses on slow, controlled isolation exercises, power training centers more on explosive, full-body movements, which are great for burning calories as well as toning muscles. Sanchez asserts that once you begin to include power training in your weekly workouts, you can expect improvements in other areas as well. "Working the whole body as a unit is great for developing an athletic look and eliminating any existing muscle imbalances. Another benefit is that this type of training really shapes and tightens your legs and glutes, since most of the exercises involve a lot of explosive lower-body actions. Targeting your fast-twitch fibers is one of the best things you can do to develop awesome legs."

POWER POTENTIAL

If you look closely at the backgrounds of present-day IFBB fitness pros, you'll notice that many of them were collegiate gymnasts. Some believe that a gymnastics background is beneficial to fitness competitors because of the skill and technical ability required to perform onstage. Sanchez, however, feels that these former gymnasts excel not only because of their technical training and superior routines but also because of the power training they've done over the years.

The plyometric and bodyweight exercises that gymnasts perform on a daily basis allow them to execute the difficult moves required in competition and handle their own bodyweight with ease, thus allowing them to gracefully execute movements that require a high degree of strength and power. In addition, this regimen has led to the shapely, lean physique rewarded by the judges. Others who've trained for years using only classical bodybuilding-style training to sculpt an aesthetically pleasing shape may never develop the explosive potential of their fast-twitch fibers.

Thus, power training is key for achieving peak athletic performance and maximum aesthetic beauty. Check out the exercises and program included here; they're sure to nourish the athlete that resides within you. Power training just might be the stimulus your body needs to break through a plateau and finally develop that pro athlete look. Now, if only you could get the salary to match!

POWER PRELIMINARIES

Before incorporating these power moves into your workout, heed the following advice from IFBB fitness pro Sanchez.

Find a coach to teach you correct form for all these exercises — preferably someone who's a certified strength and conditioning specialist (CSCS) and has experience working with athletes. It's very difficult to master these moves just by looking at them in a magazine. You need the feedback and help of a trained professional to do them correctly and safely.

If you're a beginner, start with circuit training to build up your anaerobic fitness level. This will enable you to build the base you need to eventually complete a full power workout without fatiguing prematurely. Remember, these moves involve many muscle groups at once, and they can leave you gasping for breath if you're not physically prepared to handle the workload.

Use compound moves to work your muscle groups together, which will help you develop the ability to work many muscle groups as one unit. This will better prepare you for properly executing the power exercises, which are composed of explosive, coordinated, sequential body movements.

Incorporate bodyweight movements into your workouts. Dips, chins, pull-ups and push-ups are great exercises since you must learn to handle your own bodyweight. Once you master these basics, you can move on to the more advanced gymnastics and power moves that fitness competitors regularly use in their routines.

Note: These exercises and workout program are geared toward intermediate- and advanced-level exercisers. If you're new to exercise, haven't worked out consistently in the past three months or are under a doctor's care for a medical condition, consult your physician before beginning this or any other workout program.

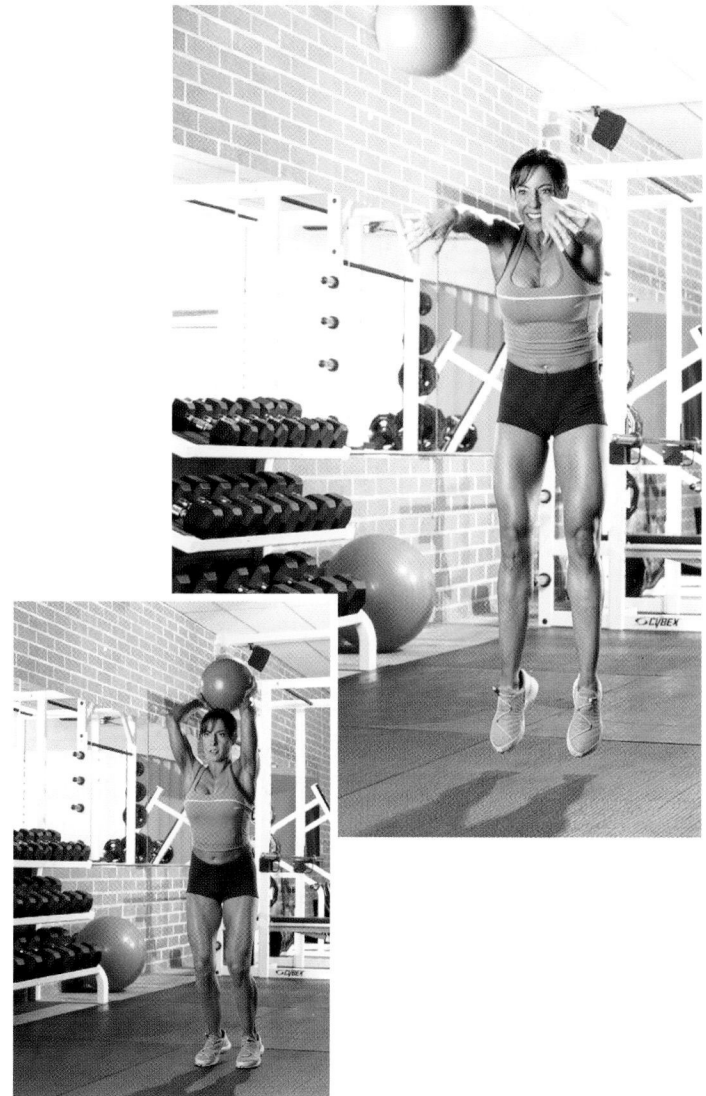

Overhead Medicine-Ball Throw

Muscle groups worked: lats, delts, pecs, traps, triceps, abs. Execution: Facing a wall or partner, stand with your feet about shoulder-width apart and hold a 4- to 8-pound medicine ball with both hands in front of your body. To begin the movement, quickly bring the ball back behind your head to "load" your muscles. At this point, your elbows should be bent at about 90 degrees, your back should be arched and your knees slightly bent. Explosively initiate the forward motion from this point by bending your knees and pushing your hips forward, allowing your upper body and arms to whip forward, firing the ball at the wall or a partner. Contract your abs hard as you release the ball. Prepare to catch the ball again, and move rapidly into the next throw. This time, pretend the ball is a hot potato — get that thing moving!

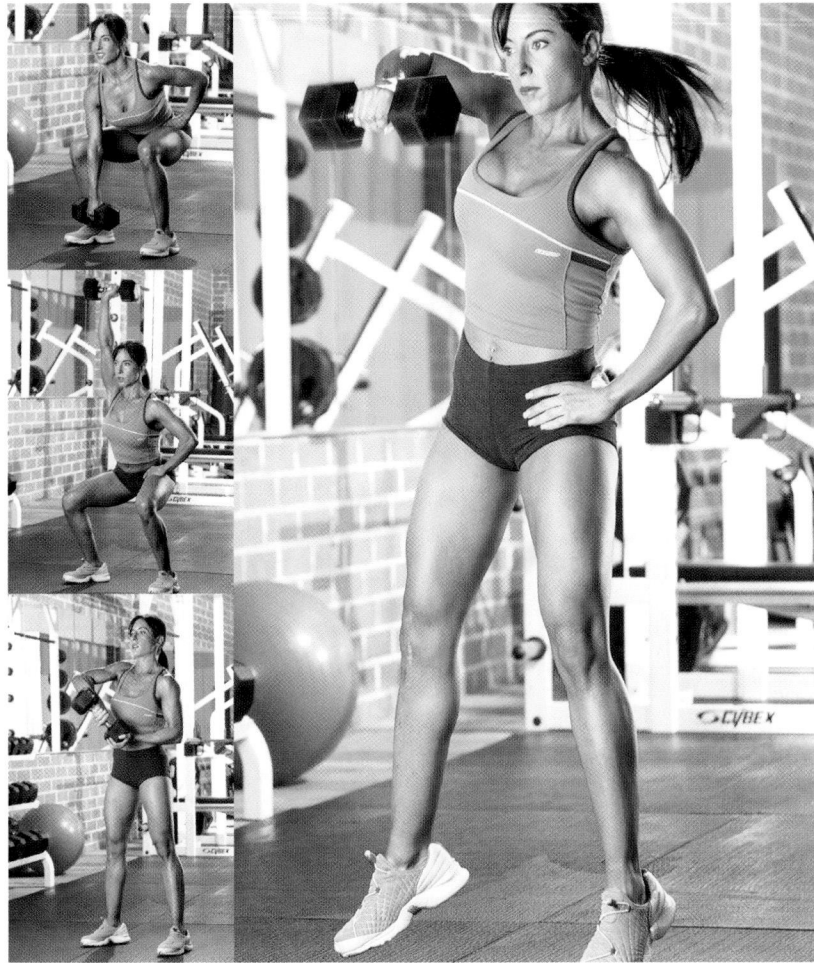

Single-Arm Dumbbell Snatch

Muscle groups worked: glutes, hamstrings, quads, calves, spinal erectors, traps, delts, triceps. Execution: With your feet slightly wider than shoulder width, bend your knees and lean forward from the hips. Grasp a dumbbell with your right hand using a pronated grip (palm facing your body), and keep your arm fully straightened. Your low back should be flat or slightly arched, your head and chest up, shoulders pulled back. From this starting position, push your hips forward powerfully and extend your knees in a jumping motion. As you drive up onto your toes, hold the dumbbell close to your thigh with your arm straight. Once your hips, knees and ankles are fully extended, shrug your shoulders and pull the dumbbell up toward your chin, allowing your elbow to bend. After you've pulled the dumbbell as high as you can, rotate your elbow under the weight quickly, bend your knees and "pull" yourself under the dumbbell. Lock your elbow with the dumbbell overhead and absorb the weight by bending your knees. Come out of the finish position by lowering the dumbbell — using your free hand for support — and standing at the same time. Repeat for reps, then switch arms.

You can either incorporate these moves into your existing workout or add one or two days of power training to your weekly regimen. IFBB fitness pro Carla Sanchez recommends the routine at right, preceded by a 10-minute warm-up of skipping or light jogging.

#11 The Power Workout

Exercise	Sets	Reps
Single-Arm Dumbbell Snatch	3	10–12
Power Clean	3	10–12
Clean High Pull	3	10–12
Tuck Jump	3	15
Lateral Hop	3	15
Overhead Medicine-Ball Throw	3	12–15
Power Push-Up	3	12–15

Cardio: Do 20–30 minutes of sprints on the treadmill or track. First, warm up with an easy jog for five minutes. Once you're warmed up, start with sprint intervals: Sprint hard for 60 seconds, then jog slowly for two minutes to recover. Repeat for the desired number of intervals. Try five to start, adding one more interval each week until you can do 10.

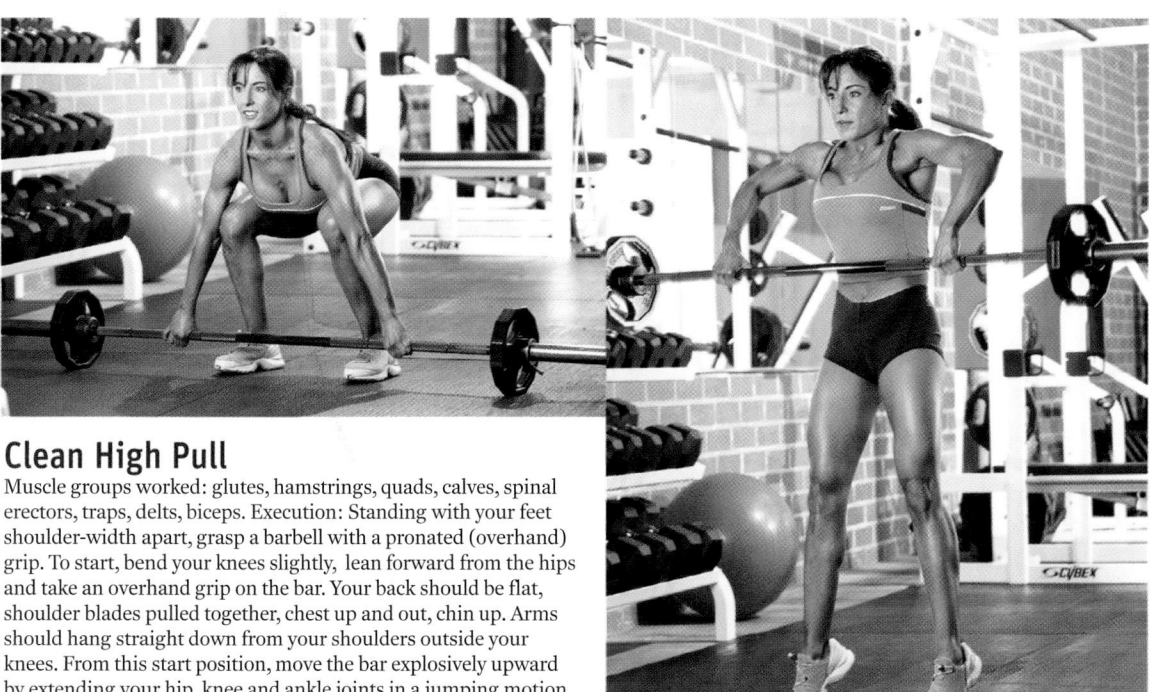

Clean High Pull

Muscle groups worked: glutes, hamstrings, quads, calves, spinal erectors, traps, delts, biceps. Execution: Standing with your feet shoulder-width apart, grasp a barbell with a pronated (overhand) grip. To start, bend your knees slightly, lean forward from the hips and take an overhand grip on the bar. Your back should be flat, shoulder blades pulled together, chest up and out, chin up. Arms should hang straight down from your shoulders outside your knees. From this start position, move the bar explosively upward by extending your hip, knee and ankle joints in a jumping motion. Keep your elbows straight, the bar close to your body, and your shoulders over the bar as long as possible to generate as much power as you can. Once you get up on your toes, shrug your shoulders and pull with your arms to finish the lift with the bar as high as possible. During this upper-body pulling action, keep your elbows out and high, as you would in an upright row. Carefully return the weight to your starting position, get set and repeat.

Lateral Hop

Muscle groups worked: glutes, abductors, adductors, hamstrings, quads, calves. Execution: In this exercise, you'll jump back and forth laterally over a small cone or low bench. You may want to practice this drill for a few weeks by jumping over a line on the ground so you don't need to worry about tripping over a raised barrier. Stand in an athletic position (knees bent, leaning forward slightly, on the balls of your feet) to the right of a low bench or small cone. Jump off both feet, pull your knees up to your chest to clear the obstacle, and land in a balanced position on the left side of the line, bench or cone. Quickly absorb the landing and explode back over the obstacle, landing back on the right side where you started. Pretend you're jumping on hot coals to limit your ground contact time — this makes the exercise more effective. Continue to jump laterally over the obstacle for the prescribed number of reps. Every time you clear the obstacle counts as one rep.

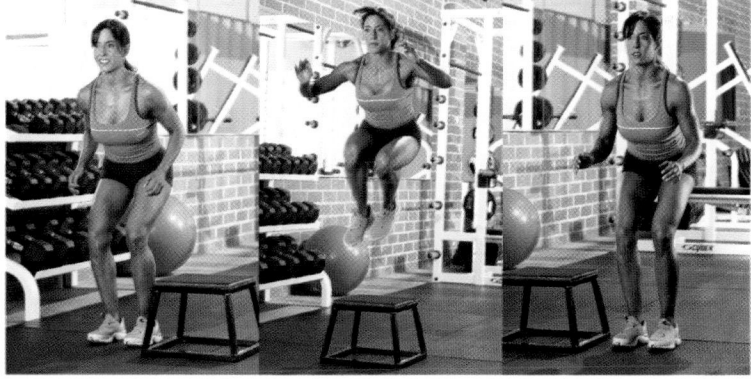

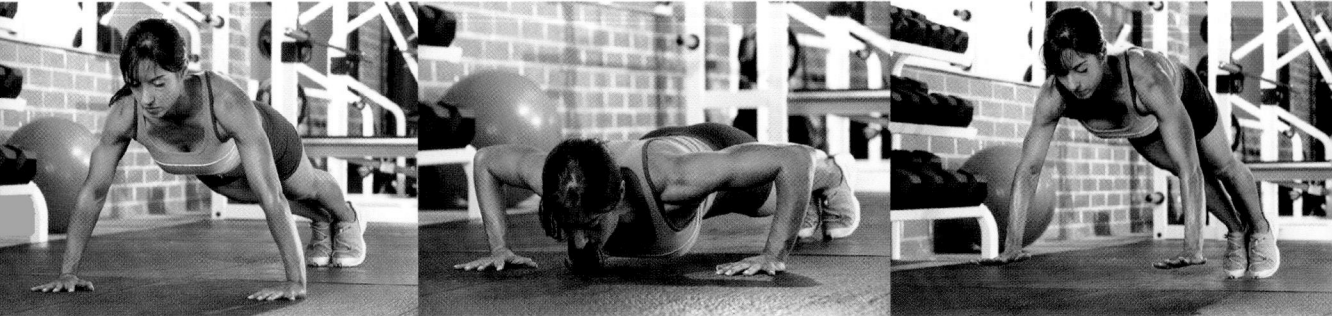

Power Push-Up

Muscle groups worked: pecs, delts, triceps. Execution: Start in a regular push-up position with your hands placed slightly wider than shoulder-width apart. Descend rapidly toward the floor, then press forcefully upward with your arms just before your body touches the ground. Continue driving up from the floor until your hands leave the ground and your upper body is airborne. Cushion the landing by bending your elbows and descend again, then quickly press up again to begin the next rep — think of hot coals being under your hands! To start, you may want to do this exercise using your knees as the ground contact point rather than your toes. This will reduce the difficulty of the movement slightly so that you can develop the proper form and build enough strength to move on to the more difficult version.

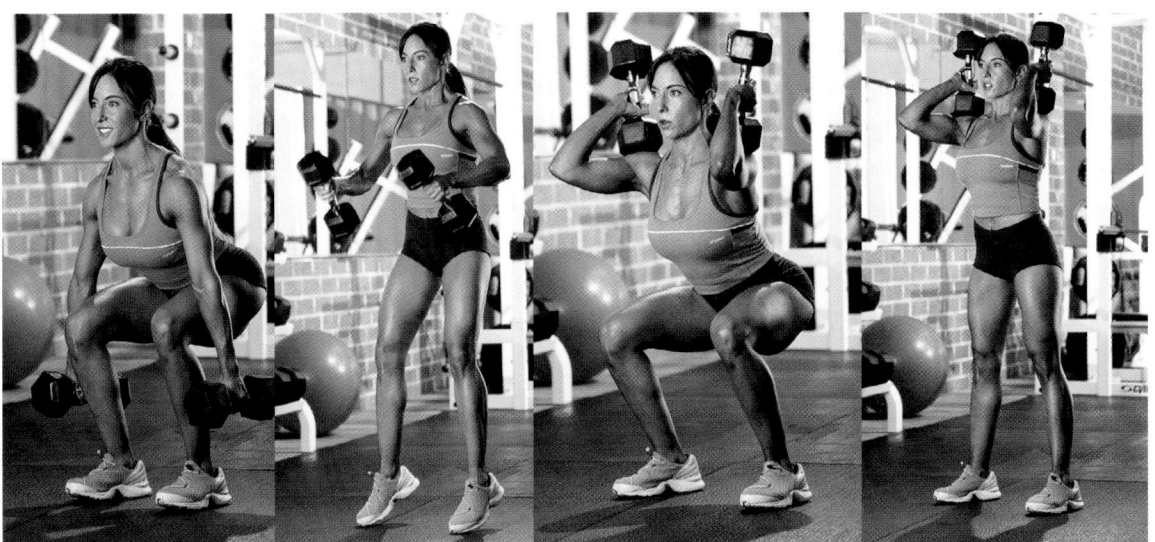

Power Clean

Muscle groups worked: glutes, hamstrings, quads, calves, spinal erectors, traps, delts, biceps. Execution: Grasp two dumbbells with a neutral grip and assume a squat position with your feet hip-width apart. From this position, move the weights explosively upward by extending your hip, knee and ankle joints in a jumping motion. Quickly rotate your elbows and arms under the dumbbells as you bring them up, pulling your body underneath the weights. Point your elbows forward or slightly up in the air after you perform the "catch" phase of the lift. Hold the weights over your shoulders in a quarter-squat position, flexing your hips and knees to absorb the weight. Finish by squatting the weights up to a standing position. Carefully return the weights to your starting position, get set and repeat. Make sure you have mastered the technique of the clean high pull before moving on to the power clean. It's crucial that you get the timing aspect of this movement down. Ideally, it will feel like the weights are moving explosively and you're just timing the bending of your arms with the momentum of the weights. Technique and timing are key. Get an experienced strength coach or trainer to teach you the basics.

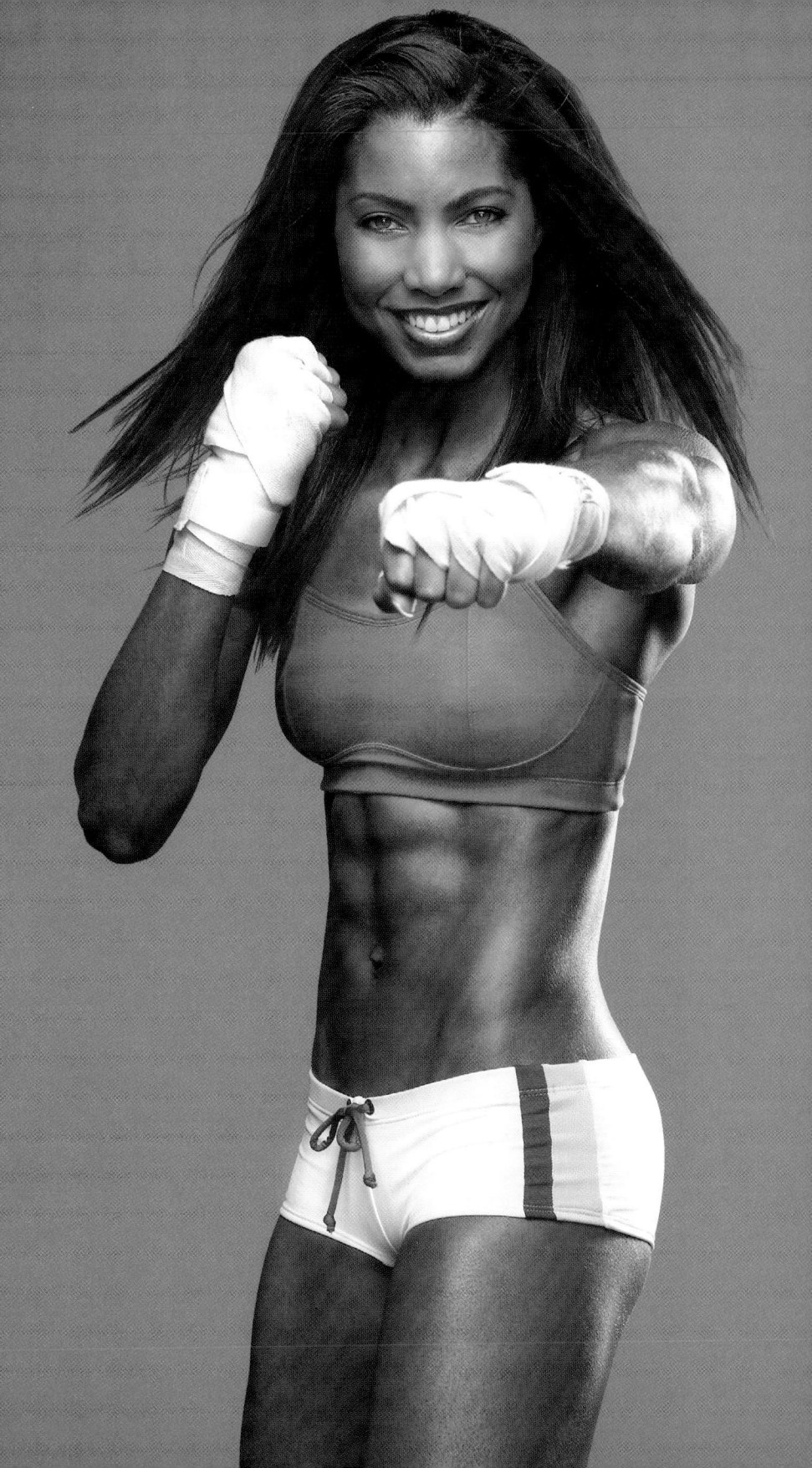

cardio

contents

You cannot beat bodyfat with weight training alone. If you really want to banish the blubber that is covering your abs (and arms and butt), you need to commit to doing heart-pounding, sweat-drenching, calorie-burning cardiovascular fitness workouts.

In this section, you will find just the routines you need to help round out your training 1-2-3 fat-burning punch.

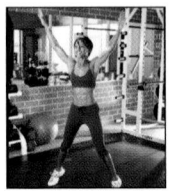
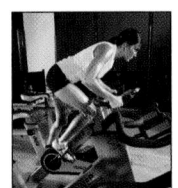
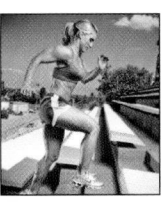

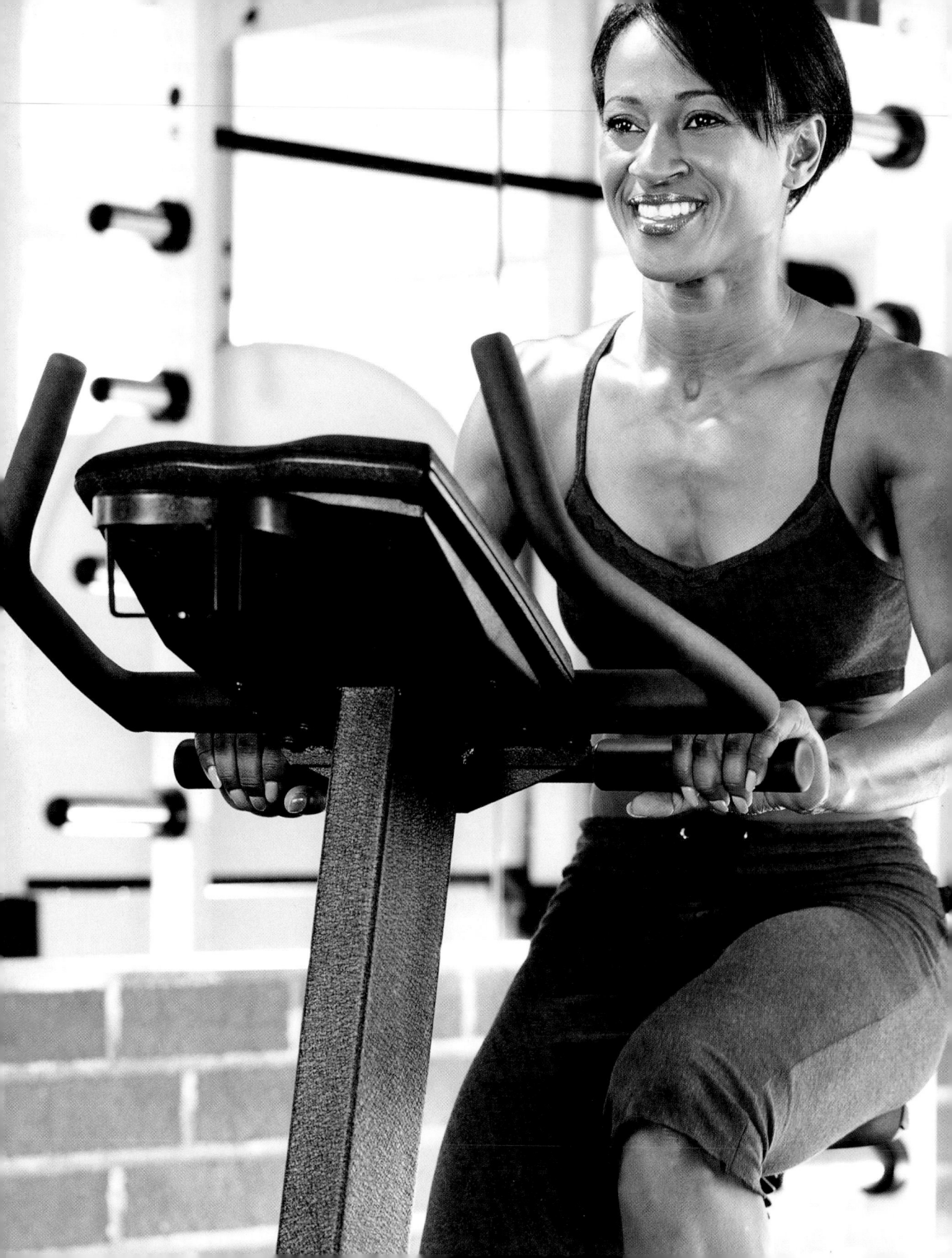

Chapter 5

Custom Cardio

Not all cardiovascular exercise is created equal. High-intensity interval training not only promotes fat-burning, but also improves cardiovascular fitness. Endurance training will also do this, as well as build your muscular endurance. Circuit training increases your heart rate to help you burn calories and build muscle strength. Here's why and how you should use each in your fitness routine.

get ready to sweat

A good workout program isn't complete without cardiovascular exercise. Aside from helping maintain a healthy heart and lungs, cardiovascular activity can also help lower bodyfat and promote a positive body image. Numerous studies link exercise with stress relief and mood regulation. So when your stress level is outrageous, your panacea comes in the form of exercise.

Don't think you need to exercise aerobically for hours on end to burn the most fat — your body is a remarkable machine, and will quickly adapt to this repeated stimulus. Who has an hour to tromp on a treadmill, anyway? To get the most bang for your buck in the shortest time, turn to interval training.

ENTER INTERVALS

Interval training involves alternating short bursts of intense activity with a session of active recovery, in which you keep moving at a less intense pace. By alternating intensity levels within a single workout, your body becomes more efficient at flushing lactic acid and toxins from your cells while simultaneously training the heart to recover faster.

As a bonus, interval training has an "afterburn" effect. This means you maintain an elevated metabolic rate for the remainder of the day. Because of the intensity, these workouts are also shorter, making them a perfect addition to a busy, modern-day schedule.

But as with sugar cookies and pumpkin pie, too much of a good thing can hurt you. Because of the high demands

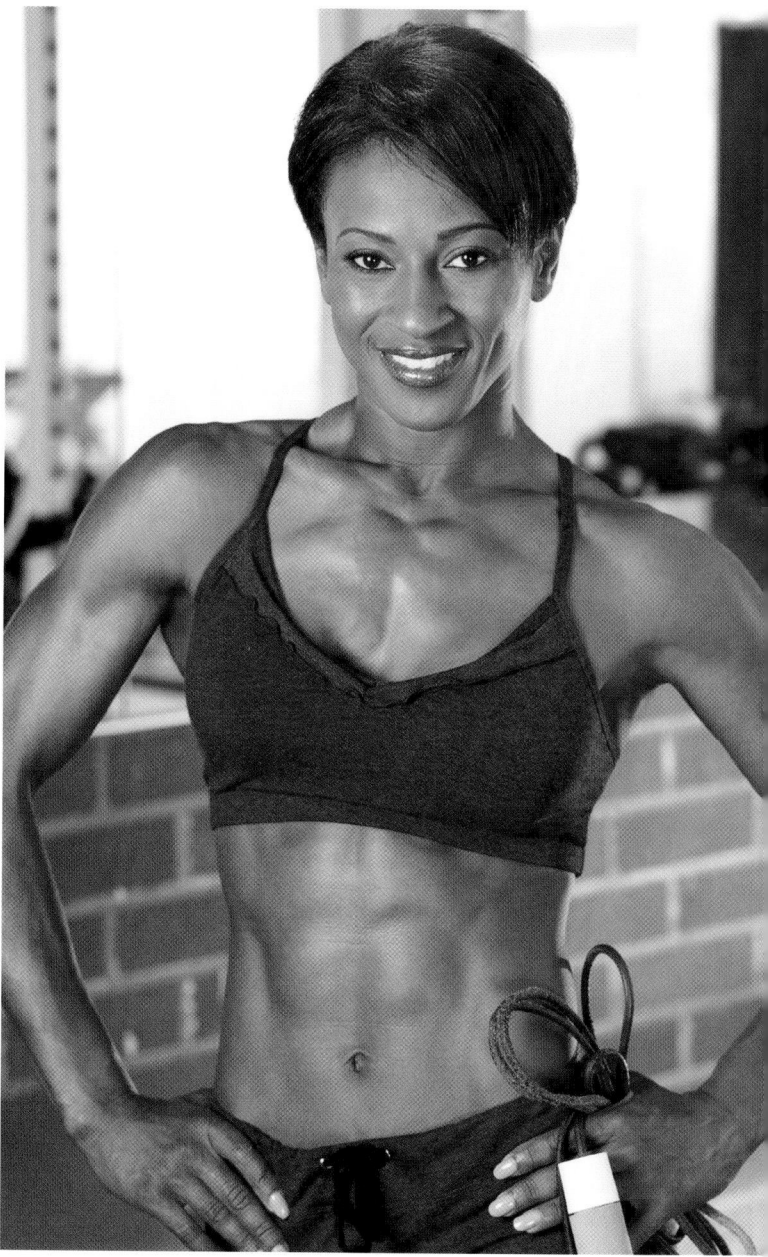

placed on the body in this type of workout, we recommend doing the more intense types of interval training no more than twice a week. For a fully rounded program, mix it in with other workouts that focus on steady-state cardio (endurance cardio, which you can do 3–5 times weekly), as well as resistance training.

CUSTOMIZE YOUR CARDIO

Hectic times (as during holidays) can be moody times, so depending on your attitude and time allotment for the day, you may want to choose one type of interval training over another. If you're down, cranky or lethargic, you'll probably want to perform the more mellow steady-state (endurance) option to re-energize your tired bod. If you're frantic, frazzled and pressed for time, consider choosing high-intensity interval training or cardio combo (circuit) training to alleviate some of your anxiety and aggression in a positive way, and get you in and out of the gym in less than 40 minutes.

#12 STEADY AS SHE GOES (ENDURANCE TRAINING)

On days when you're exhausted or even depressed, exercise may actually re-energize both your body and mind. Steady-state cardio is your friend on these days, helping to relieve stress while simultaneously burning calories and bolstering your bod. Choose an activity you enjoy and can sustain for 45–60 minutes. On a scale of 1–10, with 10 being hardest, you should aim to work at about 7 for best results. A 7 on your rating of perceived exertion (RPE) equals about 70%–75% of your maximum heart rate. Try incorporating 3–5 days of endurance training into your workout week to burn calories, increase lung capacity and improve your mood.

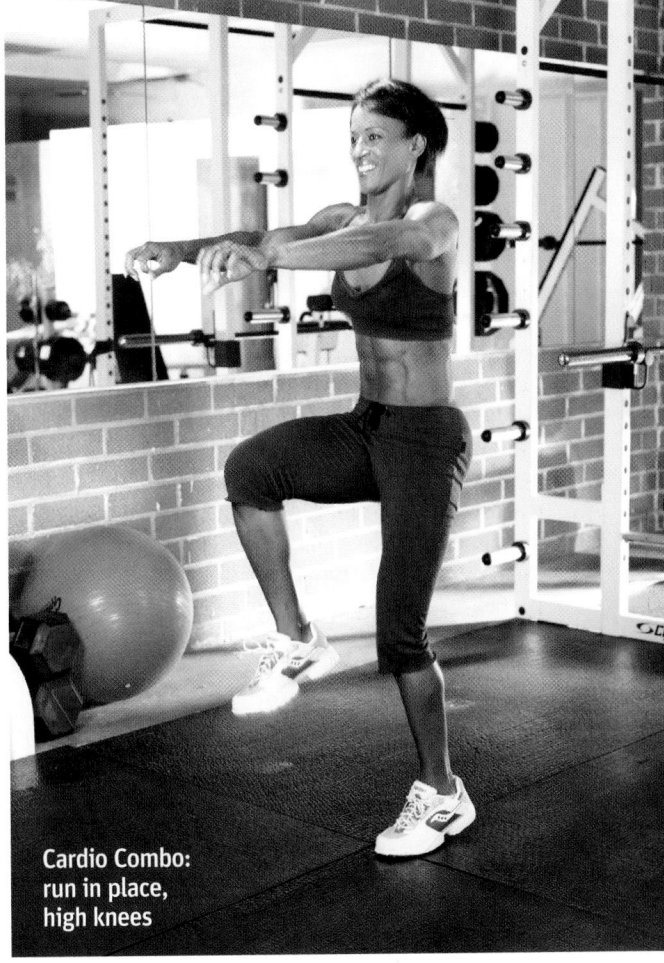

Cardio Combo:
run in place,
high knees

Target Heart Rate

220-(your age) = maximal heart rate (MHR)
MHR x 0.70 = 70% of your MHR
MHR x 0.75 = 75% of your MHR

EXAMPLE: 31-year-old woman
220-31 = 189 (MHR)
189 x 0.70 = 132
189 x 0.75 = 142
Target heart rate for steady-state cardio = 132–142 beats per minute

#13 HIIT IT! (HIGH-INTENSITY INTERVAL TRAINING)

To de-stress, perform this high-intensity interval training program (HIIT) once or twice weekly, allowing at least three days between sessions to fully recover.

Beginners should begin with 10–15-second intervals, while more advanced participants can start at 45–60 seconds. Follow each interval with at least a 1:3 ratio of work to recovery. (For example, if you do a 30-second interval, do 90 seconds of working rest.) As you advance, decrease to a 1:2 ratio of work to recovery.

Note: You may want to purchase a heart-rate monitor to use during your interval sessions. They're easy to use and will give you an accurate and instant reading of your exertion level. Write your heart-rate goals out on paper before you come to the gym so you can refer to them at a glance. If you choose not to use a monitor, go by the RPE scale of 1–10, with 10 being hardest, to determine your level of exertion. This is less accurate, but will still get the job done. During the recovery phases, you'll probably have to rely on RPE to determine your exercise intensity because your heart rate may not drop fast enough to be an accurate indicator of intensity.

Sample Program Options
Suggestions on different ways
to tackle cardio throughout the week.

ENERGIZER
Day 1	Steady State, 35–60 minutes (RPE 5–7)
Day 2	Steady State, 35–60 minutes (RPE 5–7)
Day 3	Cardio Combo (RPE 7–9)
Day 4	Off
Day 5	Steady State, 35–60 minutes (RPE 5–7)
Day 6	Cardio Combo (RPE 7–9)
Day 7	Off

FANATICAL FAT-BURNER/STRESS BUSTER
Day 1	Cardio Combo (RPE 7–9)
Day 2	Cardio Combo (RPE 7–9)
Day 3	Off
Day 4	HIIT (RPE 7–8)
Day 5	Steady State, 35–60 minutes (RPE 5–7)
Day 6	Cardio Combo (RPE 7–9)
Day 7	Off

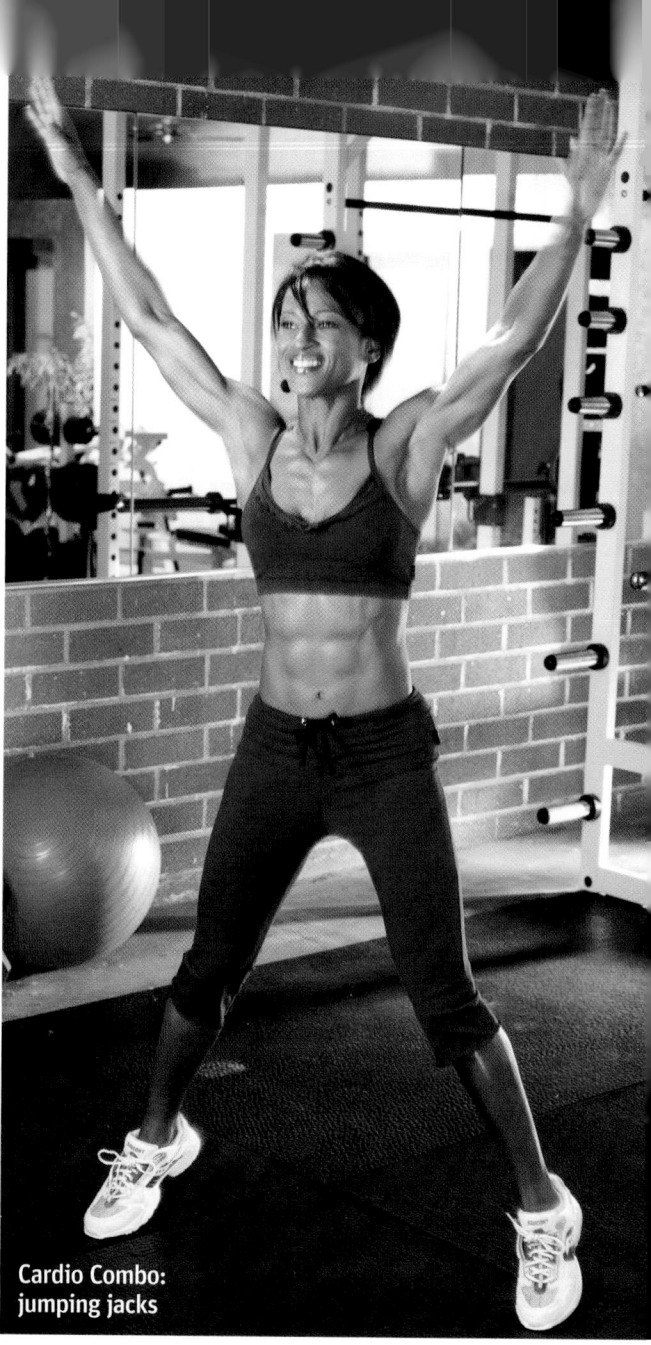

Cardio Combo:
jumping jacks

25-Minute Interval Program

TIME	RPE	%MHR
5-minute warm-up	3	
30 seconds	5-6	60
90 seconds	4-5	50
30 seconds	6-7	70
90 seconds	5-6	60
30 seconds	7-8	80
90 seconds	5-6	60
30 seconds	7-8	80
90 seconds	5-6	60
30 seconds	8-9	85
90 seconds	5-6	60
30 seconds	8-9	85
90 seconds	5-6	60
30 seconds	9	90
90 seconds	5-6	60
60 seconds	4-5	50
5-minute cool-down	3	

#14 CARDIO COMBO CRUNCH (CIRCUIT TRAINING)

This time-crunching program can get you in and out of the gym in 40 minutes or less, and will attack both cardio and weight training in one fell swoop. The idea is to elevate your heart rate with the cardio intervals and keep it relatively high while lifting weights in a circuit format to burn the most calories in the shortest period. Free-weight exercises and cardio activities that don't require machines are your best bet, as you'll never have to waste time moving around the gym or wait your turn and risk allowing your heart rate to drop.

The sample program shown at right demonstrates a total-body workout, but it can be tailored to fit your own needs. Because you're performing each weighted exercise for a full minute — it's harder than you think! — drop the poundage significantly so you can complete the exercise without stopping.

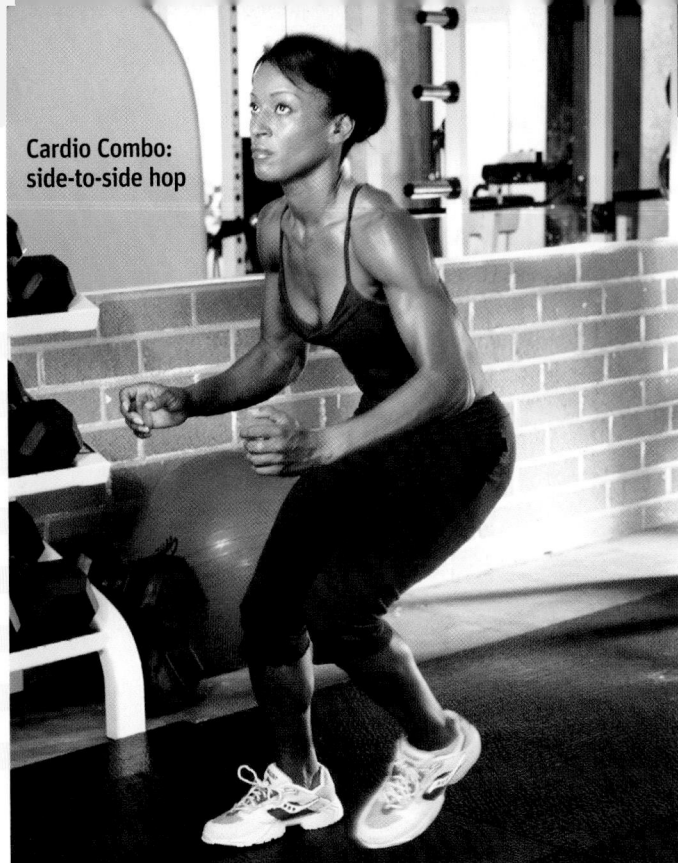

Cardio Combo: side-to-side hop

40-Minute Cardio Combo Program

5-minute cardio warm-up (RPE 4–5)*
3 minutes run in place, high knees (RPE 7–8)
1 minute lateral raise
1 minute alternating lunge
1 minute biceps curl
3 minutes jumping jacks (RPE 7–8)
1 minute overhead triceps extension
1 minute step-up
1 minute incline push-up
3 minutes jump rope (RPE 8–9)
1 minute pulldown
1 minute plié squat
1 minute overhead shoulder press
3 minutes side-to-side hop (RPE 8–9)
1 minute front raise
1 minute dip
1 minute calf raise
6 minutes abdominal crunch
5-minute cool-down and stretch*

* For your warm-up and cool-down, do whatever type of cardio you like; for example, walk or run on a treadmill or ride a stationary bike.

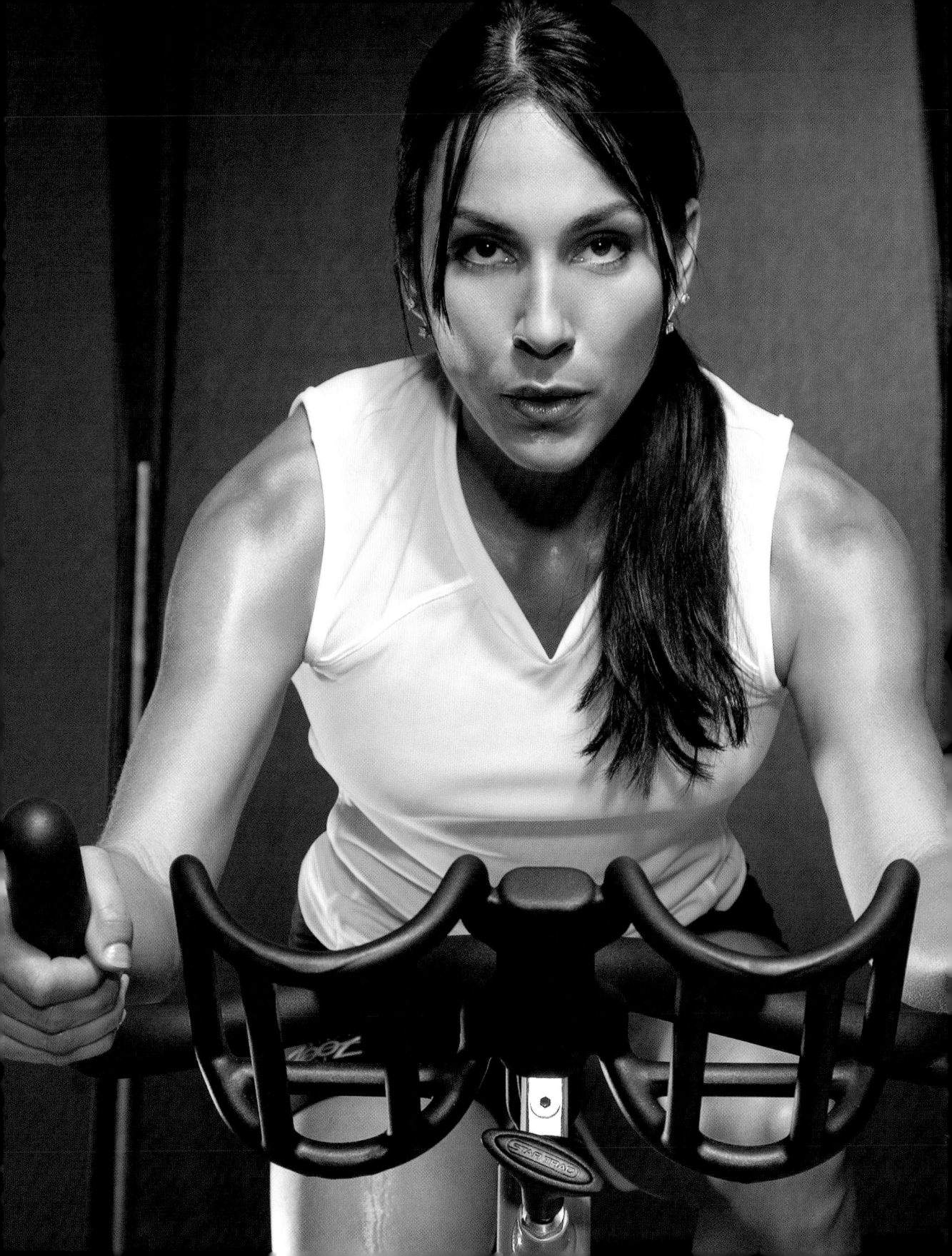

Chapter 6

Burn 300 Calories In 20 Minutes

How many times have you forgone the gym because you thought you had too little time on your hands? Perhaps you think that if you don't have at least an hour to devote to training, you should put it off until tomorrow. Tsk-tsk, banish that belief. These six high-intensity cardio routines will have you in and out of the gym fast — with big-time, fat-burning benefits to boot.

Well, consider the excuse of "not enough time" officially off-limits, because 20 minutes is all you need when your day proves hectic. On the following pages you will find six cardio routines, each guaranteed to burn 300 calories (based on a 145-pound female), designed by Jeramie R. Hinojosa, MS, senior clinical exercise specialist at East Texas Medical Center–Olympic Center Gym in Tyler, Texas. Hinojosa's workouts range from running to cycling to calisthenics to martial arts, and all can be done in the confines of your neighborhood gym or even at home with basic equipment.

"For those short on time, increasing exercise intensity with these 20-minute power bouts is an effective way to burn more calories in a short period," Hinojosa says. "Your exercise session will be more efficient and your metabolism will stay elevated long after you're done exercising."

Twenty minutes — that's all it takes for a 300-calorie-burning, fat-blasting cardio workout (and burning blubber is the whole point of this book). Then, when you have a full hour to train, you'll wonder what to do with all the extra time!

#15 Interval Program No. 1

Equipment: Treadmill

This 20-minute jaunt keeps your actual running speed constant (outside of the warm-up and cool-down), but alters the grade of incline to produce two separate gradual climbs that are six minutes in duration. The steepest, most intense part of each climb (6% incline) is also the shortest (one minute).

SPEED	INCLINE (%)	TIME (MIN.)
6.5	0	3
7	2	3
7	4	2
7	6	1
7	0	1
7	2	3
7	4	2
7	6	1
7	1	1
6.5	0	3

#16 Interval Program No. 2

Equipment: Treadmill

Here's a more gradual climb, offering one-minute plateaus between each interval. The workout peaks in the middle with one minute at an 8% incline before returning to longer, less steep climbs in the second half.

SPEED	INCLINE (%)	TIME (MIN.)
6.5	0	2
7	3	3
7	0	1
7	5	2
7	0	1
7	8	1
7	0	1
7	5	2
7	0	1
7	3	3
7	0	1
6.5	0	2

Running

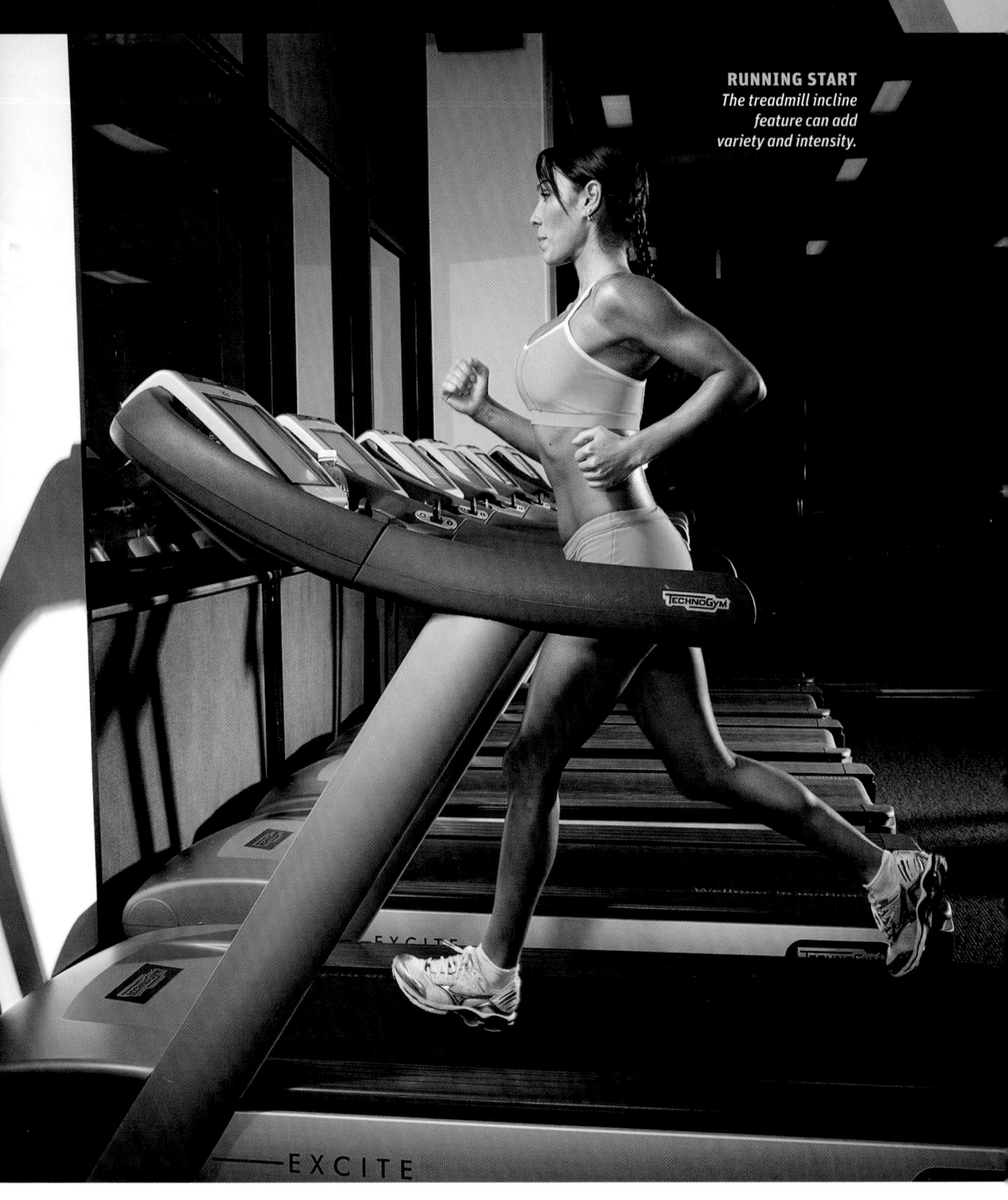

RUNNING START
The treadmill incline feature can add variety and intensity.

#17 Yellow Jersey Workout

Equipment: Indoor cycle/Spinning bike

This combination of sprints and climbs, both seated and standing, require you to constantly change the resistance/workload on the bike to the corresponding perceived exertion (or, PE; see terminology sidebar) for each phase. Regardless of intensity, smooth pedaling should be your goal throughout the ride.

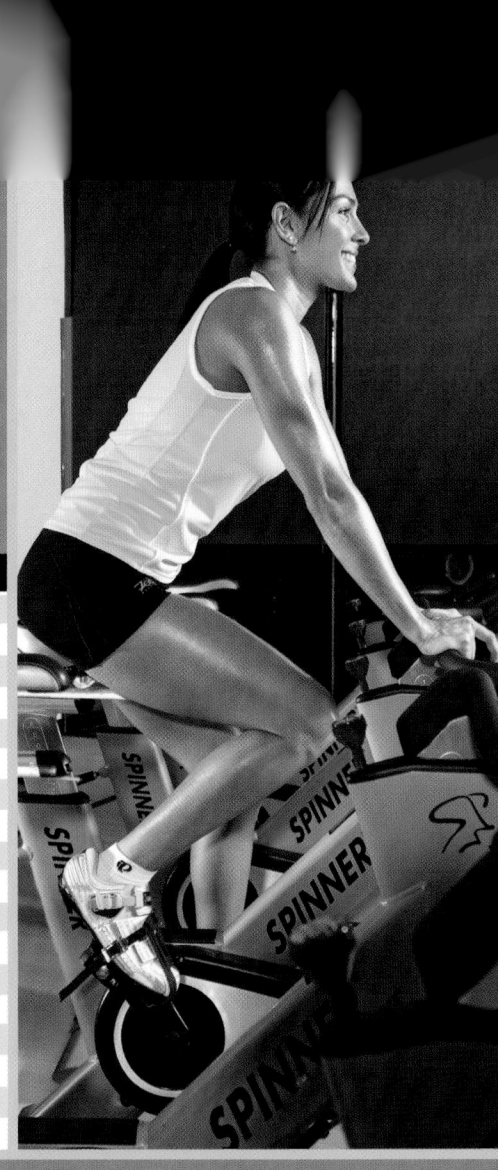

EXERCISE	TIME (MIN.)	PE
Seated Flat-Road Cycling	2	3
Seated Climb	1	6
Recovery	1	4
Out-of-Saddle Climb	1	6
Recovery	1	4
Seated Climb	1	7
Seated Flat-Road Cycling	1	3
Seated Climb	1	7
Recovery	1	4
Out-of-Saddle Climb	1	6
Recovery	1	4
Seated Acceleration	1	7
Recovery	1	5
Seated Acceleration	1	7
Recovery	1	5
Out-of-Saddle Climb	1	7
Sprint Cycling	1	9
Seated Flat-Road Cycling	2	4

SPINNING TERMS

OUT-OF-SADDLE CLIMB: Intense cycling off the seat at moderate to heavy resistance, using arms to create leverage on pedals; smooth cadence.

PERCEIVED EXERTION (PE): Level of resistance, on a scale of 1–10, as determined intuitively by the rider and controlled by turning the knob in front of the handlebars. On the scale, 1 is a resting state, 10 is maximum exertion.

SEATED ACCELERATION: Smooth and fluid increases in pedal cadence with moderate resistance over 30 seconds.

SEATED CLIMB: Intense cycling at heavy resistance while sitting back a bit in the saddle and pulling on the handlebars; abs tucked in, pushing glutes into the saddle; smooth, powerful cadence.

SEATED FLAT-ROAD CYCLING: Easy, steady cycling in the saddle at light resistance.

SPRINT: Smooth, controlled, fast cycling at a moderate intensity; focus on controlled speed.

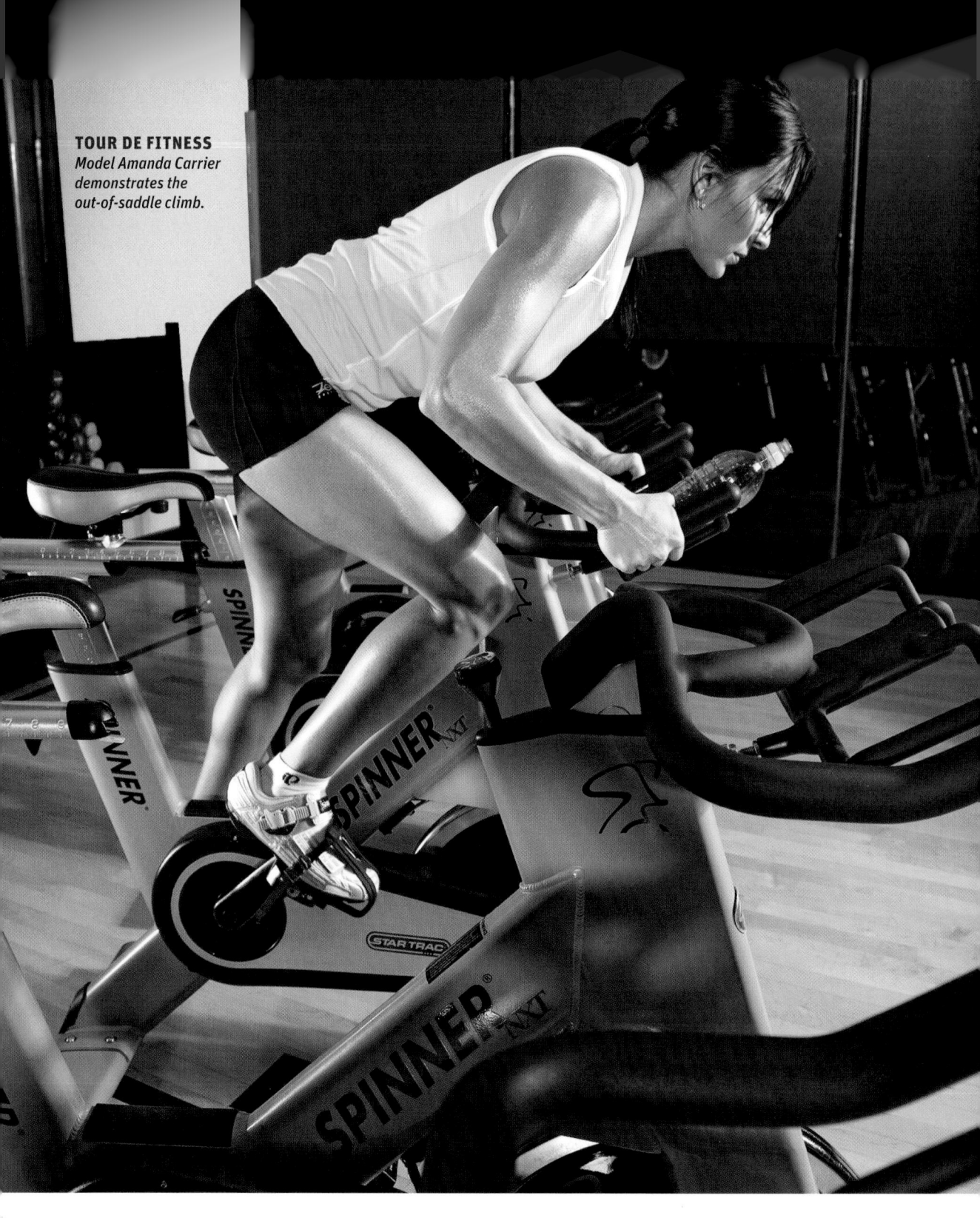

TOUR DE FITNESS
Model Amanda Carrier demonstrates the out-of-saddle climb.

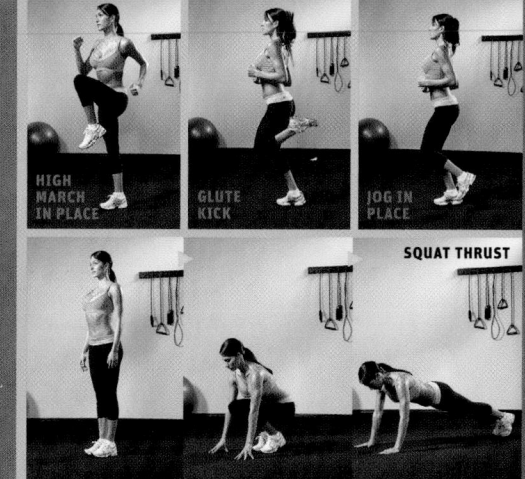

HIGH MARCH IN PLACE

GLUTE KICK

JOG IN PLACE

SQUAT THRUST

#18 Boot-Camp Blitz

Equipment: Exercise mat, step bench

This military-inspired workout may be bare-bones, but it's as effective a form of cardio as any machine can provide. Execute each exercise at a pace that elicits the corresponding PE. Move immediately from one exercise to the next, or rest a few seconds between exercises if necessary by marching in place — just don't stop moving.

EXERCISE	TIME (MIN.)	PE
March in Place (warm-up)	3	2
High March in Place	1	5
Glute Kick	1	6
Jog in Place	1	5
High March in Place	1	6
Push-Up	1	7
Squat Thrust[1]	1	6
Crunch	1	7
Split Jump[2]	1	6
Step-Up[3]	1	5
March in Place	1	4
Plank[4]	30 sec.	5
Skater's Step[5]	1	7
Reverse Crunch	1	5
Side Lunge	1	5
Plank[4]	30 sec.	5
Squat Jump[6]	1	8
March in Place (cool-down)	2	3

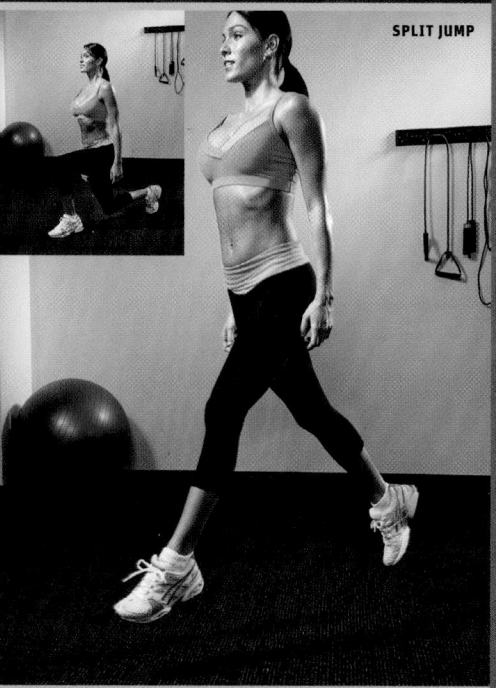

SPLIT JUMP

[1] With feet together, squat down and put your hands on the floor outside your feet. Keeping your hands on the floor, jump your feet behind you to a push-up position. Jump your feet back between your hands and stand up.

[2] Start in a lunge position, then jump and switch your feet in the air, landing in the lunge position with your feet in the opposite position.

[3] Step up and down on a 10- to 12-inch step, alternating feet.

[4] Support yourself on your forearms, fists (pinkie side down) and toes, keeping your body rigid and straight.

[5] Jump from side to side, landing on one foot and swinging your arms with each jump like a speed skater.

[6] Jump straight up in the air as high as you can, bringing your arms overhead on the leap and landing in a squat position.

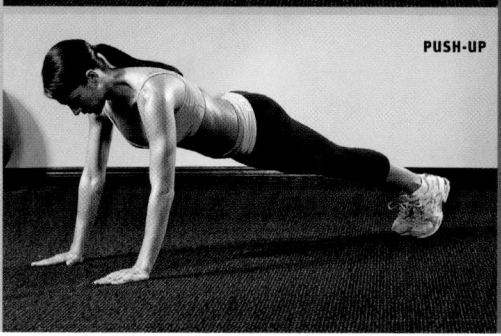

PUSH-UP

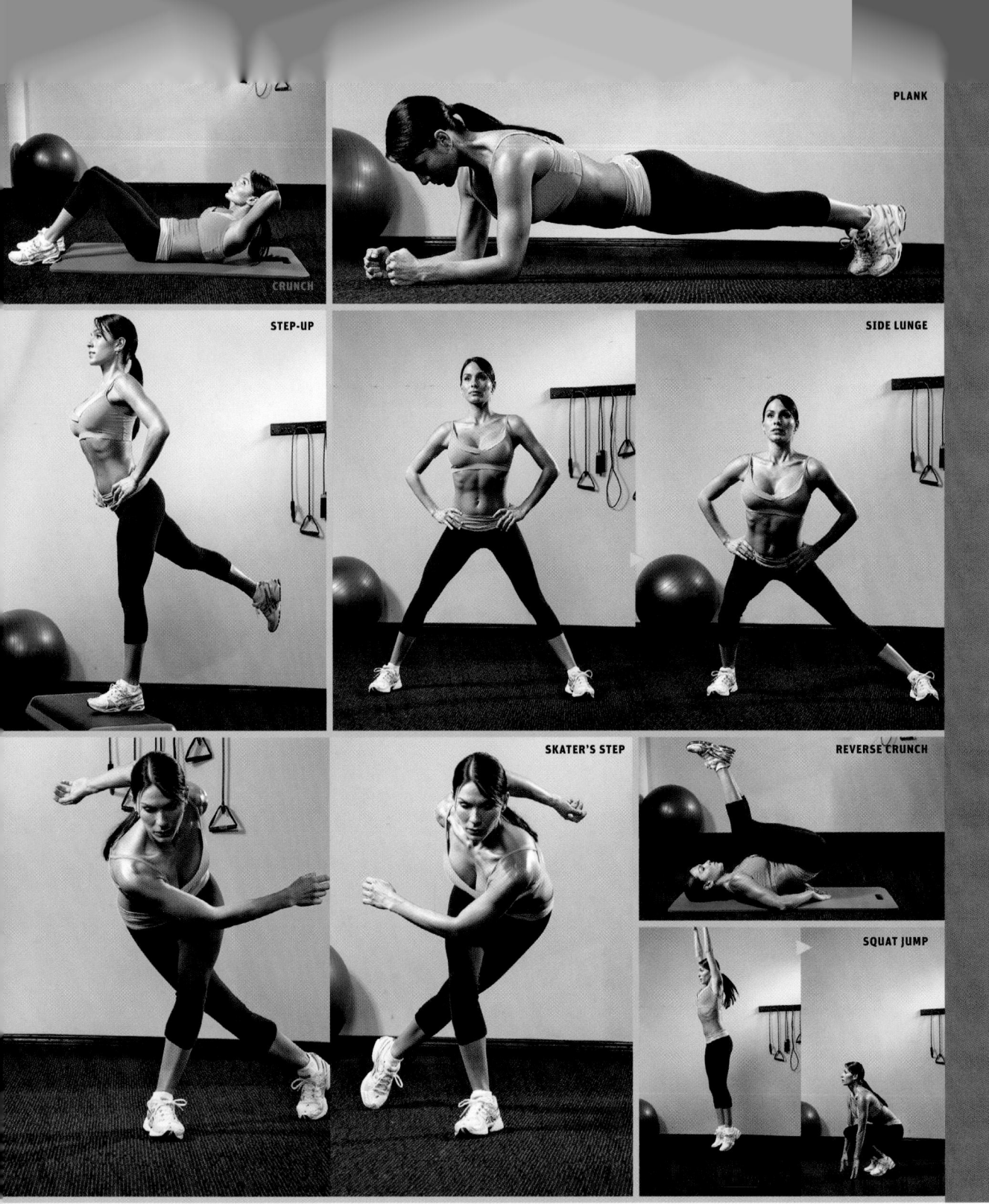

PLANK

CRUNCH

STEP-UP

SIDE LUNGE

SKATER'S STEP

REVERSE CRUNCH

SQUAT JUMP

Cardio Triathlon

#19 ## Ironwoman Workout

Equipment: Elliptical, treadmill, stationary bike.

Three pieces of gym cardio equipment, one multifaceted, calorie-torching routine. Move immediately from one machine to the next, resting only as long as it takes you to walk from the elliptical to the treadmill and the treadmill to the bike. Adjust the resistance on the elliptical trainer and bike to elicit the corresponding PE.

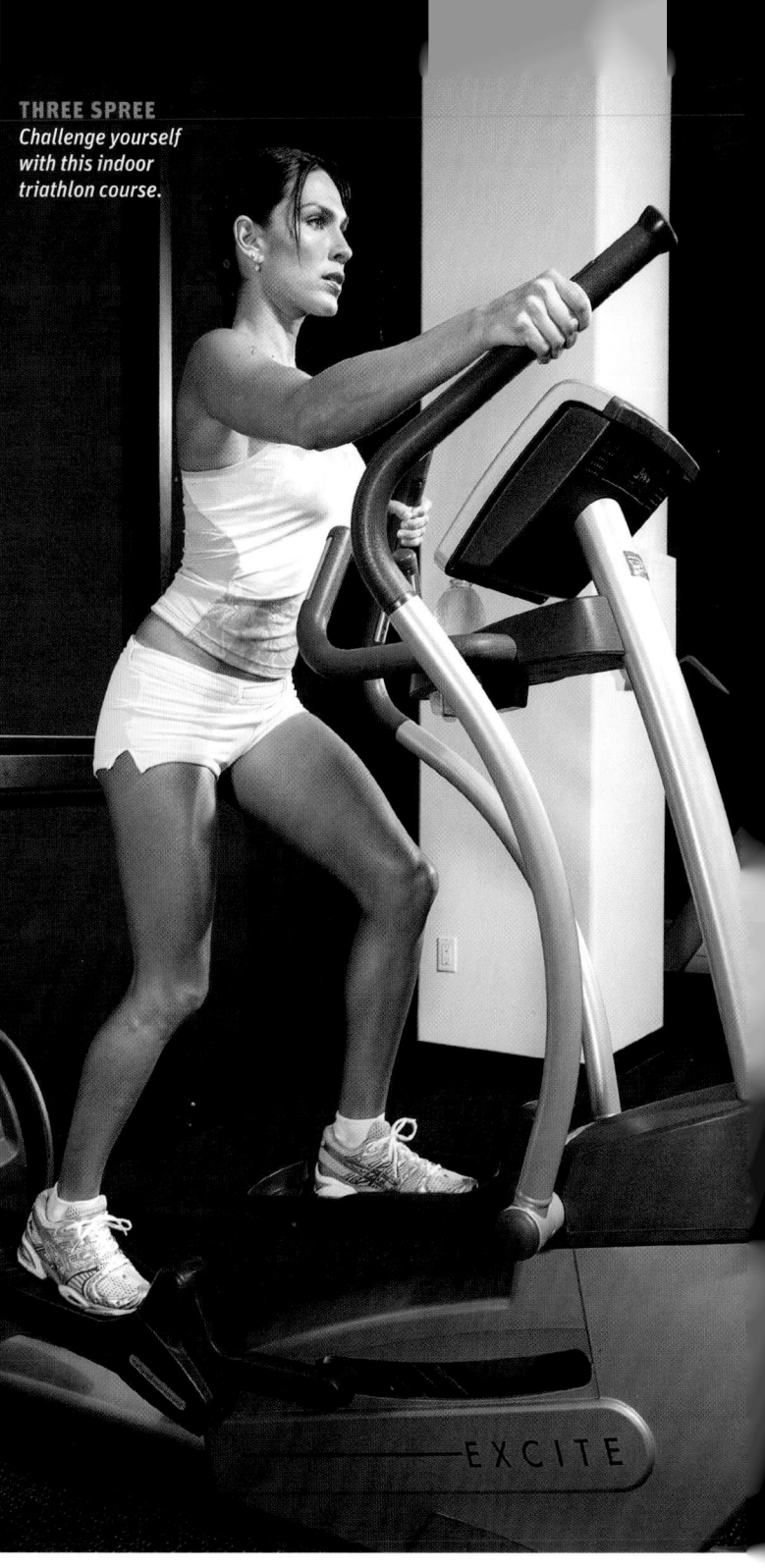

THREE SPREE
Challenge yourself with this indoor triathlon course.

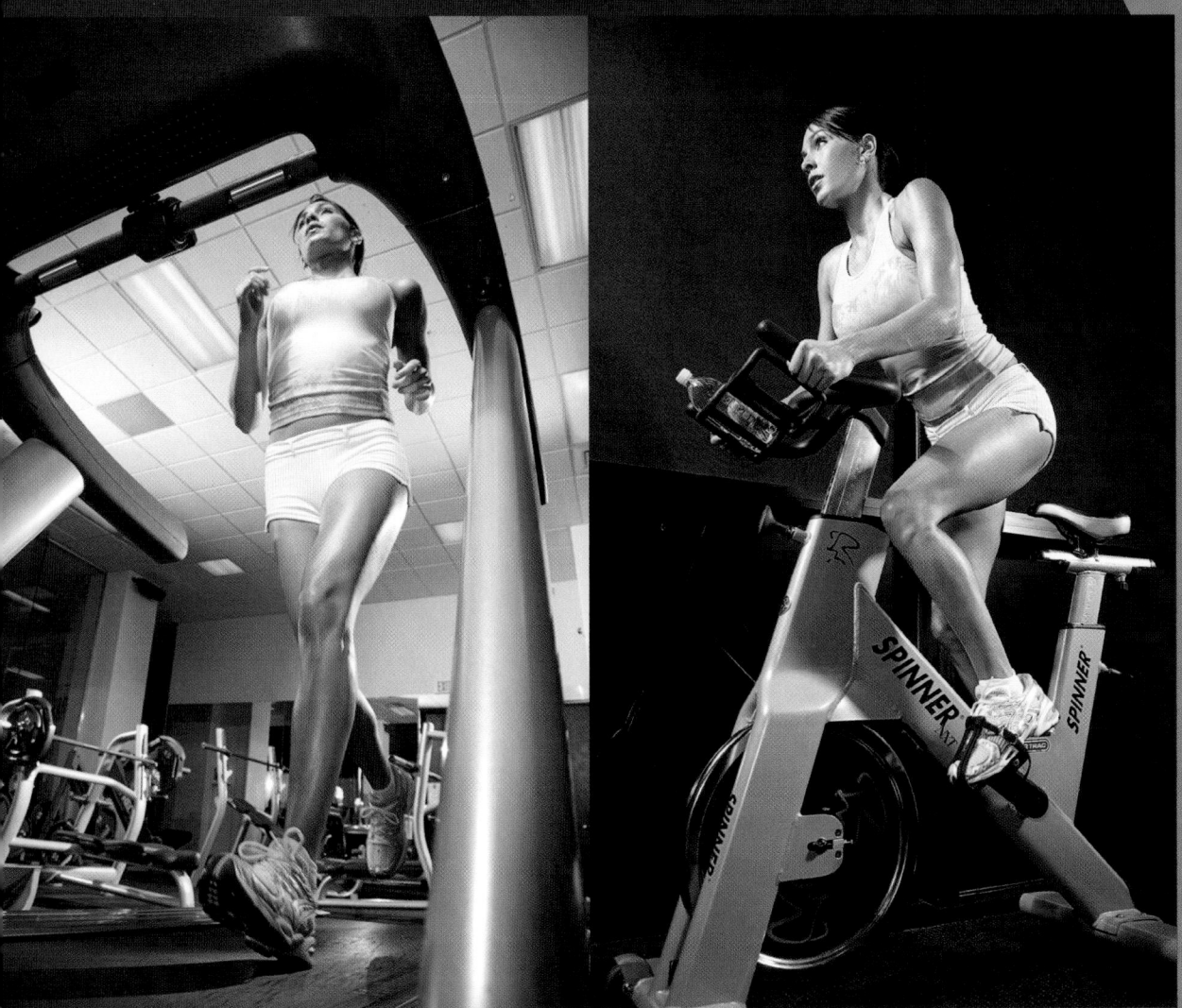

EXERCISE 1: ELLIPTICAL

Time (min.)	PE
2	5
1	8
2	5
1	8

EXERCISE 2: TREADMILL RUNNING

Time (min.)	Speed	Incline (%)
2	7	0
1	7	3
1	7	6
1	7	9
1	7	0

EXERCISE 3: INDOOR CYCLE*

Exercise	Time (min.)	PE
Seated Climb	1	6
Seated Flat-Road Cycling	1	4
Out-of-Saddle Climb	1	6
Seated Flat-Road Cycling	1	4
Sprint	30 sec.	8
Seated Flat-Road Cycling (recovery)	1	4
Sprint	30 sec.	8
Seated Flat-Road Cycling (cool-down)	2	4

*See explanation of cycling terms on page 76.

#20 Kickboxing Craze

Equipment: Jump rope, open floor space

Martial artists are some of the fittest athletes in the world — very lean and strong, not bulky. Throughout this workout, keep up your punching, kicking and jumping pace so that your PE stays between 6 and 8; rest a few seconds between exercises and combinations if necessary by marching in place, but don't stop moving.

>> Warm up by jumping rope (double bounce on each jump) for three minutes. (L) means left hand, (R) means right hand.

JUMPING-JACK COMBO

Exercise	Time (min.)	PE
Jumping Jack, Jab (L), Jumping Jack, Jab (R)	1	6–8
Jumping Jack, Front Kick (L), Jumping Jack, Front Kick (R)	1	6–8
Jumping Jack, Uppercut (L), Jumping Jack, Uppercut (R)	1	6–8
Jumping Jack, Side Kick (L), Jumping Jack, Side Kick (R)	1	6–8
Jumping Jack, Cross (L), Jumping Jack, Cross (R)	1	6–8
Jump Rope (alternate step)	2	jogging speed

KICKBOXING COMBO 1

Exercise	Time (min.)	PE
Knee Raise (L), Roundhouse (L), Cross (R), Jab (L)	1	6–8
Knee Raise (R), Roundhouse (R), Cross (L), Jab (R)	1	6–8
Uppercut (L), Hook (R), Front Kick (L), Back Kick (R)	1	6–8
Uppercut (R), Hook (L), Front Kick (R), Back Kick (L)	1	6–8
Jump Rope (alternate step)	2	jogging speed

KICKBOXING COMBO 2

Exercise	Time (min.)	PE
Squat, Side Kick (L)	1	6–8
Squat, Side Kick (R)	1	6–8

>> Cool down by jumping rope (double bounce on each jump) for two minutes.

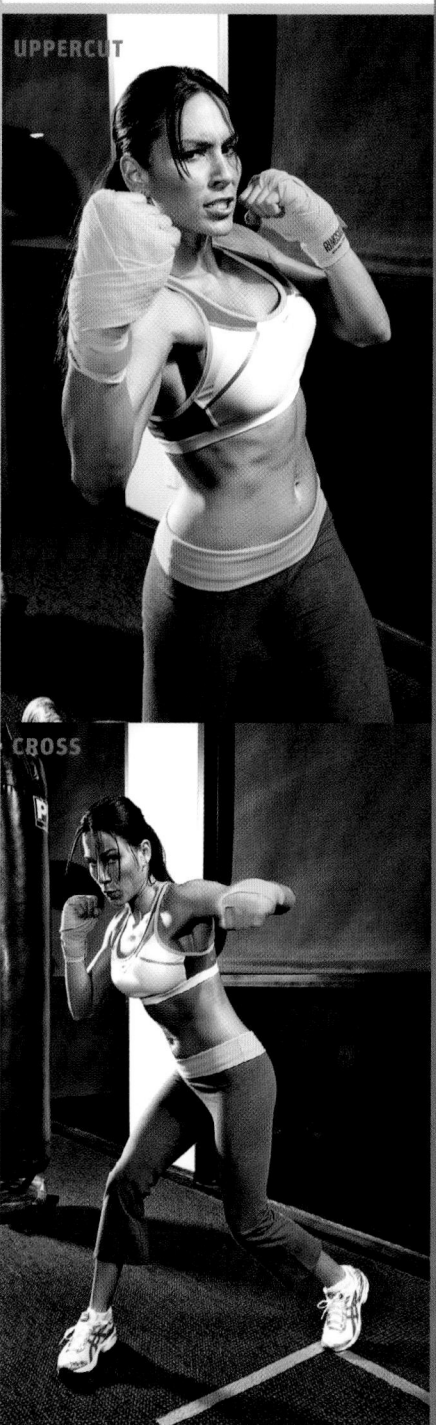

UPPERCUT

CROSS

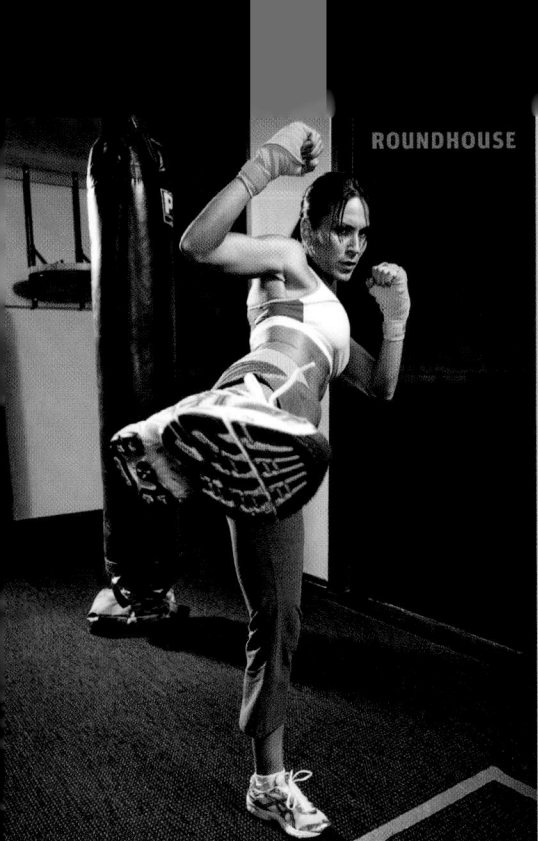

ROUNDHOUSE

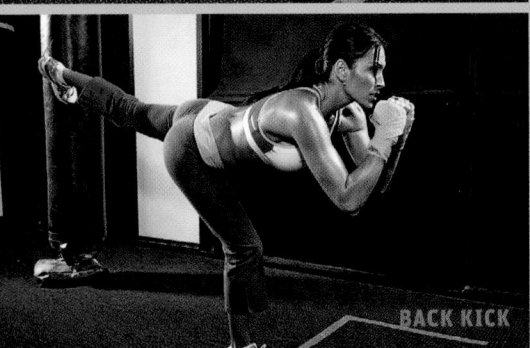

BACK KICK 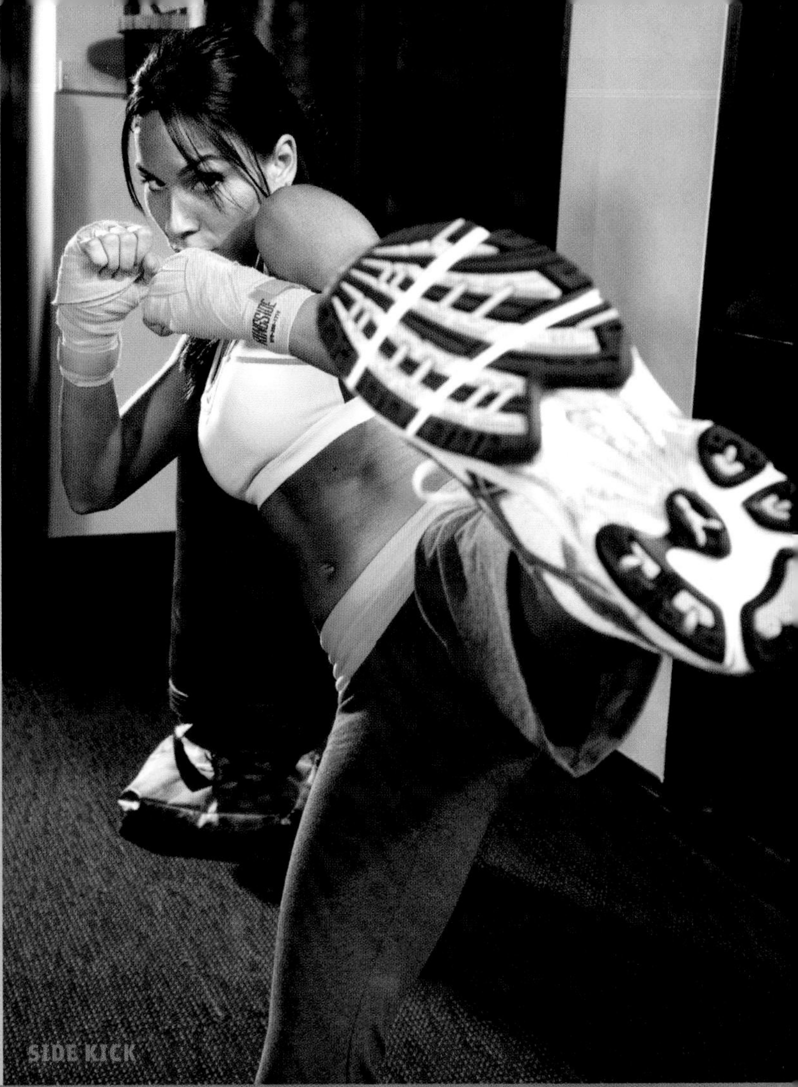   SIDE KICK

MARTIAL ARTS TERMS

BACK KICK: A kick executed by extending at the hip and extending the knee rearward; similar to the front kick, but in the opposite direction.

CROSS: A punch thrown from the rear hand across the body while twisting your hips.

FRONT KICK (NOT SHOWN): A kick in front of the body; flex at the hip and extend at the knee.

HOOK (NOT SHOWN): A punch thrown from the leading hand by jabbing your elbow forward as the forearm stays flexed and parallel to the floor.

JAB (NOT SHOWN): A straight, arm-length punch thrown from the leading hand.

ROUNDHOUSE: Similar to the side kick, but the toes of the kicking leg are pointed.

SIDE KICK: A kick executed to the side, beginning with a knee raise to the side and extending the knee; the heel of the kicking leg is pushed out.

UPPERCUT: A punch executed from the hip in an upward motion; the elbow is flexed as you jab straight up.

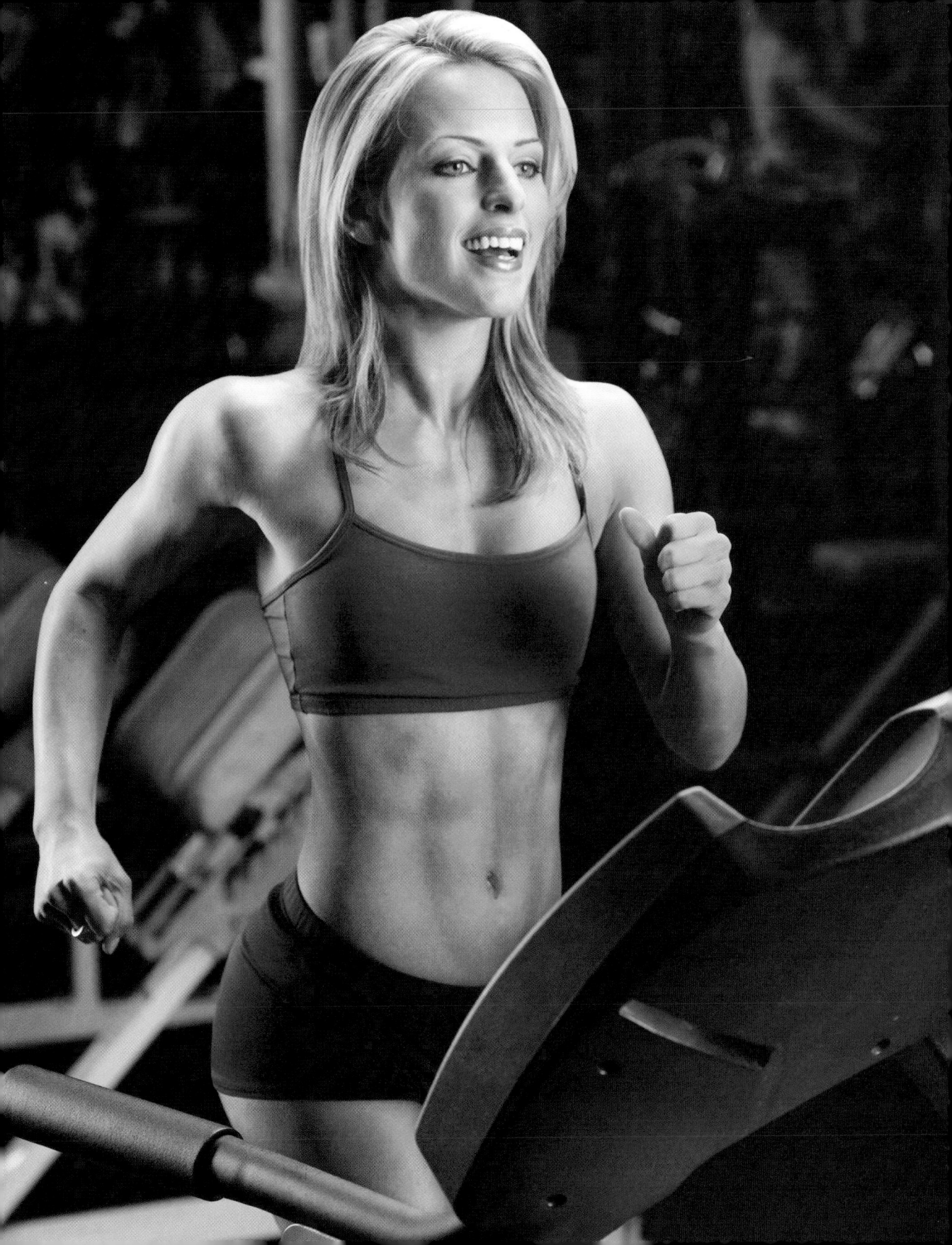

Chapter 7

5 Cardio Workouts You Should Be Doing

Want to boost your metabolism and burn fat faster? Amp up your intensity to increase your EPOC, or excess postexercise oxygen consumption. EPOC represents the energy required to recover from exercise, says Chris Scott, PhD, exercise physiologist at the University of Southern Maine Human Performace Laboratory (Portland).

"When exercise ends, it takes time and energy for muscle cells to return to resting levels. Recovery can also be expensive: Depleted glucose and fat stores need to be refilled, accumulated cell products need to be removed and protein levels need to be built back up. All this requires energy," Scott says. And the more rebuilding to be done, the greater the rate of EPOC, which in turn means more calories (using fatty tissue as fuel) are being burned after your workout.

One primary factor in determining EPOC is exercise intensity, says Scott; another is duration — just not to the same extent. Numerous studies support this idea, such as a *Journal of Strength and Conditioning Research* study done by Cedarville University (Ohio) researchers. When women performed either a weight-training or a cardio session, both of which burned the same amount of calories and were similar in intensity, the subjects experienced similar EPOC responses.

It's well known that lower-intensity aerobic exercise burns fat, but that doesn't mean your workouts should be a walk in the park. "Intense exercise is associated with a tremendous amount of fat break-down," Scott says. "The higher the exercise intensity, the greater the amount of carbo-hydrate burned. But the energy requirements of recovery, especially an active recovery, need to be considered. To be sure, muscle uses mostly carbs during weight training, but all the fat that's bro-ken down during exercise is subsequently used to fuel recovery. EPOC primarily depends on fat and lactic acid as fuel. In fact, the recovery from EPOC is almost all aerobic and a terrific oxidizer of fat."

That said, the programs featured here vary in level of intensity and duration but all have a high EPOC. Whatever your pref-erence, there's a workout geared to you.

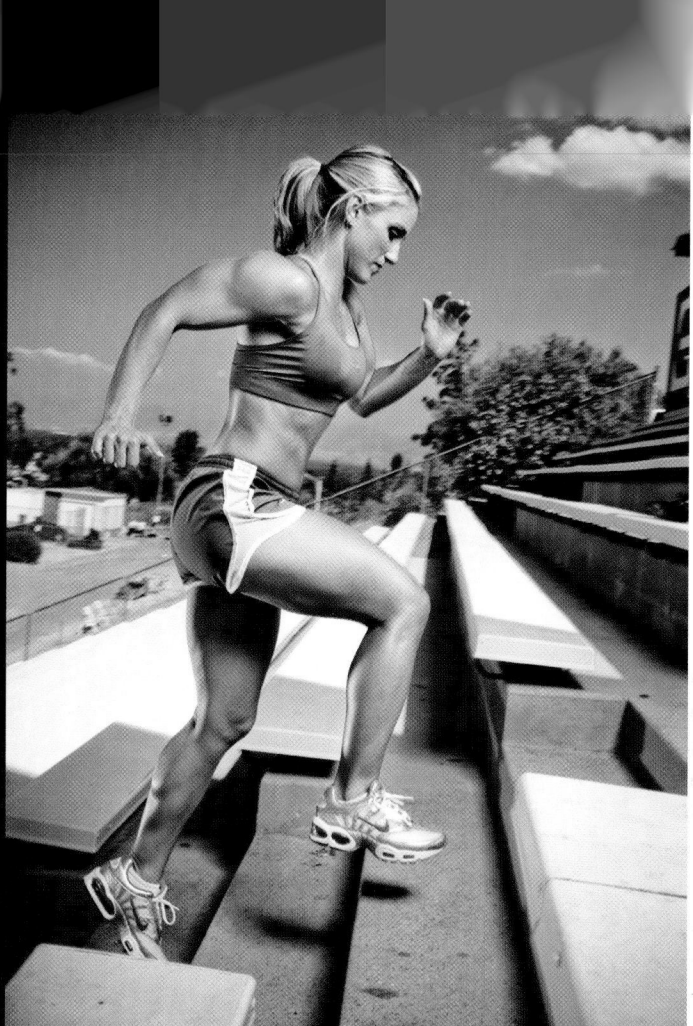

#21 EPOC PROGRAM 1:
Keep Up the Tempo

Run, walk or bike at a steady pace that has you working at 80%–90% of your maximum heart rate (MHR) or 6–7 intensity rating. (To cal-culate your MHR, subtract your age from 220; see "What Is Intensity Rating?" on page 89.)

Duration: 30–60 minutes

Intensity: High (6–7 intensity rating)

Why it works: University of New Hampshire (Durham) researchers examined the effects of constant walking at 70% intensity on a tread-mill for 20, 40 and 60 minutes with three hours of recovery. While EPOC was elevated in each of the three trials as compared to the con-trol, it was significantly higher after the 60-minute bout of exercise. More specifically, the 60-minute-duration EPOC measurement was approximately twice that of the 20- and 40-minute durations.

#22 EPOC PROGRAM 2:
Slow and Steady

Go the distance doing the activity you like — biking, running, walking — at a light to moderate pace.

Duration: 60–80 minutes

Intensity: Light to moderate (about 3 intensity rating)

Why it works: Researchers at the Laboratory of Nutrition and Exercise Physiology at Nakamura Gakuen University (Fukuoka, Japan) examined the EPOC effects after moderate exercise. Subjects performed 30 or 60 minutes of exercise on separate days of 60% VO_2 max (maximal oxygen consumption), which equates to about 70%–75% MHR. Results indicated that longer-duration exercise results in a greater and longer EPOC. More specifically, EPOC lasted for 116 minutes after the 60-minute bout compared to 46 minutes for the 30-minute workout.

In a separate study, University of Victoria (Canada) researchers found similar results and concluded that increasing work time elevates energy cost during and after exercise.

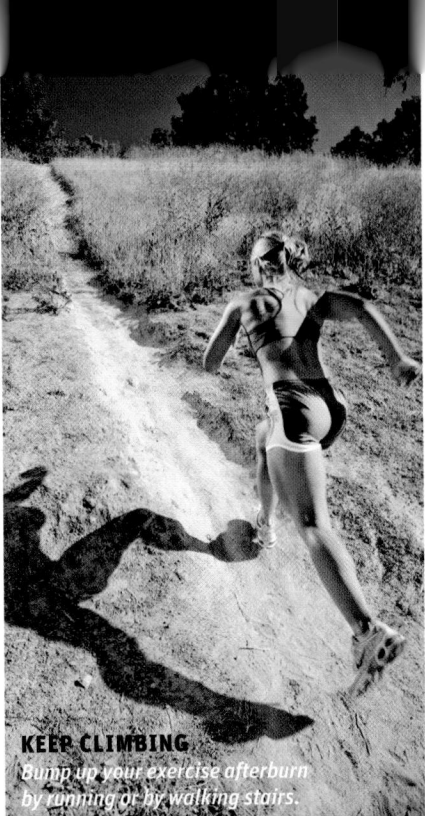

KEEP CLIMBING
Bump up your exercise afterburn by running or by walking stairs.

#23 EPOC PROGRAM 3:
Cross-Train

Can't commit to just one activity? With this workout, you don't have to. Mix up your cardio activities by doing 2–4 bouts of high-intensity exercise that are 15–20 minutes each. Or switch between weight training and cardio, but keep the intensity high. Rest up to five minutes between each bout, or walking to your next machine will do.

Duration: 30–80 minutes

Intensity: High (6–7 intensity rating)

Why it works: Want to save time in the gym? Researchers at Brigham Young University (Provo, Utah) found that workouts in which resistance training followed aerobic activity exhibited greater EPOC than workouts that are resistance only, running only or resistance training followed by running.

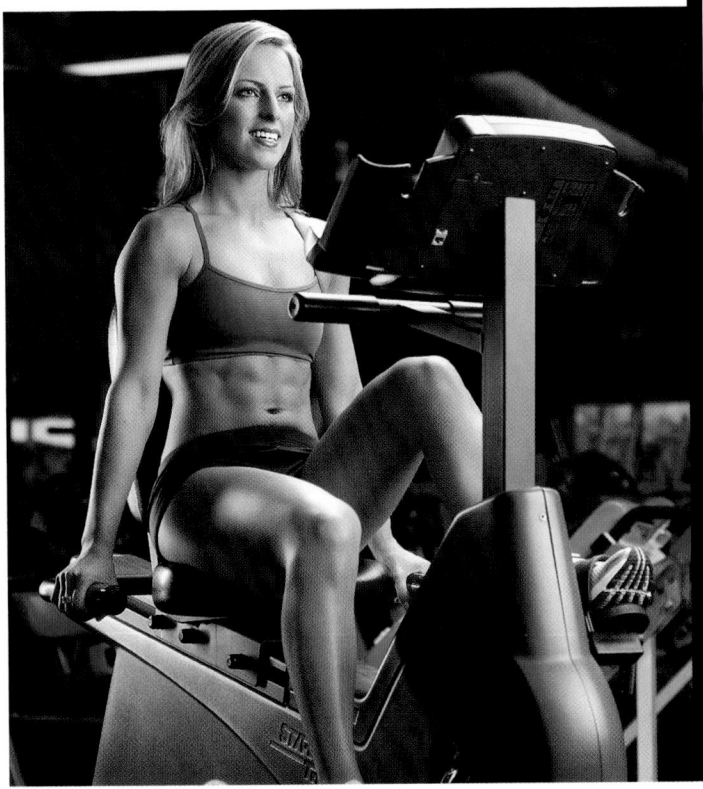

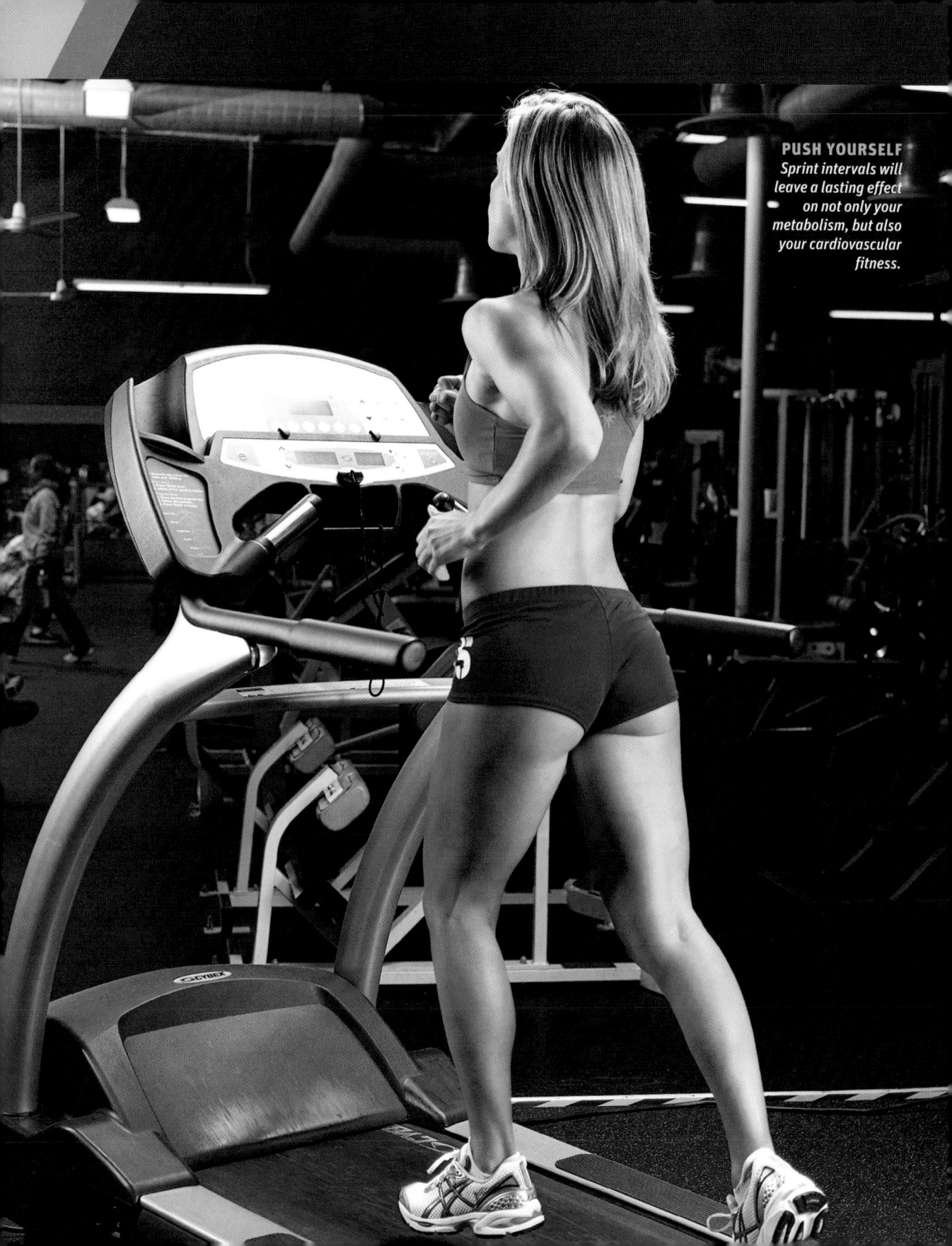

#24 EPOC PROGRAM 4:
Supramaximal Interval Training

Think 15–20 one-minute all-out sprints with 2- to 5-minute walks in between.
Duration: 60–80 minutes
Intensity: High (7–9 intensity rating)
Why it works: When researchers at Flinders University of South Australia (Adelaide) compared continuous running for 30 minutes at 70% VO2 max (about 80% MHR) and interval running of 20 one-minute intervals at 105% VO_2 max (100%-plus MHR) with two-minute rest periods, the latter was the EPOC winner. The supramaximal interval training had double the EPOC levels as its continuous-exercise counterpart. In another study, Norwegian scientists found that supramaximal training of three two-minute bouts of exercise followed by three-minute rest periods produced EPOC for up to four hours.

#25 EPOC PROGRAM 5:
Circuit Training

Perform one weight-training exercise per bodypart at 20 reps per minute (slow and controlled on both the up and down portions of the rep) with a weight load that's 60% of your one-rep max. Run to each station and complete the circuit three times, resting only 20 seconds between each.
Circuit: Leg press, biceps curl, bench press, triceps pulldown, lat pulldown, crunch, lateral raise
Duration: 30 minutes
Intensity: Moderate to high (4–7 intensity rating)
Why it works: Circuit training that consists of three sets of eight exercises resulted in a higher EPOC within 30 minutes of exercising as compared to an equivalent-intensity treadmill workout, according to researchers at Shippensburg University (Pennsylvania) in the journal *European Journal of Applied Physiology*. The duration of your resting period may also impact your EPOC after circuit training, say Southeastern Louisiana University (Hammond) researchers. They found that a higher EPOC occurred when subjects rested 20 seconds between circuits than when they took 60-second rest periods.

WHAT IS INTENSITY RATING?

>> How to gauge your exercise intensity
Besides heart rate and the amount of oxygen you consume during exercise (VO_2 max), determining your exertion is as easy as quantifying it with an intensity rating. No fancy watches or lab appointments are necessary; perceived exertion is simply how hard you feel your body is working based on the physical sensations you experience — increased heart rate, breathing rate, sweating and muscle fatigue. Although this is a subjective measure, your exertion rating can provide a fairly good estimate of your actual heart rate during physical activity. This allows you to adjust the intensity (and, as a result, improve the benefits) of your workout.

>> How to use the Intensity Rating Scale
Perception of exertion should reflect how heavy and strenuous the exercise feels, combining all sensations of physical stress, effort and fatigue.

Use the scale below as your guide. Choose the number that best describes your level of exertion, as it will give you a good idea of the intensity level of your activity, and you can use this data to speed up or slow down your movements to reach your desired range. Most important, concentrate on how you feel instead of what the actual workout load is. If you get hung up on numbers, time, weight or your treadmill neighbor, you won't be able to get an honest assessment.

INTENSITY RATING	DESCRIPTION
0	Complete rest
1	Very weak
2	Weak
3	Moderate
4	Somewhat hard
5-6	Hard
7-9	Very hard
10	Extremely hard (almost maximal)
10+	Exhaustion

nutrition

Sure, you could get rid of pesky, unwanted pounds with weight training and cardio alone, but you need good nutrition to say bye-bye to them faster. In this section, you will learn the building blocks of eating for fat loss. There are tips to drop pounds in a jiffy, a two-week eating plan to make losing weight a no-brainer and snacks to power your efforts in the gym.

contents

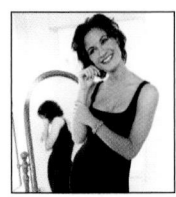
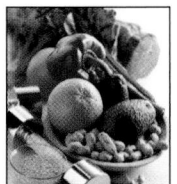
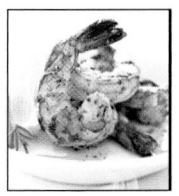

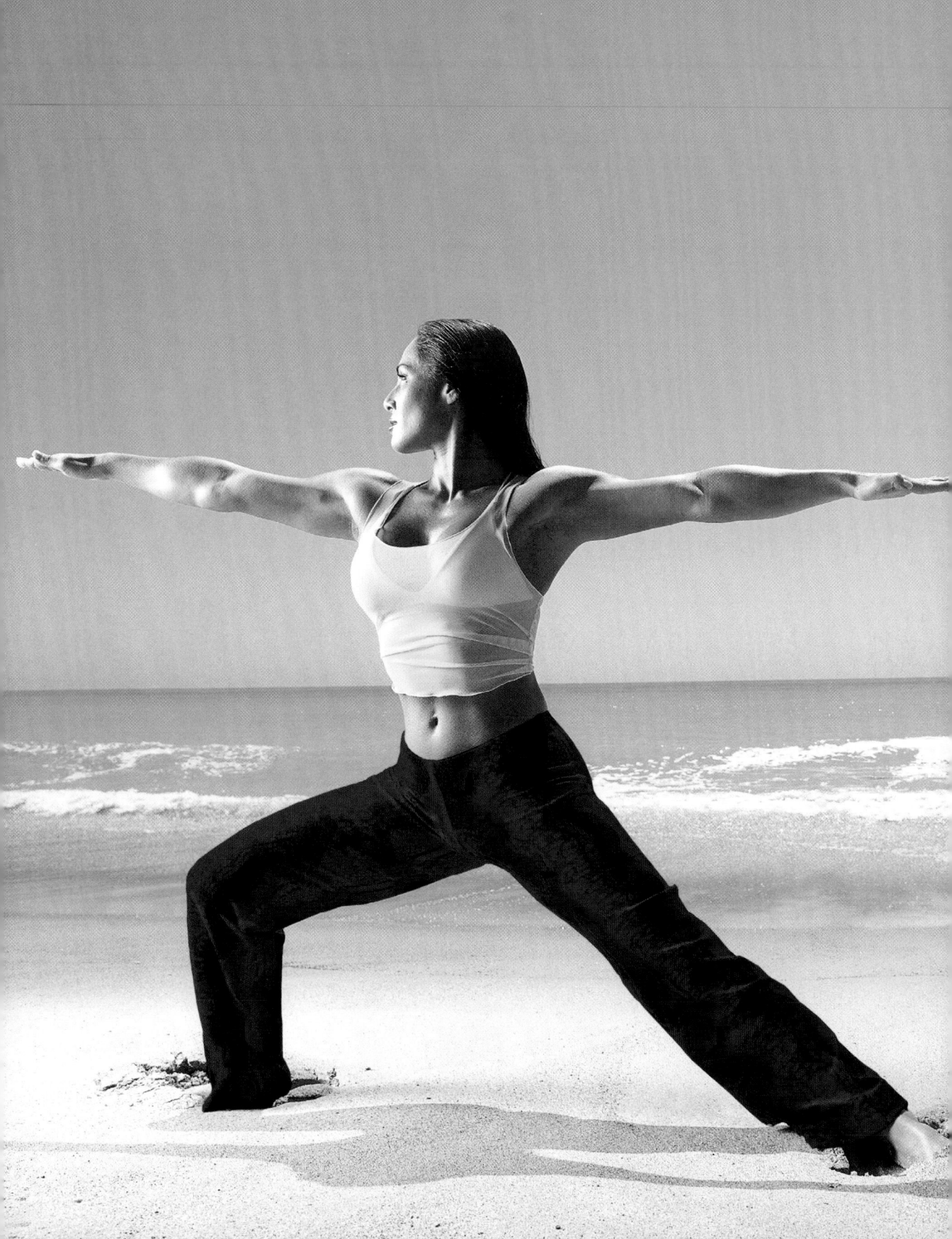

Chapter 8

Countdown To Looking Leaner

Diet is everything. The way that you eat determines not only how well you will perform in the gym, but also how well your jeans fit or how you will look when you put on your bathing suit.

Luckily there are some simple things that you can do when you want to look great in no time flat. Following the tips on the next pages will help.

Thirty days and counting. It's not the best way to shape up, but here you are, a month away from a vacation, a wedding or other photo-op moment, and you need to shed some fat fast. Help! We went to those in the know — fitness pros Angel Friend, Lisa Lowe, Cynthia Bridges and Lena Johannesen, as well as nutrition consultants Todd Swinney and Mike Davies — for advice. They all stress that quick-fix diets are no substitute for staying in shape year-round, but they also know that, hey, bodyfat happens. Here's what you can do to ditch it without going to dangerous extremes.

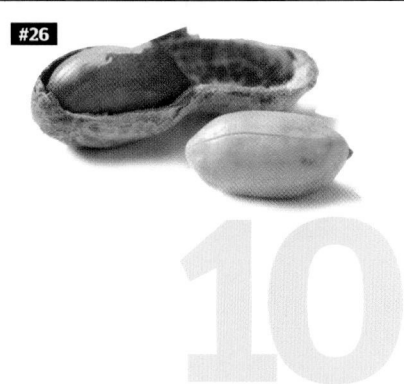

#26

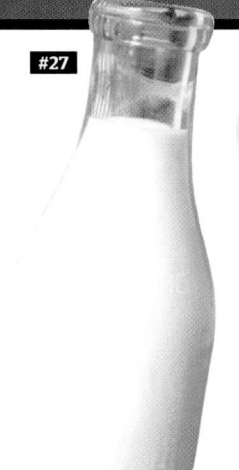

#27

9 CUT BACK ON ALL SIMPLE CARBS.

Simple carbs, such as fruit juices, candy and fruit, can add up quickly to push you over your daily calorie requirements, especially when you drink those calories. Swinney even recommends limiting dairy products, which contain lactose (milk sugar). Instead, focus on complex carbs for energy. They'll be more satiating and provide you with energy for your workouts without encroaching on your fat-loss goals.

10 CUT BACK ON ALL HIGH-FAT FOODS.

Swinney, a certified sports nutritionist and personal trainer in Maryland, works with pro fitness competitor Stacy Simons on her diet. He recommends avoiding red meat, egg yolks, butter and margarine, nuts and nut butters, oils and anything known to be high in fat. "Keep your fat intake under 25 grams a day," agrees Davies, whose clients include IFBB fitness pros Jen Hendershott and Adela Garcia. Although it's not wise to live on such a low-fat diet, doing it for a month shouldn't cause adverse health effects.

#28

8 ELIMINATE ALL PROCESSED AND REFINED FOODS.

That includes some types of bread, pasta, bagels and cereals. "Choose more nutrient-dense carbohydrates like brown rice, potatoes, sweet potatoes, beans and old-fashioned oatmeal," Swinney advises. They'll be absorbed more slowly and the higher fiber content should help satisfy you more. Again, your emphasis at this time should be to replace simple carbs and refined foods with less-processed complex carbs for energy.

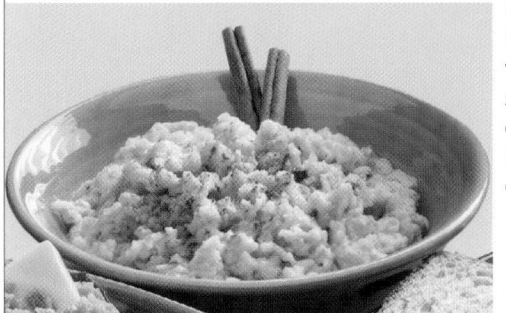

7 LIMIT TOTAL CARBOHYDRATE INTAKE. #29

"One thing that helped me most recently is dropping almost all starchy carbs," says Friend, who makes her home in Las Vegas. Optimal carb intake will vary by individual; you may need two or even three small portions of starchy carbohydrates daily to keep your motor revved. "The trick is to lower carb calories just enough to lose bodyfat without crushing your energy levels," Swinney explains. There's a very fine line between success and failure, so make small adjustments, not huge ones.

Johannesen, a Southern California transplant from Norway, fills out her meals with antioxidant-rich green vegetables and salads with no or low-fat dressing. Cutting carbs will also usher fluids out of your system and reduce bloat that masquerades as fat.

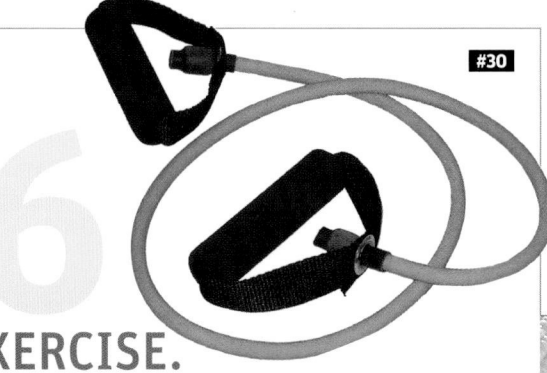

> Focus your efforts around complex carbs for energy. They'll be more satiating and provide you with energy for your workouts without encroaching on your fat-loss goals.

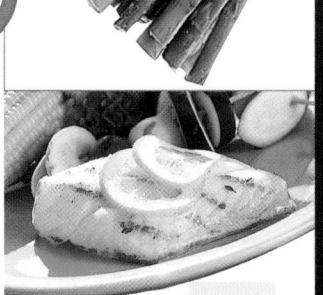
#31

6 EXERCISE.

Not a diet strategy per se, but we couldn't omit this important advice! "Break your cardio up into two 30–45-minute sessions per day at least five days per week," Davies advises. "And keep up your weight training for shape and tone."

If you can't manage double sessions, Bridges, another Southern California fitness pro, recommends 30 minutes of cardio at up to 80% of your maximum heart rate each day. Check first with your doctor about strenuous exercise, especially if you're just beginning or have any type of health condition.

Friend reports great results with cross-training. "Instead of just getting on a treadmill for an hour, get on it for 20 minutes, then do an elliptical for 20 and a rower for 20. It makes cardio a lot more interesting and fun, too."

"Running tends to lean you out the fastest," Johannesen adds. Other good choices are bicycling, incline treadmill walking, the elliptical trainer, swimming and hiking. Your weight workout needn't be long, but should be relatively intense to raise your thermic effect of activity, which includes your postworkout calorie burn.

5 EAT LEAN PROTEIN WISELY.

"Ingesting protein tends to increase your metabolic rate to a greater extent than either carbs or fats," Swinney states. The "A" list includes skinless chicken and turkey breast, egg whites, tuna, other white fish and shellfish such as shrimp, scallops, lobster and crab. Dividing your protein among five smaller meals per day also helps keep cravings at bay.

Quick Fixes Quickly Fade

Although these tips are intended to help you reach the pinnacle of physical perfection, they might be counterproductive if used too often. The human body is a finely tuned instrument designed to survive stressful conditions. Over the long haul, there's no way to trick your body. Calorie reductions below your daily requirement, no matter how small, will cause your metabolism to slow down. It doesn't matter what supplements you take, or how much exercise you do to try to offset this slowdown — you just can't beat your own physiology.

Before considering any quick-fix solution, remember this: A lean individual who loses more than about 1 pound per week is burning up lean muscle as fuel. Losing water, or dehydrating your body, means you're reducing your relative lean body mass and increasing your relative fat mass. Over time, that means you must keep cutting calories to avoid gaining more fat, which in turn further slows your metabolism. Pretty soon, you'll have conditioned your body to become a fat-storing machine, rather than a fat-burning machine. No matter how you spin it, quick-fix, extreme dieting can only make you fatter in the long run.

DRINK UP! WATER, THAT IS.

Water contributes to feelings of fullness and assists in the fat-burning process. If you're eating more protein and exercising more, you'll need more water than you normally would. Aim for 3 quarts of water or more a day. Try drinking 1 quart before, during and after your exercise session, 1 in the morning and 1 in the afternoon.

#32

Before considering any quick-fix solution, remember this: A lean individual who loses more than about 1 pound per week is burning up lean muscle as fuel.

ROTATE YOUR CALORIES.

Lowe, a fitness model in Northern California, points out, "It takes a bit of calculating, but for me it's the best way to shed weight quickly and it works." To get in shape for a couple of her last pro contests, she rotated between eating 1,500 calories over four meals daily for three consecutive days, then bumped it up to 1,900 calories for one day. "It's all about staying within your daily calorie budget. Don't skip meals, but take calories away from your total number of meals throughout the day," she adds. "I was shocked. I was still eating my chicken and turkey, but I could eat tortillas, cereal and bagels — the things everybody backs away from. If the discipline isn't there to stay with a typical precontest diet, it's just not going to work."

Depending on your bodytype, activity level and current calorie consumption, reduce anywhere from 300–500 calories on your low days. Avoid going too low on calories, however, or your resting metabolic rate will drop. If your energy suffers, try only two low-calorie days between higher-calorie days.

#33

2 SUPPLEMENT.

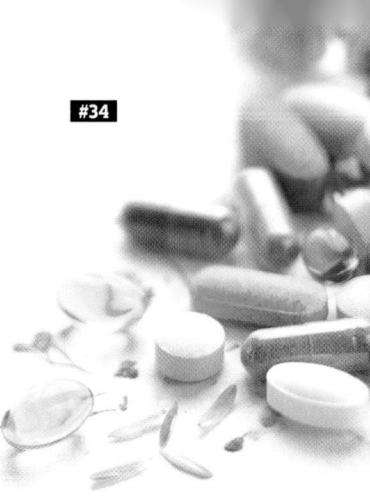

#34

A good multivitamin-mineral tops Johannesen's list to help cover nutritional needs during a reduced-calorie phase. Vigorous exercise can result in mineral loss via sweat and urine, and deficiencies can hinder endurance. Bridges likes to include L-carnitine, coffee or green tea (taken before exercise, it can boost endurance and intensity), a mild herbal thermogenic, glutamine (helpful in higher-stress times) and protein powder. "Sometimes I'll use something called PMS Tea, which is a mild herbal diuretic, to drop a bit more water the last day or two before the event," she remarks.

Friend adds flax-oil capsules, 2,000 milligrams twice a day, to the mix, or you can substitute a tablespoon of flaxseed oil on a salad, or add ground flaxseed to a protein shake or oatmeal.

1 ELIMINATE OR REDUCE CONDIMENTS.

"Another way to lose weight is to shed extra water, so I refrain from using condiments that are higher in sodium content," Friend notes. Beware of mustard, ketchup, barbecue sauce, steak sauce, seasonings and fat-free salad dressings, which can be high in sugars or sodium, contributing to water retention. Read labels carefully, and when eating out, ask for your food to be prepared without seasonings, oils or sauces.

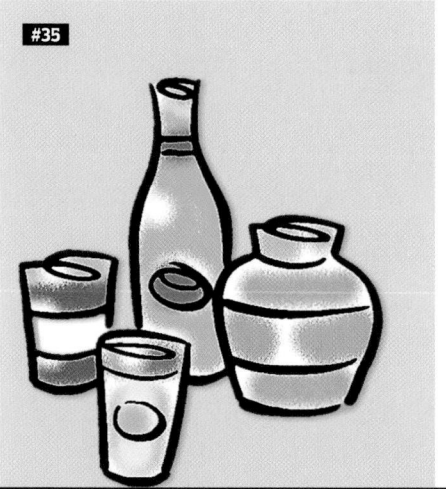

#35

BLAST OFF!

Your big event is here. Enjoy — you've earned it! But come tomorrow, continue the fitness lifestyle so you maintain your fantastic improvements.

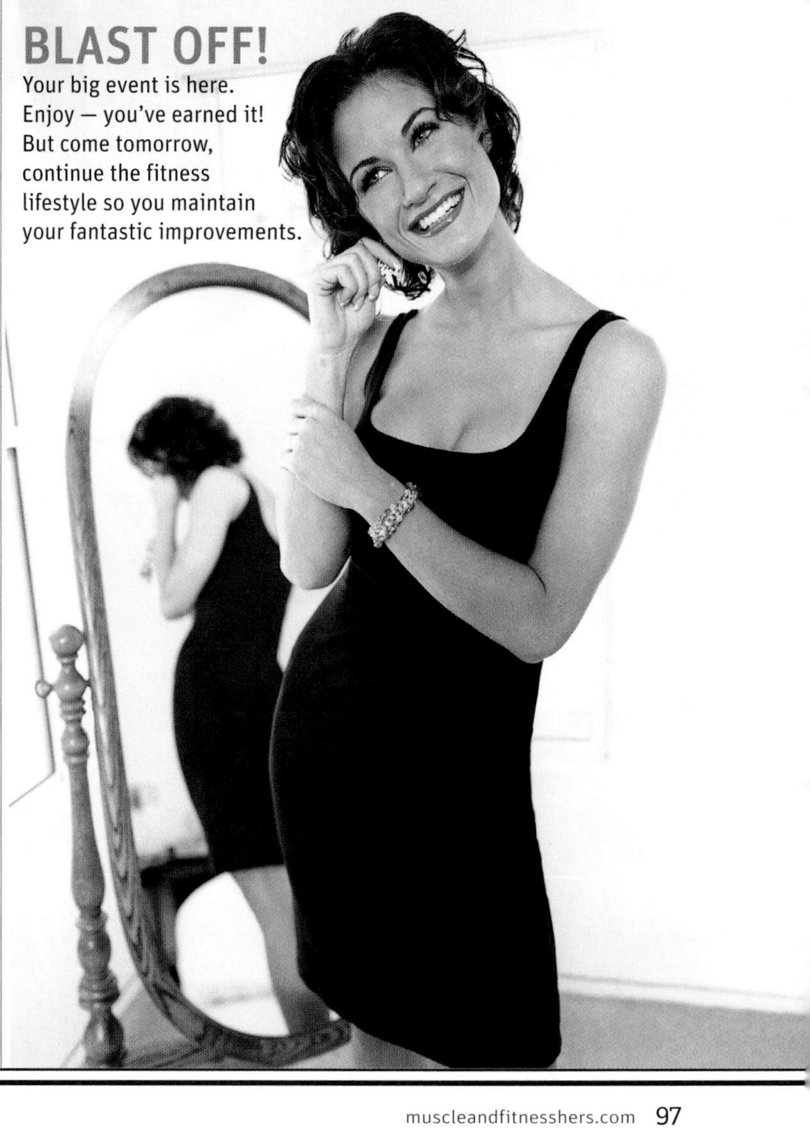

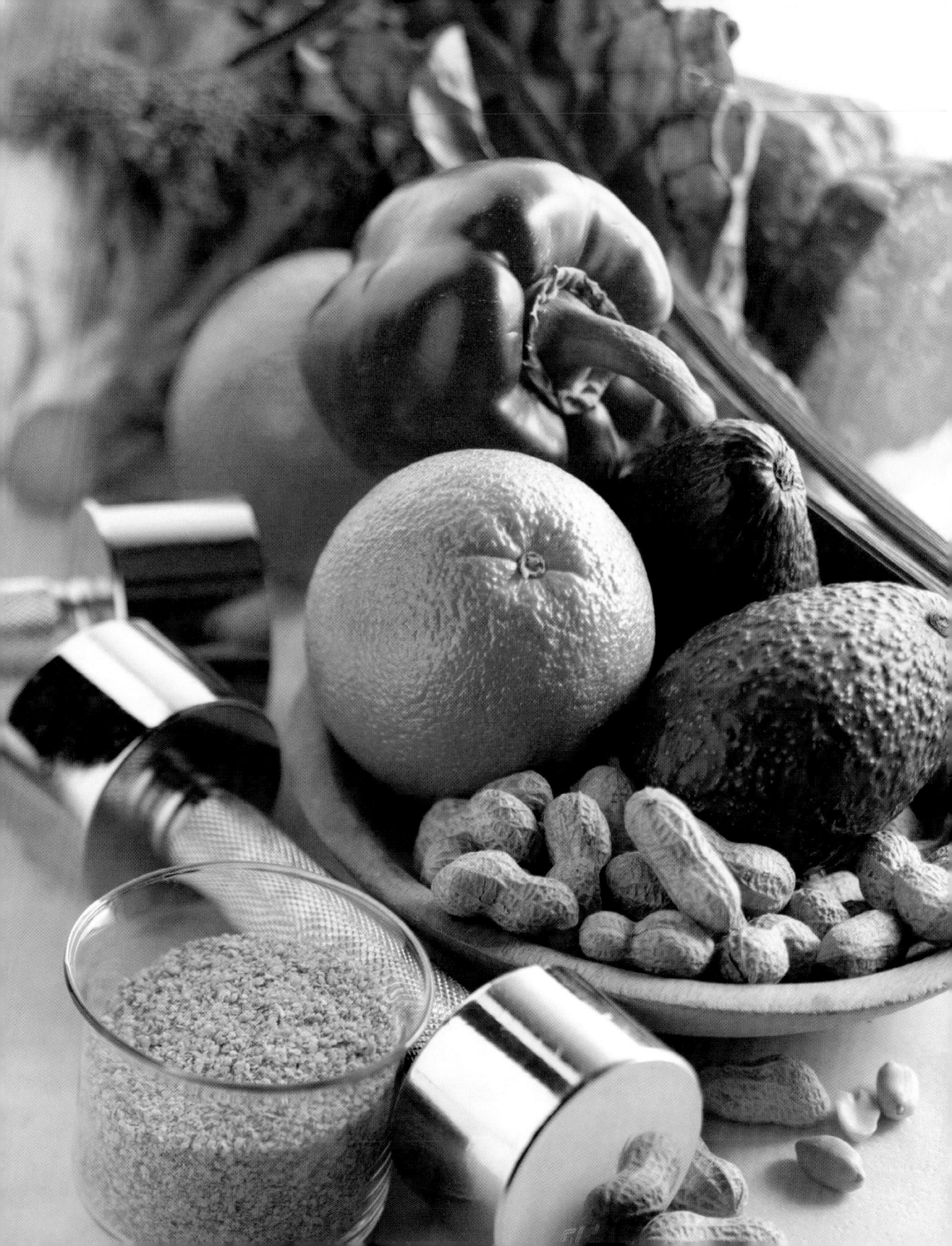

Chapter 9

The Ultimate No-Brainer Diet

You're probably wondering how to send those extra ten pounds packing. Here's the answer. We have taken out all the work of developing a meal plan that has the right mix of carbohydrates, protein, fat and fiber. The following two-week meal plan will help you safely and effectively get into shape without lots of stress, worry or even much effort. All you have to do is a little cooking and some good eating.

It's important that you keep in mind that healthy eating doesn't have to be difficult or time consuming. In fact, we have made it very simple for you. Just follow the 14-day meal plan we've developed specifically for you — the active woman who wants to lose weight and maintain lean muscle mass, but still has to keep up with a hectic schedule.

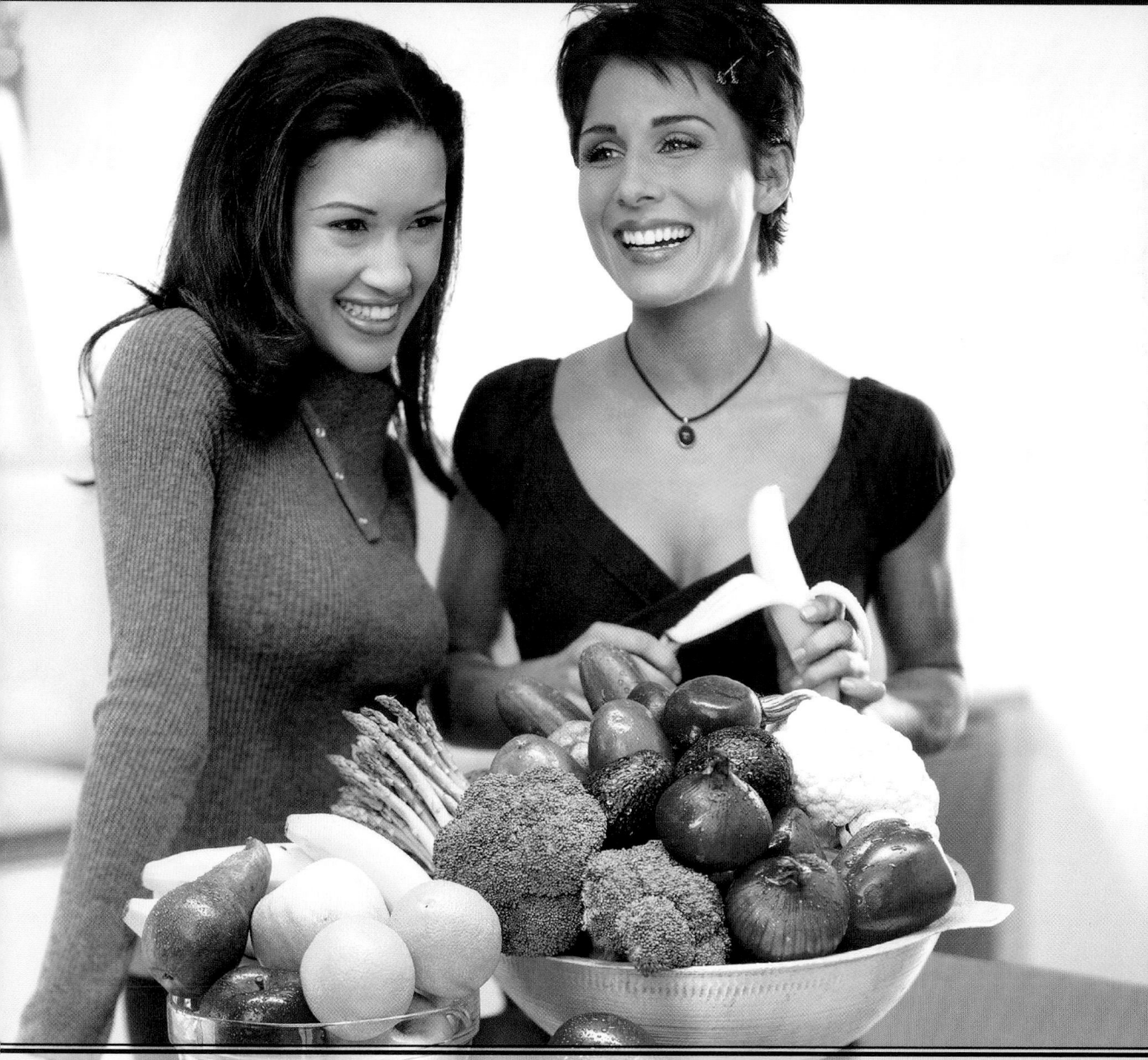

speedy black-bean burritos

8 oz. chicken breast meat (uncooked)
15-oz. can black beans, drained
½ cup salsa
3 Tbsp. uncooked bulgur wheat
Leaf lettuce
1 tomato
4 flour tortillas

Slice chicken thinly and sauté in a lightly oiled pan until thoroughly cooked. Remove from pan and set aside. Combine black beans, salsa and bulgur in a saucepan; simmer gently five minutes, stirring occasionally. Add chicken and heat 1–2 minutes. Remove from heat, cover and let stand five minutes. Meanwhile, shred 1 cup lettuce and dice tomato. Heat a tortilla in an ungreased skillet until warm and soft, then spread a line of the bean mixture down center of tortilla. Top with lettuce, tomato and additional salsa, if desired. Roll tortilla around filling, then repeat with remaining tortillas. Makes 4 burritos.

NUTRITION FACTS (per burrito): *240 calories, 15 g protein, 27 g carbohydrate, 8 g fat, 6 g fiber*

lunch, day 3

1 Speedy Black-Bean Burrito
1½ cups tossed salad
2 Tbsp. reduced-fat dressing
1 cup 1% milk

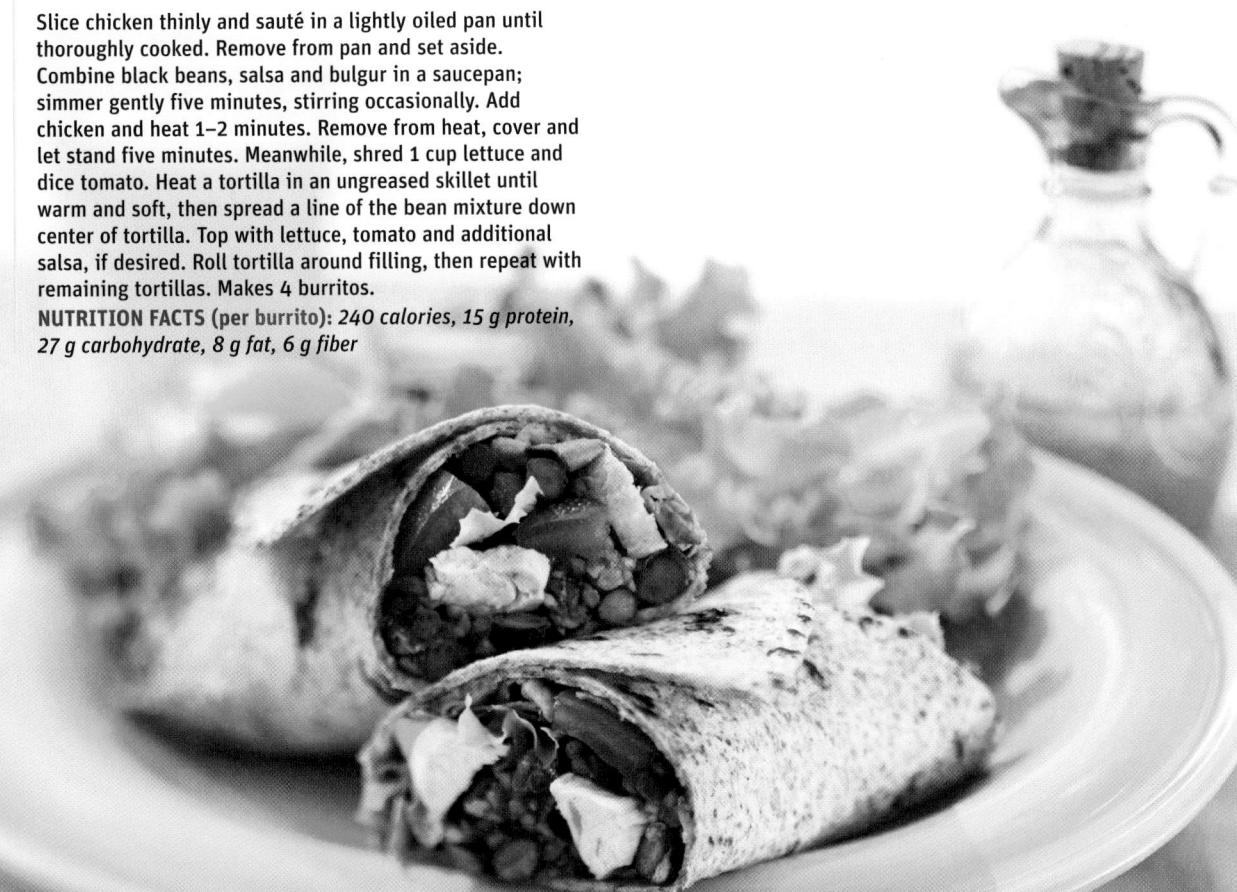

Follow the meal plan for two weeks and then begin again. Remember, weight loss doesn't happen overnight. A loss of 1–2 pounds per week is ideal since this will allow you to maintain lean muscle and lose bodyfat; a very-low-calorie diet would cause you to lose muscle mass along with the bodyfat. Muscle is tied to your metabolism, so a well-planned and well-executed program is much more sensible than extreme plans. Anyway, you can follow such meal-skipping, extreme-calorie-cutting, energy-depriving plans for only a short period before you get fed up!

the guidelines

Numbers are based on a moderately active woman who weighs about 140 pounds. She weight trains 2–3 times a week and does cardio three times a week. Strive for these daily totals:

Recommendation		Basis
Calories	Approximately 1,600 calories	Suggestion for weight loss of 1–2 pounds per week (range of 1,500–1,700 calories daily)
Carbs	200–260 grams	Based on 50%–65% of calories
Protein	75–95 grams	Based on 0.55–0.68 gram per pound (1.2–1.5 grams per kg) of bodyweight
Fat	35–55 grams	20%–30% of calories
Fiber	25–35 grams	General recommendations for health

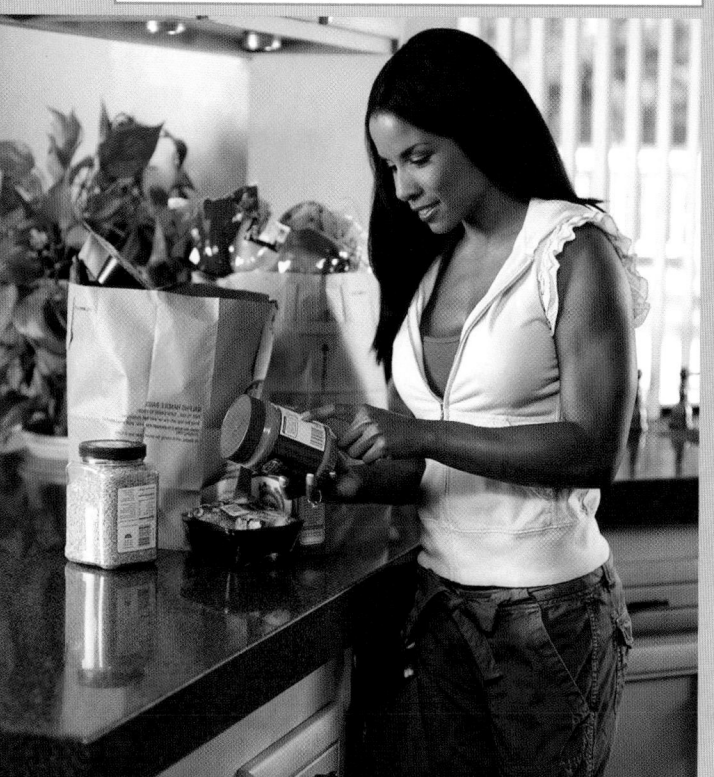

week one

day one #36

BREAKFAST:
1½ oz. oatmeal (from half-cup dry) w/ 1 cup 1% milk
1 small banana

SNACK:
1 serving Made-From-Scratch Applesauce (see recipe on page 103)

LUNCH:
2 slices whole-wheat bread
2 Tbsp. reduced-fat peanut butter
1½ cups tossed salad w/ 1 Tbsp. low-cal Italian dressing
1 cup 1% milk

SNACK:
3 cups light microwave popcorn

DINNER:
3 oz. broiled swordfish
1 cup cooked broccoli florets
1 cup rice pilaf

SNACK:
1 cup fat-free lemon yogurt

DAILY TOTALS: *1,675 calories, 83 g protein, 243 g carbohydrate, 41 g fat, 28 g fiber*

day two #37

BREAKFAST:
2 oz. Total Raisin Bran w/ 1 cup 1% milk
1 medium banana

SNACK:
1½ oz. low-fat, low-salt crackers (or 1½ servings)

LUNCH:
5 oz. turkey
2 slices rye bread
1 tsp. fat-free mayonnaise (see Tarragon Turkey Dijon recipe on page 107 for sandwich variation)
1½ cups tossed salad w/ 1 Tbsp. low-cal Italian dressing

SNACK:
1 medium orange

DINNER:
3 oz. baked chicken breast
1 small potato, baked with skin
1½ cups tossed salad w/ 1 Tbsp. balsamic vinaigrette

SNACK:
1 cup 1% milk

DAILY TOTALS: *1,600 calories, 97 g protein, 230 g carbohydrate, 33 g fat, 20 g fiber*

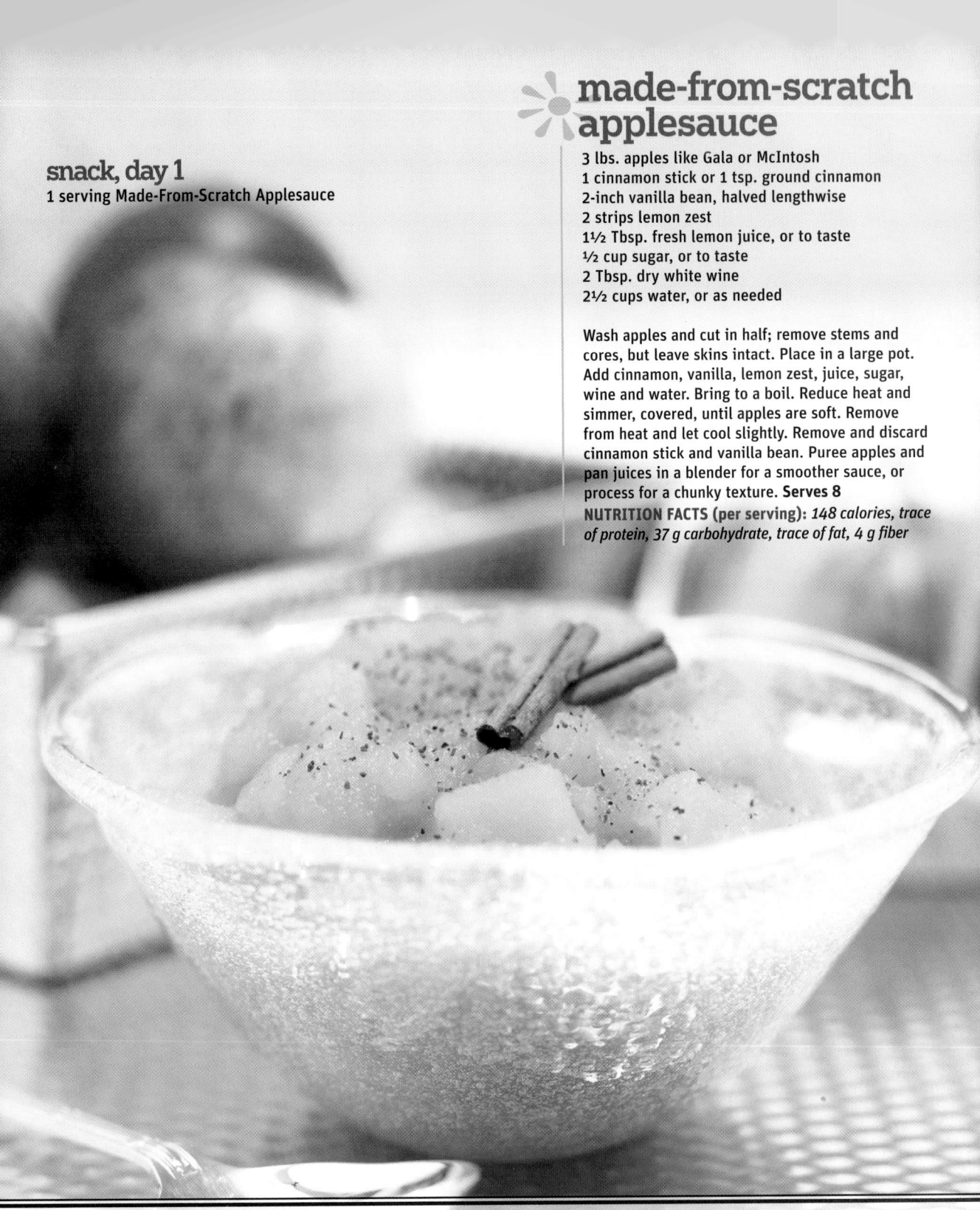

snack, day 1
1 serving Made-From-Scratch Applesauce

made-from-scratch applesauce

3 lbs. apples like Gala or McIntosh
1 cinnamon stick or 1 tsp. ground cinnamon
2-inch vanilla bean, halved lengthwise
2 strips lemon zest
1½ Tbsp. fresh lemon juice, or to taste
½ cup sugar, or to taste
2 Tbsp. dry white wine
2½ cups water, or as needed

Wash apples and cut in half; remove stems and cores, but leave skins intact. Place in a large pot. Add cinnamon, vanilla, lemon zest, juice, sugar, wine and water. Bring to a boil. Reduce heat and simmer, covered, until apples are soft. Remove from heat and let cool slightly. Remove and discard cinnamon stick and vanilla bean. Puree apples and pan juices in a blender for a smoother sauce, or process for a chunky texture. **Serves 8**

NUTRITION FACTS (per serving): *148 calories, trace of protein, 37 g carbohydrate, trace of fat, 4 g fiber*

BREAKFAST:
1½ oz. Grape-Nuts cereal w/ 1 cup 1% milk
1 cup blueberries
SNACK:
1 medium apple
LUNCH:
Speedy Black-Bean Burrito (see recipe on page 101)
1½ cups tossed salad w/ 2 Tbsp. reduced-fat dressing
1 cup 1% milk
SNACK:
1 cup low-fat fruit yogurt
DINNER:
3 oz. ground turkey breast patty, grilled
1 medium whole-wheat roll
3 oz. baked french fries
SNACK:
1 granola bar
DAILY TOTALS: *1,570 calories, 74 g protein, 222 g carbohydrate, 43 g fat, 22 g fiber*

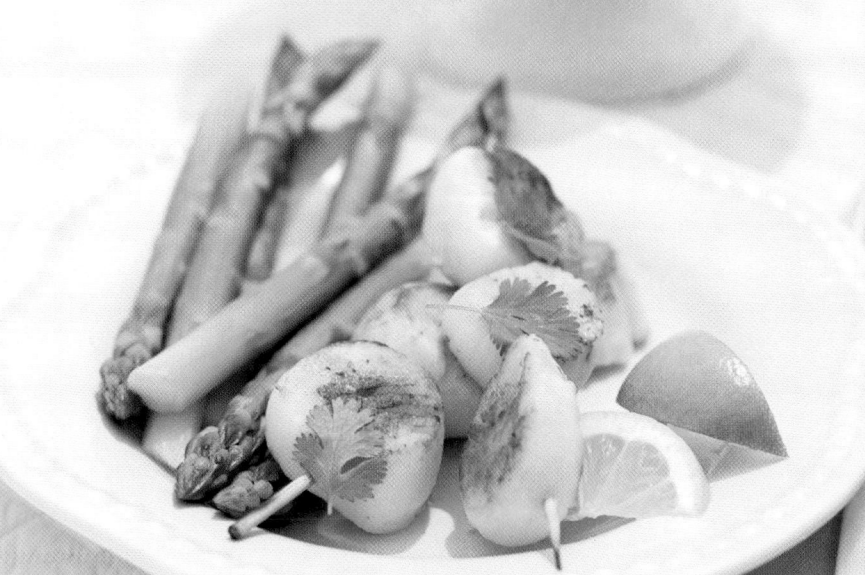

dinner, day 6
3 oz. broiled scallops
½ cup couscous
1 cup cooked asparagus

day four #39

BREAKFAST:
1¼ oz. All-Bran cereal w/ 1 cup 1% milk
8 oz. grapefruit juice
SNACK:
3 medium prunes or other dried fruit
LUNCH
2 slices multigrain bread
2½ Tbsp. reduced-fat peanut butter
1 cup 1% milk
SNACK:
15 animal crackers
DINNER:
2 small slices thin-crust pizza with light cheese
1½ cups tossed salad
1 Tbsp. low-fat creamy Italian dressing
SNACK:
1 cup low-fat peach yogurt
DAILY TOTALS: *1,590 calories, 63 g protein, 228 g carbohydrate, 47 g fat, 29 g fiber*

day five #40

BREAKFAST:
1 small or ½ large whole-wheat bagel
1 tsp. fruit preserves or jam
½ cup fresh fruit cup
1 cup 1% milk
SNACK:
½ small cantaloupe
LUNCH:
2 oz. tuna, canned in water, drained
2 slices seven- or nine-grain bread
1 tsp. fat-free mayonnaise
SNACK:
1 oz. Cheerios
DINNER:
1 slice light vegetable quiche (frozen entree)
1½ cups tossed salad
1 Tbsp. low-cal Italian dressing
SNACK:
1 cup low-fat raspberry yogurt
DAILY TOTALS: *1,484 calories, 65 g protein, 207 g carbohydrate, 44 g fat, 20 g fiber*

day six #41

BREAKFAST:
1 Low-Fat Carrot Muffin
 (see recipe on page 108)
1 cup 1% milk
1 large peach
SNACK:
1 cup strawberries
LUNCH:
1½ cups chef's salad (with 3 oz. lean poultry
 or meat and 1 oz. grated low-fat cheese)
1 Tbsp. reduced-fat dressing
1 small (4-inch-round) whole-wheat pita
SNACK:
3 cups light microwave popcorn
DINNER:
3 oz. broiled scallops
½ cup couscous
1 cup cooked asparagus
SNACK:
1 cup low-fat fruit yogurt
DAILY TOTALS: *1,650 calories, 95 g protein, 236 g carbohydrate, 36 g fat, 23 g fiber.*

day seven #42

BREAKFAST:
1½ oz. oatmeal (from half-cup dry)
1 cup 1% milk
1 medium banana
SNACK:
1½ oz. low-fat onion-flavored crackers
LUNCH:
2 oz. low-fat cheese
½ cup baby carrots
4 half-stalks celery
1 high-fiber English muffin
1 cup low-fat pineapple-flavored
 cottage cheese
SNACK:
1 cup low-fat mixed-fruit yogurt
DINNER:
1 small vegetable egg roll
1 cup vegetable lo mein
½ cup stir-fry vegetables (prepared
 with minimum oil)
SNACK:
1 oz. Cheerios or other high-fiber cereal
DAILY TOTALS: *1,747 calories, 73 g protein, 250 g carbohydrate, 35 g fat, 26 g fiber*

week two

day eight #43

BREAKFAST:
2 oz. Fiber One cereal
½ large banana
1 cup low-fat fruit yogurt
SNACK:
1 medium orange
LUNCH:
1 cup vegetarian lentil soup (canned)
1 whole-wheat dinner roll
1½ cups tossed salad w/ 1 Tbsp. low-cal
   Italian dressing
1 cup 1% milk
SNACK:
3 Dutch pretzels
DINNER:
1 serving low-fat vegetarian lasagna (frozen entree)
1½ cups tossed salad w/ 1 Tbsp. low-cal Italian
dressing
SNACK:
½ cup light ice cream
DAILY TOTALS: *1,490 calories, 66 g protein,
239 g carbohydrate, 30 g fat, 36 g fiber*

day ten #45

BREAKFAST:
1½ oz. Cracklin' Oat Bran cereal w/ 1 cup 1% milk
1 medium pear
SNACK:
1 cup diced pineapple
LUNCH:
½ cup hummus (garbanzo bean spread)
1 9-inch flour tortilla
¼ cup cooked eggplant
¼ cup cooked zucchini
¼ cup cooked summer squash
1 cup 1% milk
SNACK:
1 granola bar
DINNER:
1 cup cooked linguini pasta
4 oz. broiled shrimp, topped with lemon and pepper
1 cup cooked broccoli florets
SNACK:
½ cup light chocolate pudding made with 1% milk
DAILY TOTALS: *1,628 calories, 75 g protein,
251 g carbohydrate, 36 g fat, 25 g fiber*

day nine #44

BREAKFAST:
½ high-fiber English muffin
1 Tbsp. reduced-fat peanut butter
1 cup 1% milk
4 oz. fresh orange juice
SNACK:
8 cinnamon graham crackers
LUNCH:
1½ cups Greek salad with 1 oz. feta cheese
1 Tbsp. low-fat creamy Italian dressing
1 6-inch whole-wheat pita
1 cup 1% milk
SNACK:
4 Tbsp. seedless raisins
DINNER:
3 oz. chicken breast, simmered in 4 oz. tomato
   sauce with green peppers, onions and mushrooms
1½ cups tossed salad w/ 1 Tbsp. low-fat French
   dressing
SNACK:
1 cup low-fat fruit yogurt
DAILY TOTALS: *1,620 calories, 75 g protein,
218 g carbohydrate, 50 g fat, 20 g fiber*

day eleven #46

BREAKFAST:
1½ oz. oatmeal w/ 1 cup 1% milk
2 Tbsp. seedless raisins
SNACK:
1 medium peach and ½ cup raspberries
LUNCH:
2 oz. tuna, canned in water, drained
2 slices whole-wheat bread
1 tsp. fat-free mayonnaise
1 cup baby carrots
¾ cup low-fat cottage cheese
1 cup 1% milk
SNACK:
1 cup low-fat fruit yogurt
DINNER:
3 oz. pork loin chop
1 cup long-grain brown rice
1½ cups tossed salad w/ 1 Tbsp. low-cal
   Italian dressing
SNACK:
½ oz. baked tortilla chips
DAILY TOTALS: *1,640 calories, 90 g protein,
228 g carbohydrate, 41 g fat, 26 g fiber*

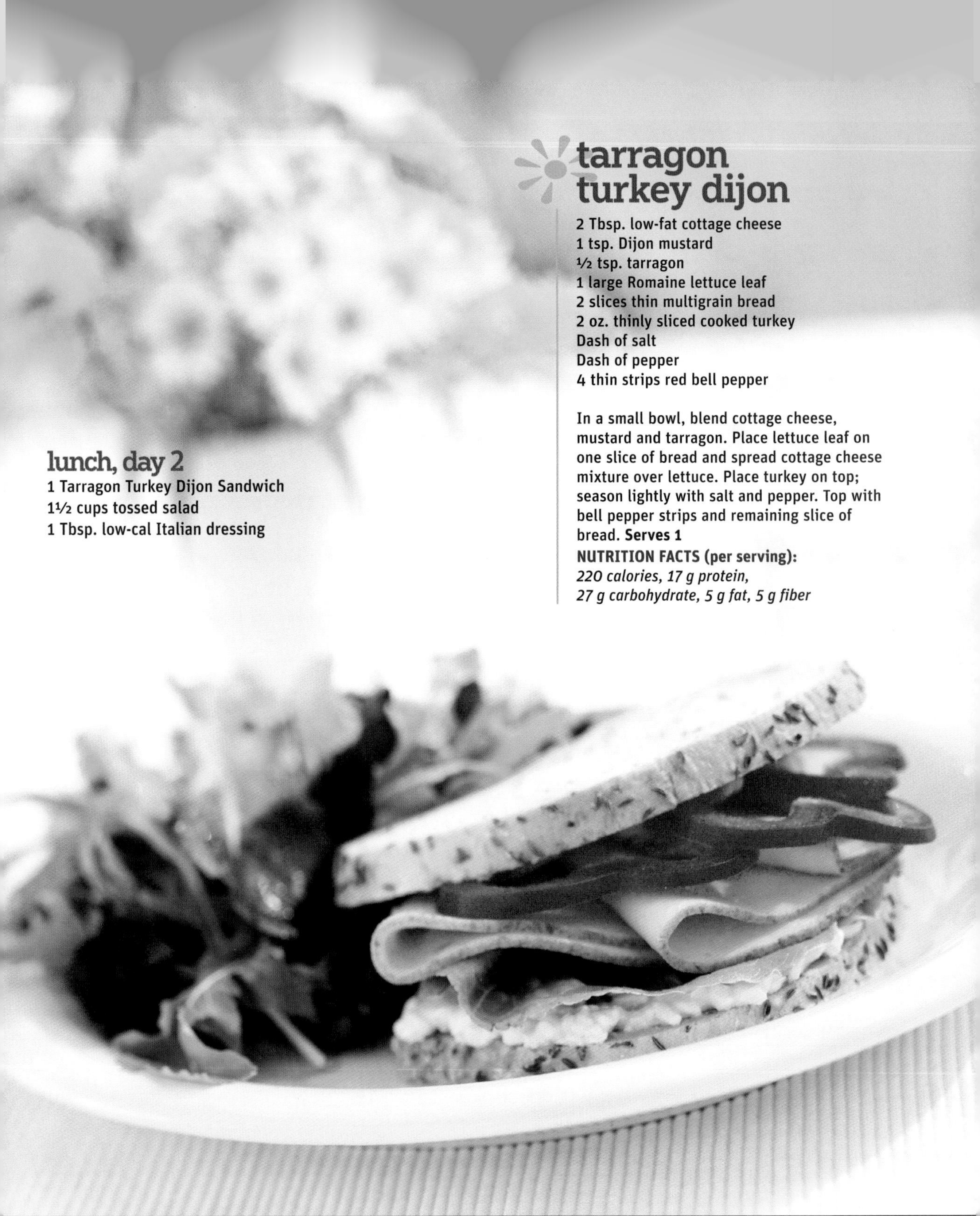

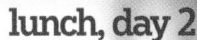

tarragon turkey dijon

2 Tbsp. low-fat cottage cheese
1 tsp. Dijon mustard
½ tsp. tarragon
1 large Romaine lettuce leaf
2 slices thin multigrain bread
2 oz. thinly sliced cooked turkey
Dash of salt
Dash of pepper
4 thin strips red bell pepper

In a small bowl, blend cottage cheese, mustard and tarragon. Place lettuce leaf on one slice of bread and spread cottage cheese mixture over lettuce. Place turkey on top; season lightly with salt and pepper. Top with bell pepper strips and remaining slice of bread. **Serves 1**
NUTRITION FACTS (per serving):
220 calories, 17 g protein,
27 g carbohydrate, 5 g fat, 5 g fiber

lunch, day 2

1 Tarragon Turkey Dijon Sandwich
1½ cups tossed salad
1 Tbsp. low-cal Italian dressing

breakfast, day 6

1 Low-Fat Carrot Muffin
1 cup 1% milk
1 large peach

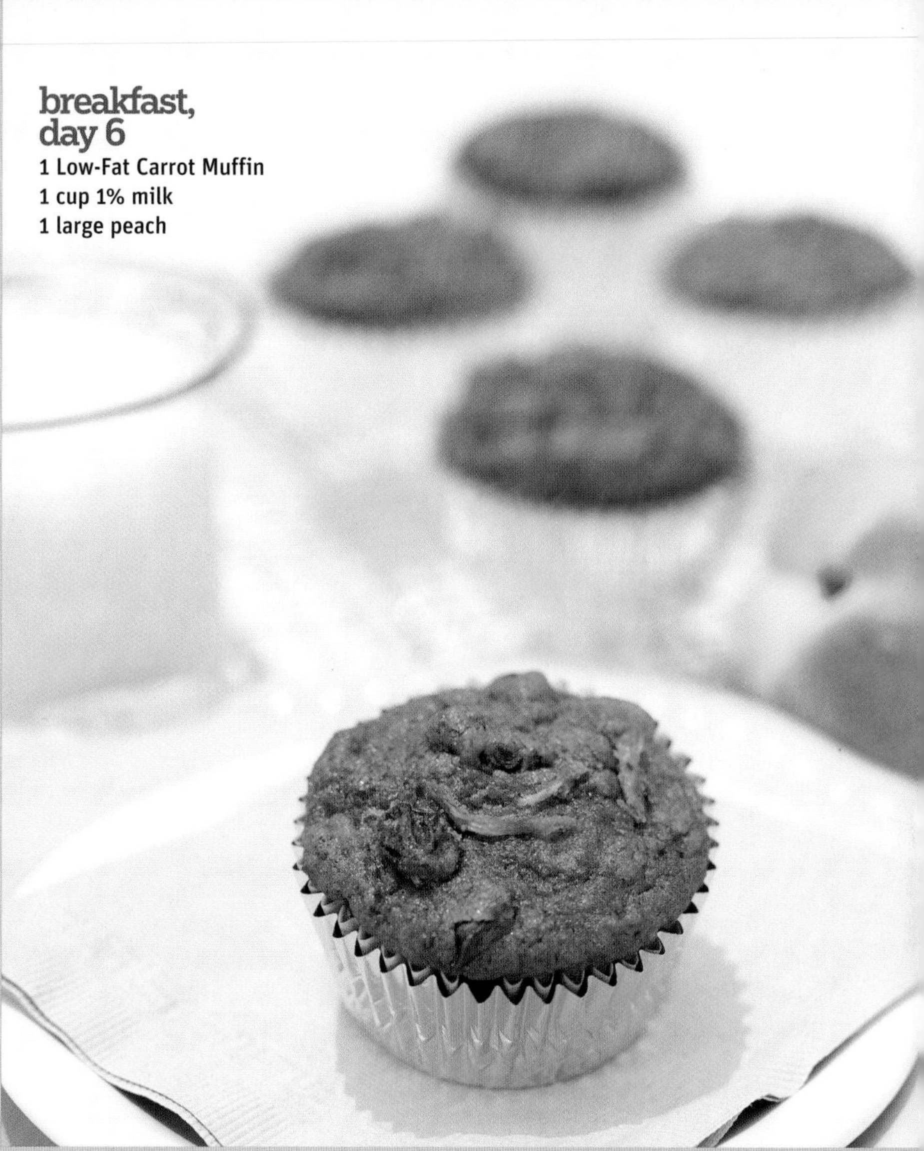

low-fat carrot muffins

2 cups whole-wheat flour
⅔ cup ready-to-eat bran flakes
2 tsp. baking powder
1 tsp. ground cinnamon
½ tsp. grated nutmeg
1½ cups skim milk
1½ cups shredded carrots
½ cup raisins
½ cup egg substitute
½ cup honey
2 Tbsp. canola oil
2 Tbsp. molasses

Preheat oven to 375 degrees F. In a large bowl, combine flour, bran flakes, baking powder, cinnamon and nutmeg. In a separate bowl, combine milk, carrots, raisins, egg substitute, honey, oil and molasses. Stir liquid ingredients into dry ingredients until just blended. Be careful not to overmix. Spray muffin tins with nonstick spray or use paper muffin cups. Fill cups about three-quarters full. Bake for 20–25 minutes or until a toothpick inserted into the center of the muffins comes out clean. Makes 12–14 muffins. **NUTRITION FACTS (per muffin):** *170 calories, 5 g protein, 26 g carbohydrate, 5 fat, 5 g fiber*

day twelve

#47

BREAKFAST:
2 medium whole-wheat pancakes w/ 2 Tbsp. light syrup
1 cup strawberries
1 cup 1% milk
SNACK:
1 medium banana
LUNCH:
1 cup chunky vegetable soup (canned)
2 slices whole-wheat bread
2 Tbsp. reduced-fat peanut butter
1 cup 1% milk
SNACK:
1 oz. Fruit 'n Fibre cereal
DINNER:
1 chicken wrap with beans (9-inch flour tortilla,
   2 oz. cooked chicken, ½ cup black beans)
1½ cups tossed salad, added to wrap
1 Tbsp. low-fat French dressing
SNACK:
1 cup low-fat cherry yogurt
DAILY TOTALS: *1,683 calories, 70 g protein,
254 g carbohydrate, 43 g fat, 24 g fiber*

day thirteen

#48

BREAKFAST:
1 large egg, scrambled
½ high-fiber raisin English muffin
1 cup 1% milk
4 oz. fresh orange juice
SNACK:
8 medium dried apricots
LUNCH:
2 slices low-fat deli turkey breast
2 slices pumpernickel bread
1 tsp. mustard
1½ cups tossed salad w/ 1 Tbsp. Dijon vinaigrette
SNACK:
1 cup low-fat lemon yogurt
DINNER:
3 oz. broiled swordfish
1 medium potato, baked with skin
1 cup cooked peas
1 cup 1% milk
SNACK:
1 medium low-fat oatmeal cookie
DAILY TOTALS: *1,460 calories, 82 g protein,
202 g carbohydrate, 36 g fat, 25 g fiber*

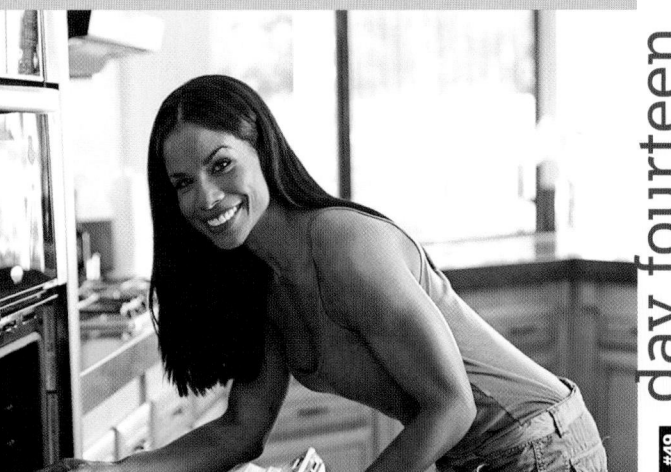

day fourteen

#49

BREAKFAST:
1½ oz. Fruit 'n Fibre cereal w/ 1 cup 1% milk
½ large banana
SNACK:
1 cup low-fat blueberry yogurt
LUNCH:
2 slices whole-wheat bread
2 slices low-fat American cheese
1 tsp. mustard
1 cup baby carrots
1 cup 1% milk
SNACK:
3 cups light microwave popcorn
DINNER:
3 oz. 90% lean ground beef patty, grilled,
   served on ½ hamburger bun
3 oz. baked french fries
1½ cups tossed salad w/ 1 Tbsp. low-cal
   Italian dressing
SNACK:
1 cup blueberries
DAILY TOTALS: *1,700 calories, 84 g protein,
250 g carbohydrate, 41 g fat, 24 g fiber*

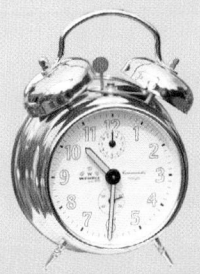

your eat-lean-for-life guide

Eat a variety of foods that you like. Eating many different foods ensures that you get all the nutrients (and non-nutrient compounds) you need for optimal health without getting too much of things that may not be as nutritious. Including a variety of foods in your diet also prevents boredom — by increasing the number of nutritious foods you choose from, you increase the likelihood that you will stick to healthful eating.

Snack. Snacking is a great way to "take five" and relieve stress. Always have nutritious snacks on hand to munch on. Choose nutrient-dense foods to fill in the gaps in your diet. If, for example, you have difficulty meeting your daily calcium requirements, choose low-fat yogurt, pudding, cheese or milk for snacking. Snacking helps you refuel and prevents you from becoming so hungry that you overeat.

Plan. Plan what, when, where and how. Schedule time to eat, just like you schedule meetings. Busy lives mean planning and compromising, and you can compromise on time without skimping on nutritional quality. Plan breakfast meetings, and develop a list of lunches and snacks you can eat at your desk or while you're on the go.

Be an educated eater. Learn the basics of good nutrition, label-reading and dining out. Being an educated eater means you have the knowledge necessary to make informed choices no matter how crunched for time you become. Look at reliable websites for sound nutrition information; some of these include www.eatright.org of the American Dietetic Association, www.nutritiondata.com of the USDA and www.navigator.tufts.edu of Tufts University.

Don't skip meals. Skipping meals not only causes you to miss nutrients important for your health and performance but it can also lead to overeating. You become so hungry that "anything goes" (into your mouth) and all good intentions go out the window. Oftentimes you end up eating the first thing you can grab, which may not be very nutritious.

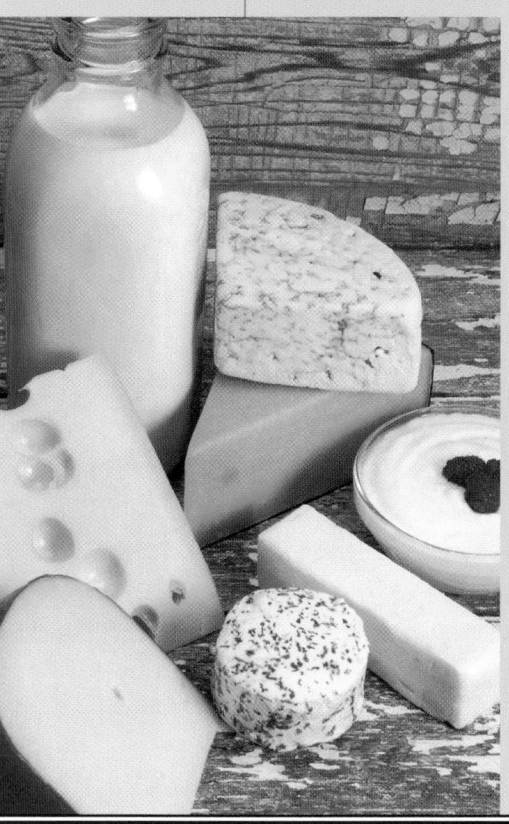

Be creative. Think of time-saving eating opportunities, such as: planning meals that can be used as leftovers, lunches you can eat at your desk, snacks you can munch on when you're on the go, crockpot meals that cook on their own during the day, and other dinners you can fix in 10 minutes or less. Keep in mind that dinner doesn't have to be hot to be nutritious, and breakfast or lunch can be leftovers from a previous meal.

Be flexible. Things don't always work out the way we plan them to. Be prepared and have an alternative or two. Don't give up or give in, and always try to make the best of bad situations.

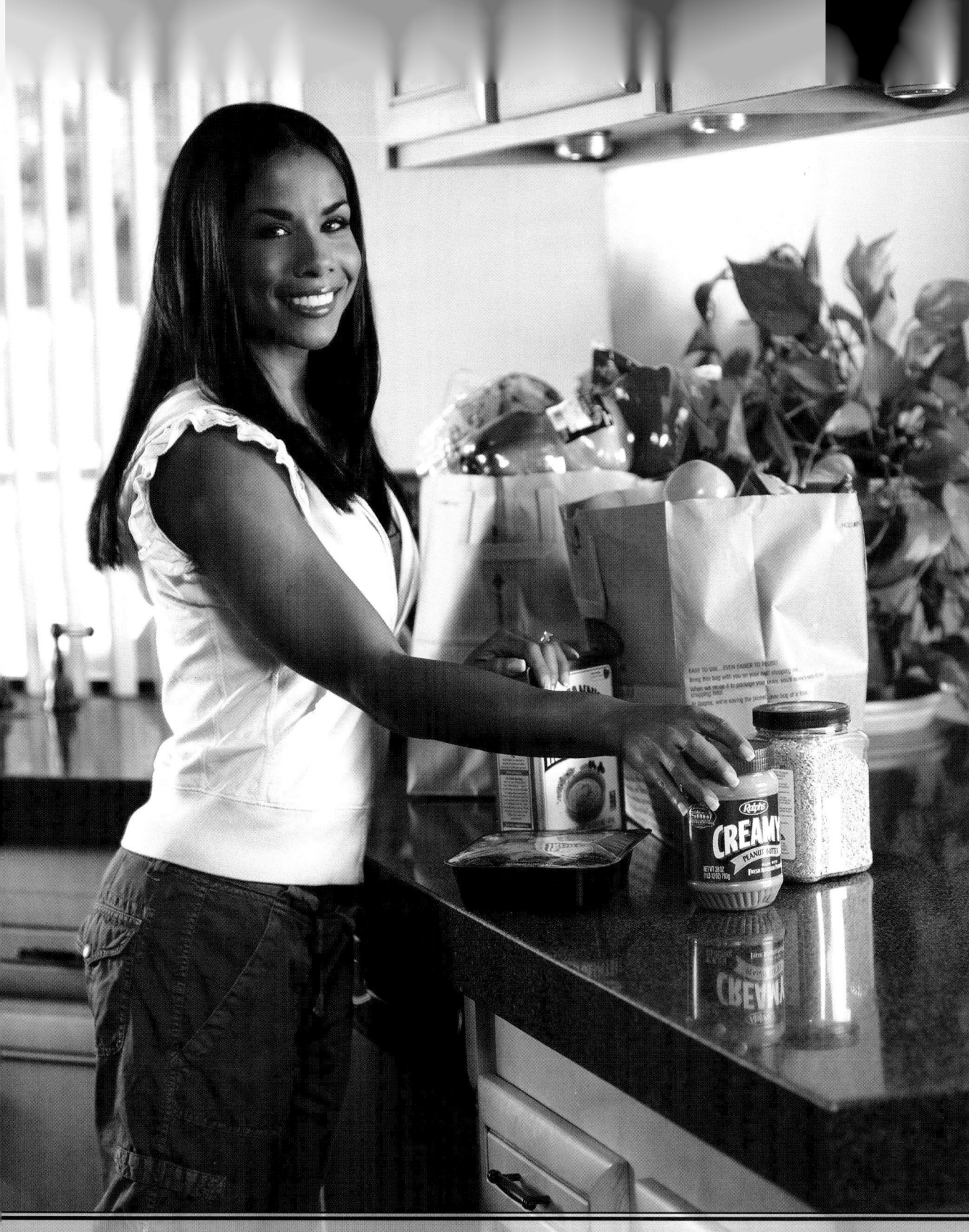

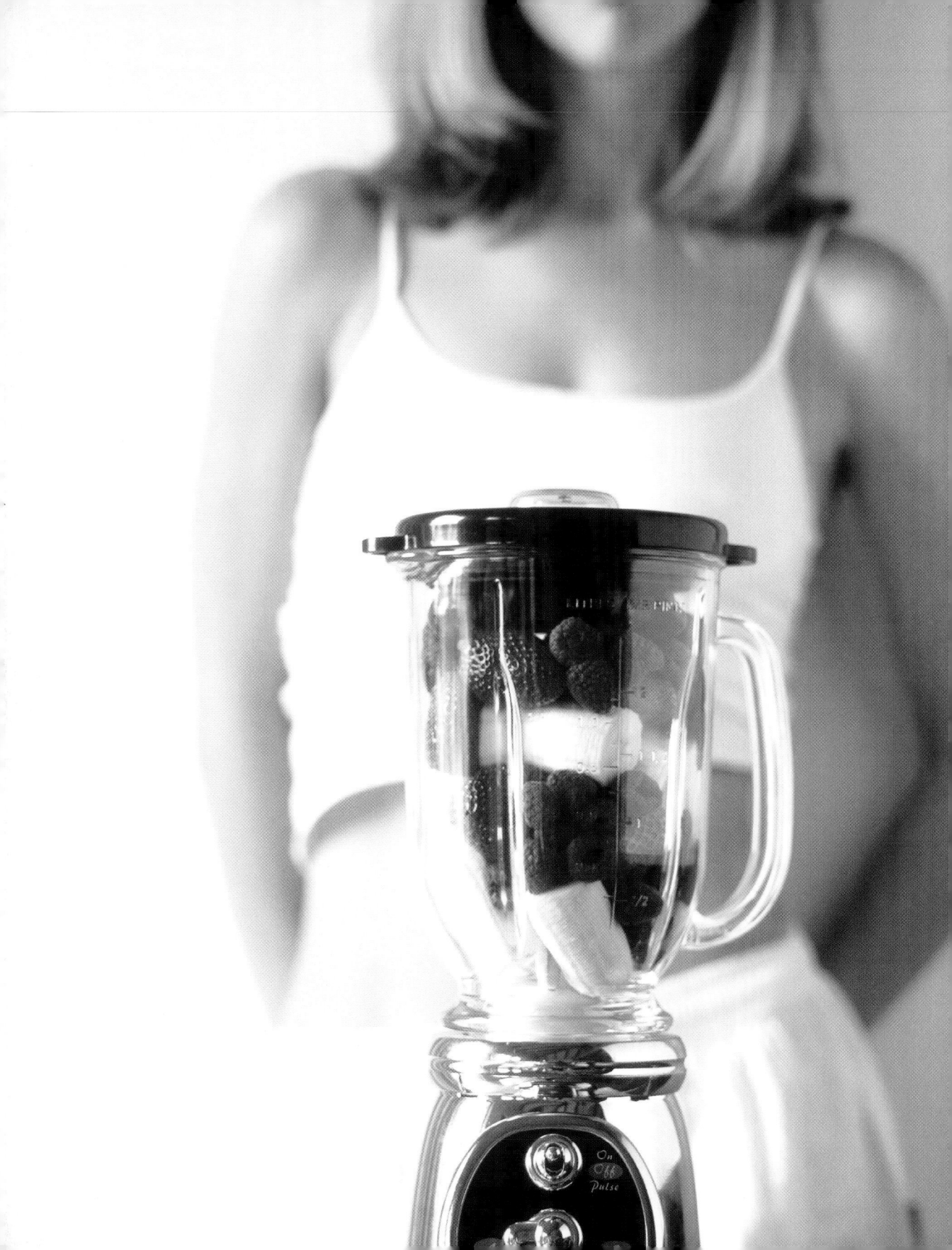

Chapter 10

Fill Your Tank

If you've ever thought that it was best to work out on an empty stomach, this is the chapter for you. The mistaken notion that exercising before breakfast (or any other major meal) will help you burn fat ends here. Food fuels your body so you can work out harder. Without it, you're signaling your body to hold on to the fat you're trying to burn since it thinks it is facing conditions of famine.

If you've ever left the gym feeling weak or felt fatigued during your workout, take a look at what you ate beforehand. Nutrition is the cornerstone of training success, and there's no more critical time than the hour or so prior. Research shows that having the right amount and types of protein and carbs before your workouts will not only help you go longer and be stronger, but will help you recover and prepare for your next session. Whether you're just hitting the weights, heading out for a run or pumping iron *and* the pedals, we give you the snacks to fuel your workout right.

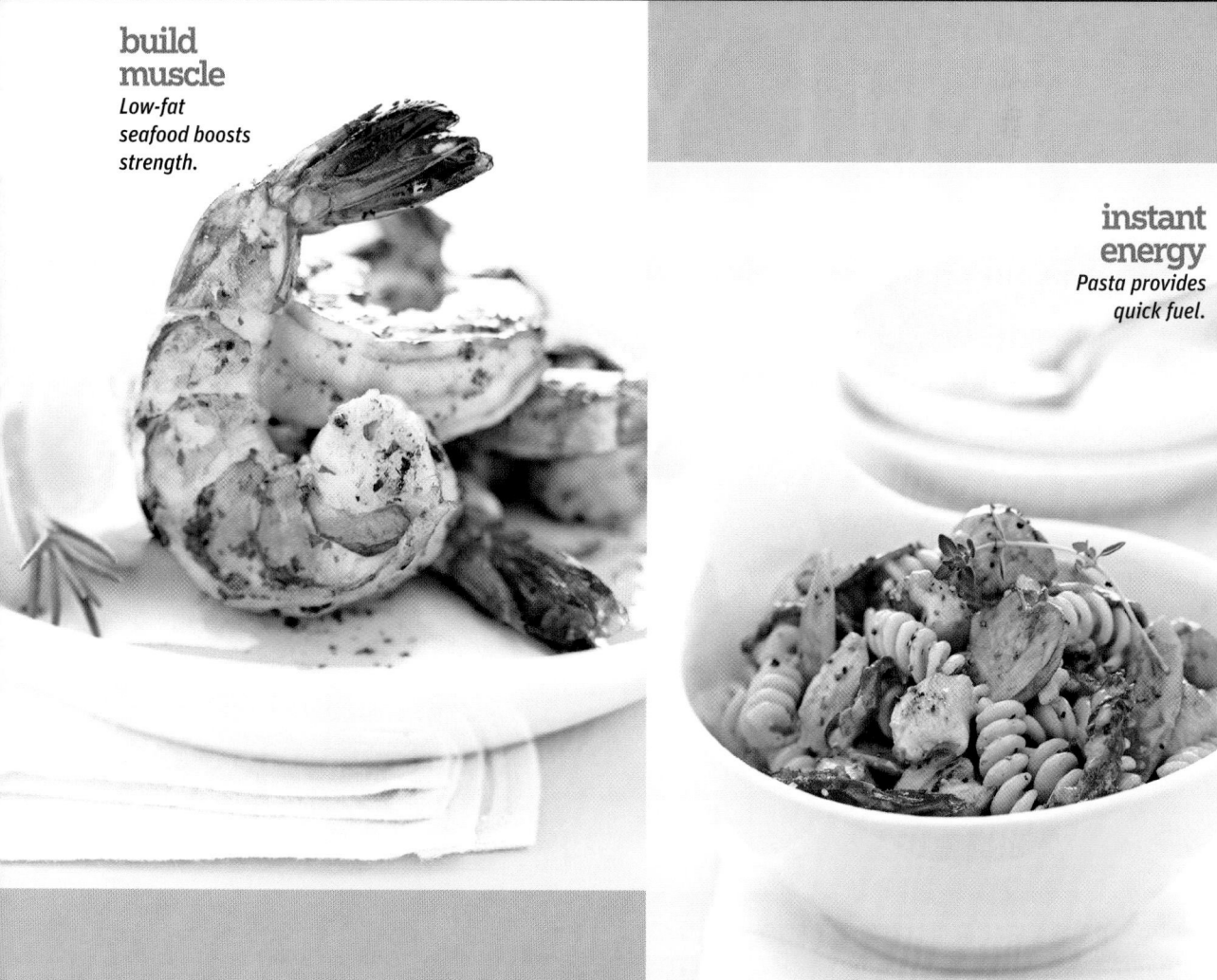

build muscle
Low-fat seafood boosts strength.

instant energy
Pasta provides quick fuel.

STRENGTH WORKOUT

To ensure that your body has enough fuel to optimally drive the muscle-building and recovery process, you need to take in the right kind of nutrients 60 minutes or so before you step into the gym. To prepare for your strength workout, ingest about 0.1 gram of protein per pound of bodyweight and 0.2 gram of carbs — so for a 130-pound woman, that equates to about 13 grams of protein and 26 grams of carbs. In general, 10–15 grams of protein and 25–30 grams of carbs should fit the bill for most women.

Choose moderate- to fast-digesting (read: low-fat) sources of protein, such as egg whites, low-fat fish, turkey breast, chicken breast, whey protein and soy protein. Carbs should be low-glycemic and slow-digesting to prevent insulin surges, which could limit fat-burning during the workout. Whole grains, fruit, brown rice and oatmeal are excellent choices.

STRONG SNACKS

Try one of these seven snacks an hour or so before you hit the weights.

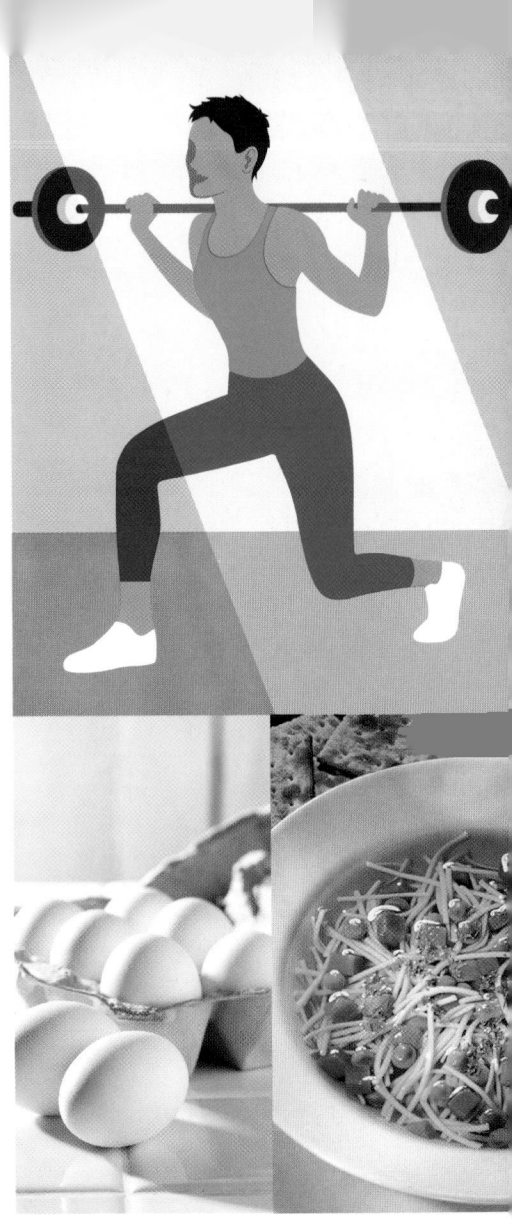

FOOD	PROTEIN (G)	CARBS (G)
1½ oz. canned tuna w/ 1 Tbsp. fat-free mayo on 9 whole-wheat crackers **#50**	14	28
2 large scrambled egg whites 1 cup cooked oatmeal **#51**	14	25
¾ scoop whey or soy protein blended in water w/ 1 medium banana **#52**	16	28
2 oz. deli chicken breast 2 slices whole-wheat bread **#53**	16	26
2 oz. boiled shrimp ½ cup cooked brown rice **#54**	14	24
2 cups chicken noodle soup 3 whole-wheat crackers **#55**	13	27
2 hard-boiled egg whites 1 whole-wheat English muffin **#56**	14	27

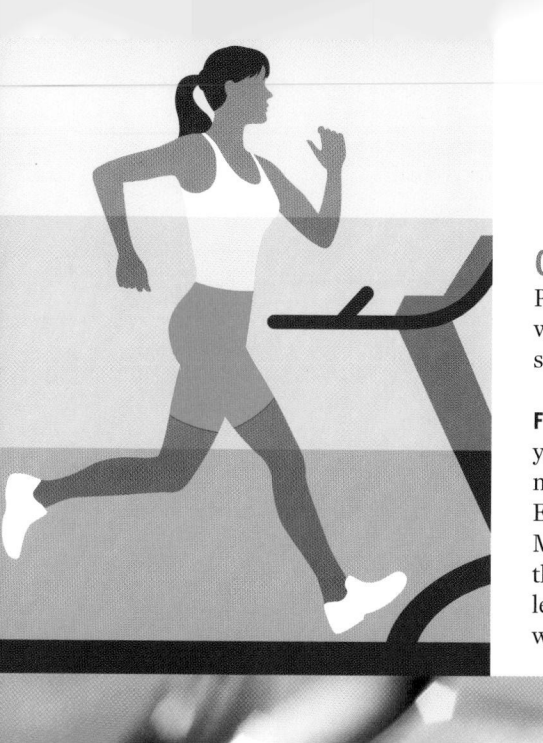

CARDIO WORKOUT

People do cardio for different reasons; some do it for health, others for weight control or weight loss. Why you do it will influence what you should eat before you train.

For performance. If you want to up the ante and go longer or faster in your chosen cardio discipline, then you need ample amounts of low- to moderate-glycemic carbs, such as raisins, popcorn and apple juice. Endurance athletes tend to concentrate on these types of carbs. Multiple scientific studies have concluded that adding some protein to the mix can help athletes trying to improve stamina. Endurance athletes should also ingest about 0.1 gram of protein per pound of bodyweight and increase their carb intake to about 0.4 gram per pound in their preworkout meal. That is 13 grams of protein and 52 grams of carbs for a 130-pound woman; getting 10–15 grams of moderate- to fast-digesting protein and 40–60 grams of carbs will do the trick for most. Protein choices should be those that digest quickly since the amino acids (the building blocks of protein) will be used by your muscles for fuel during the workout. Again, look to low-fat options for protein sources.

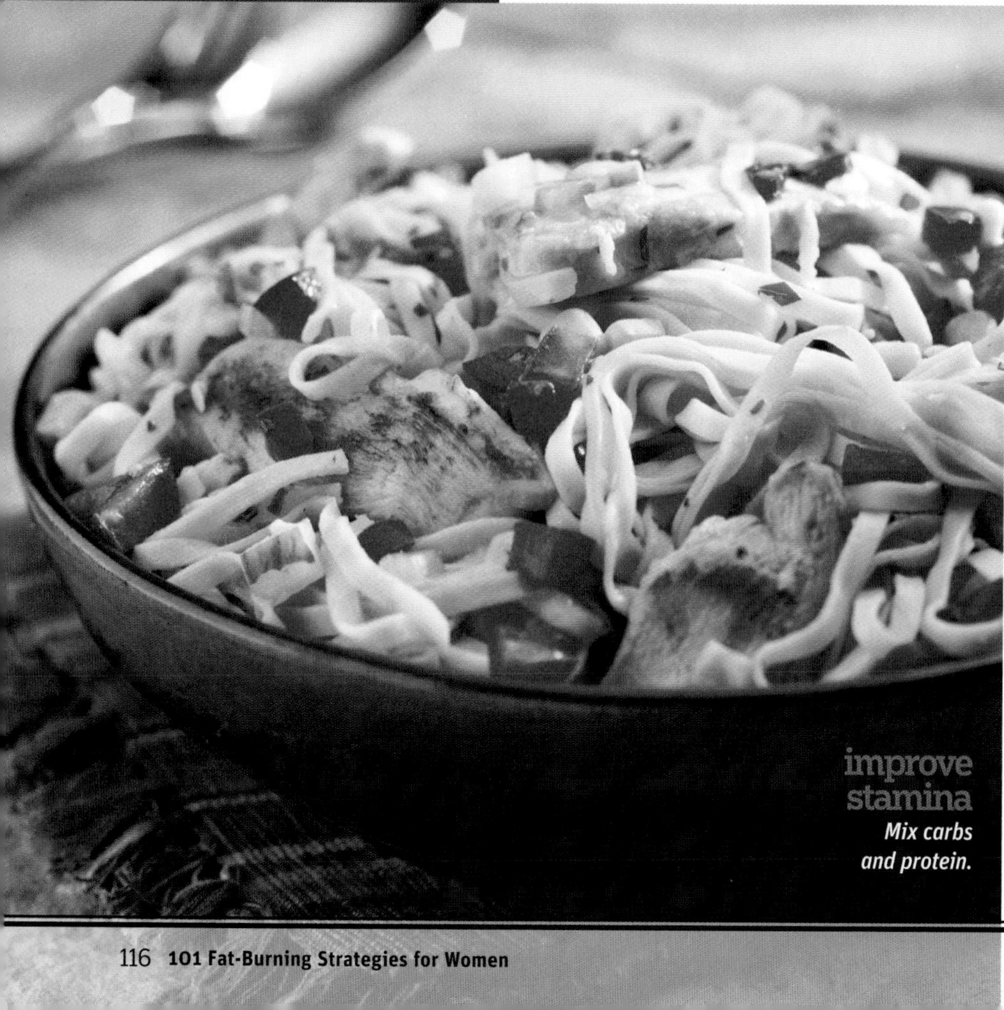

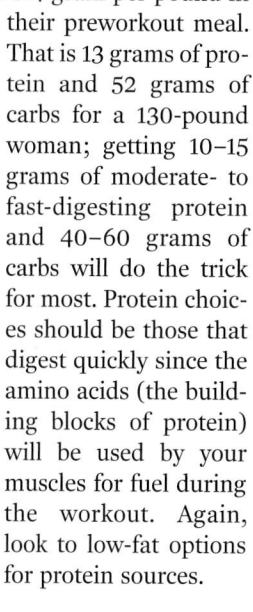

improve
stamina
*Mix carbs
and protein.*

LONG-LASTING SNACKS

An hour before your marathon cardio sessions, get adequately fueled with any of these snacks.

FOOD	PROTEIN (G)	CARBS (G)
1½ oz. canned tuna w/ 1 Tbsp. fat-free mayo on 4 slices pumpernickel bread **#57**	18	50
½ scoop whey protein blended in water w/ ⅔ cup blueberries 1 whole-wheat English muffin w/ 1 Tbsp. low-sugar preserves **#58**	17	50
2 oz. deli turkey breast 1 large whole-wheat pita 1 cup whole strawberries **#59**	17	48
2 oz. chopped chicken breast 1 cup cooked whole-wheat pasta w/ ½ cup marinara sauce **#60**	19	51

For fat-burning. If your main cardio goal is to burn fat — lots of it — then avoid carbs altogether. Multiple research studies show that when you don't eat carbs before aerobic exercise, more bodyfat is burned. But that doesn't mean you should run on an empty stomach. Japanese researchers reported in the journal *Perception and Motor Skills* that when athletes consume only amino acids before aerobic exercise, they burn even more fat than when they drink water alone. Reach for snacks that deliver about 5–10 grams of fast-digesting protein.

LEAN SNACKS

An hour before your get-lean cardio sessions, choose one of these.

FOOD	PROTEIN (G)	CARBS (G)
½ scoop whey protein blended in water **#61**	10	0
2 hard-boiled large egg whites **#62**	8	0
1½ oz. canned light tuna **#63**	10	0

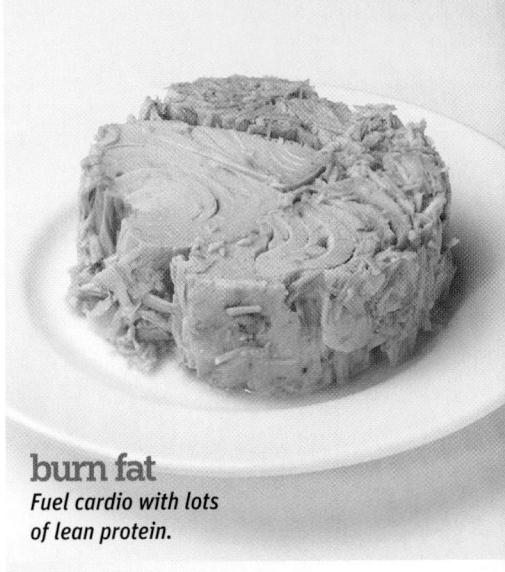

burn fat
Fuel cardio with lots of lean protein.

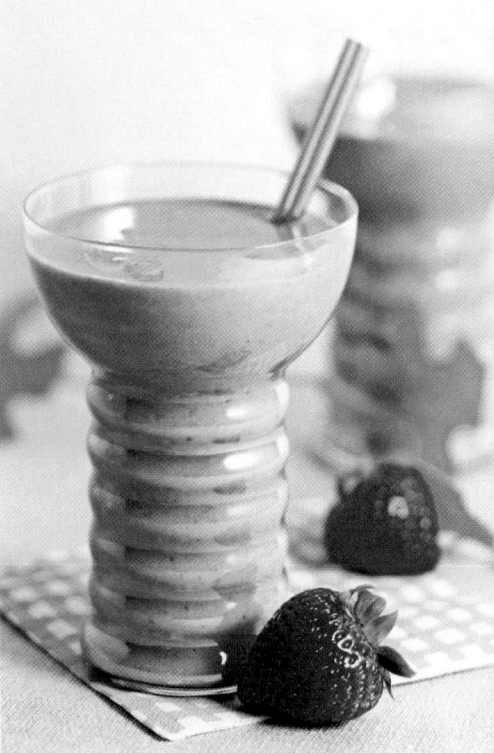

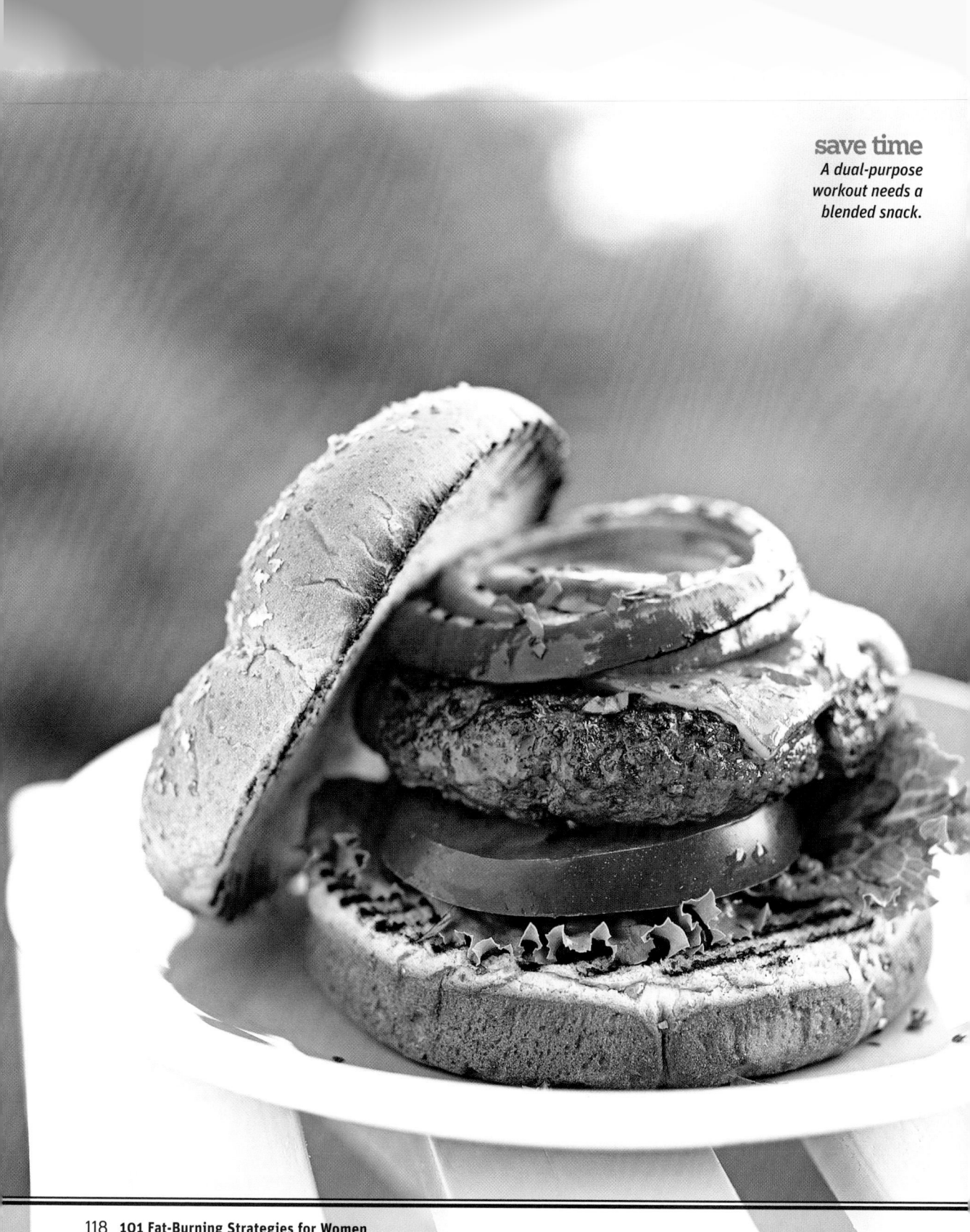

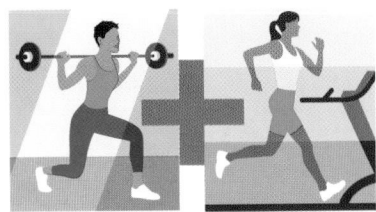

STRENGTH + CARDIO WORKOUT

If you're saving time by combining cardio and strength workouts, the nutritional makeup of your preworkout meal stays the same as when you just lift weights (0.1 gram of protein and 0.2 gram of carbs per pound of bodyweight), but the type of protein can vary. Since these dual-purpose workouts tend to last longer, you can reach for slower-digesting protein sources such as dairy, beef and even nuts, as you'll have more time before the amino acids are needed for fuel during the cardio and to support muscle recovery after the training session. Also choose slow-digesting carb sources, such as fibrous fruits and vegetables and whole grains.

DUAL SNACKS

If you're weight-training and doing cardio, munch on these an hour or so before your workout.

FOOD	PROTEIN (G)	CARBS (G)
8 oz. fat-free plain yogurt w/ 1 cup sliced strawberries #64	14	28
3 oz. 95% lean beef patty 1 whole-wheat hamburger bun 2 Tbsp. ketchup #65	20	30
2 whole large poached eggs 1 whole-wheat English muffin #66	18	28
½ cup fat-free cottage cheese mixed w/ 2 cups sliced pineapple #67	14	23
2 Tbsp. peanut butter 2 slices whole-wheat bread #68	14	32
1 cup skim milk ½ cup Special K cereal #69	12	23
¼ scoop whey or soy protein blended in 1 cup skim milk w/ ½ cup blueberries #70	14	24

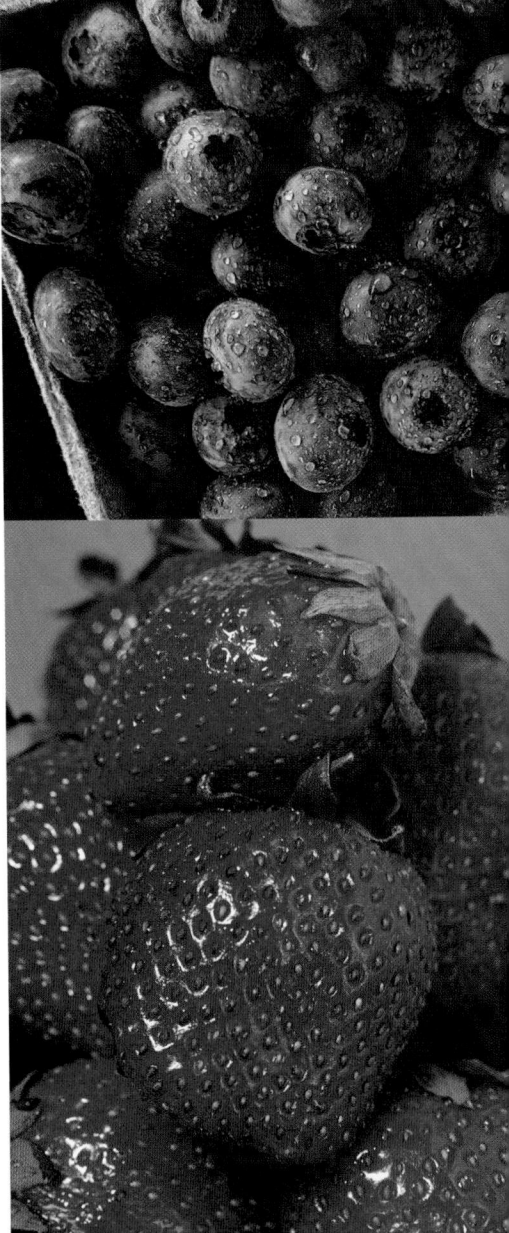

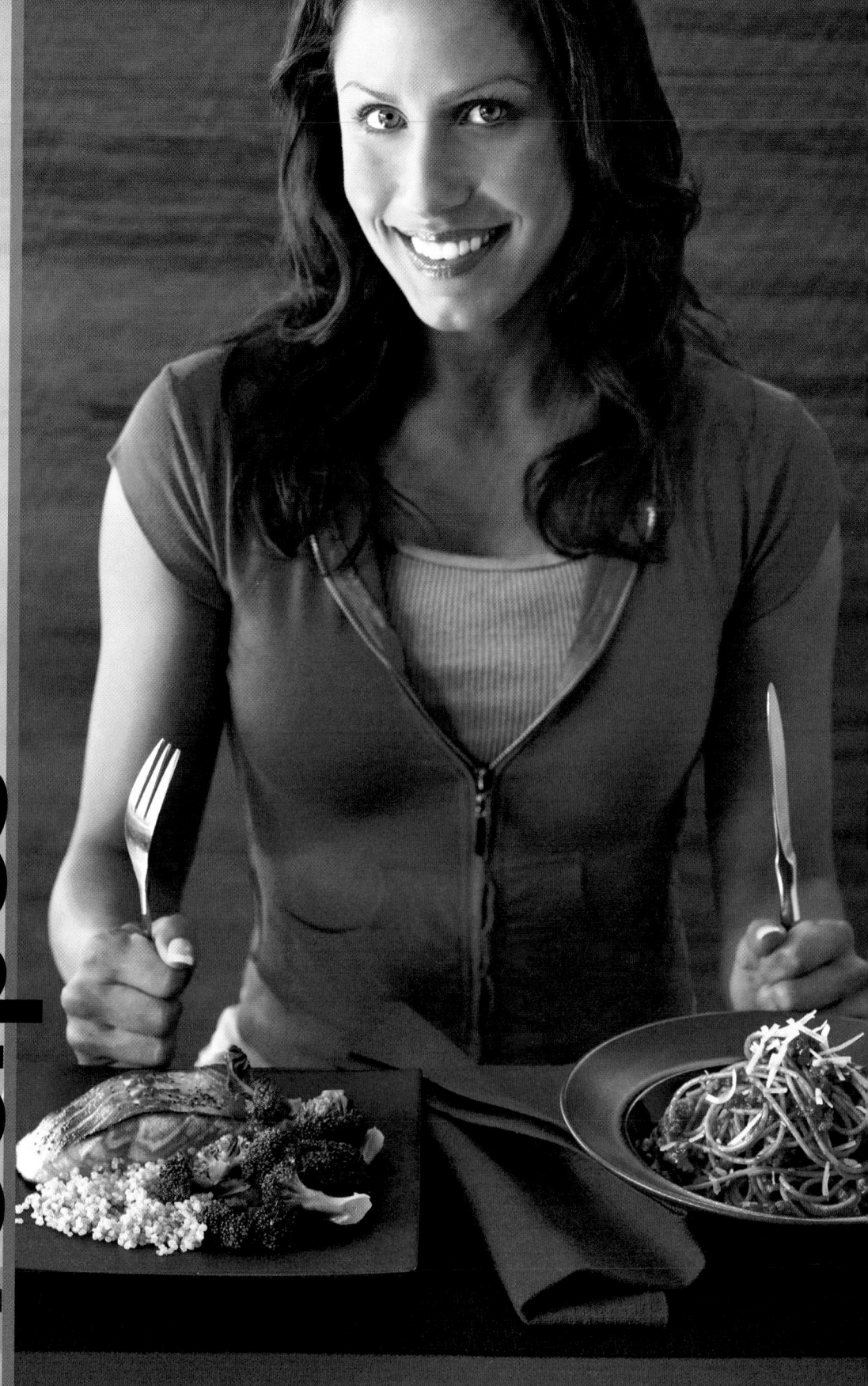

recipes

contents

One cannot get a lean physique by eating chicken breast alone. Although this section does have a few recipes for fitness' favorite feast, it also has a slew of other great-tasting, easy-to-make recipes that will help you in a snap. You can no longer complain that you don't know what to eat to achieve what you want — your best body yet.

 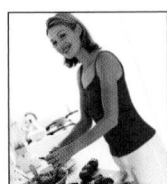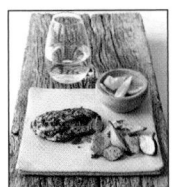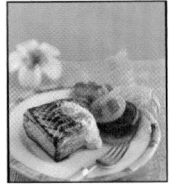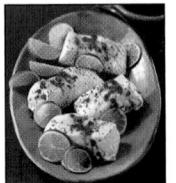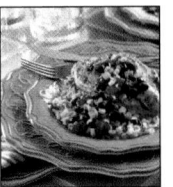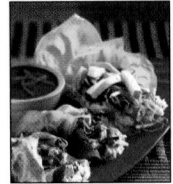

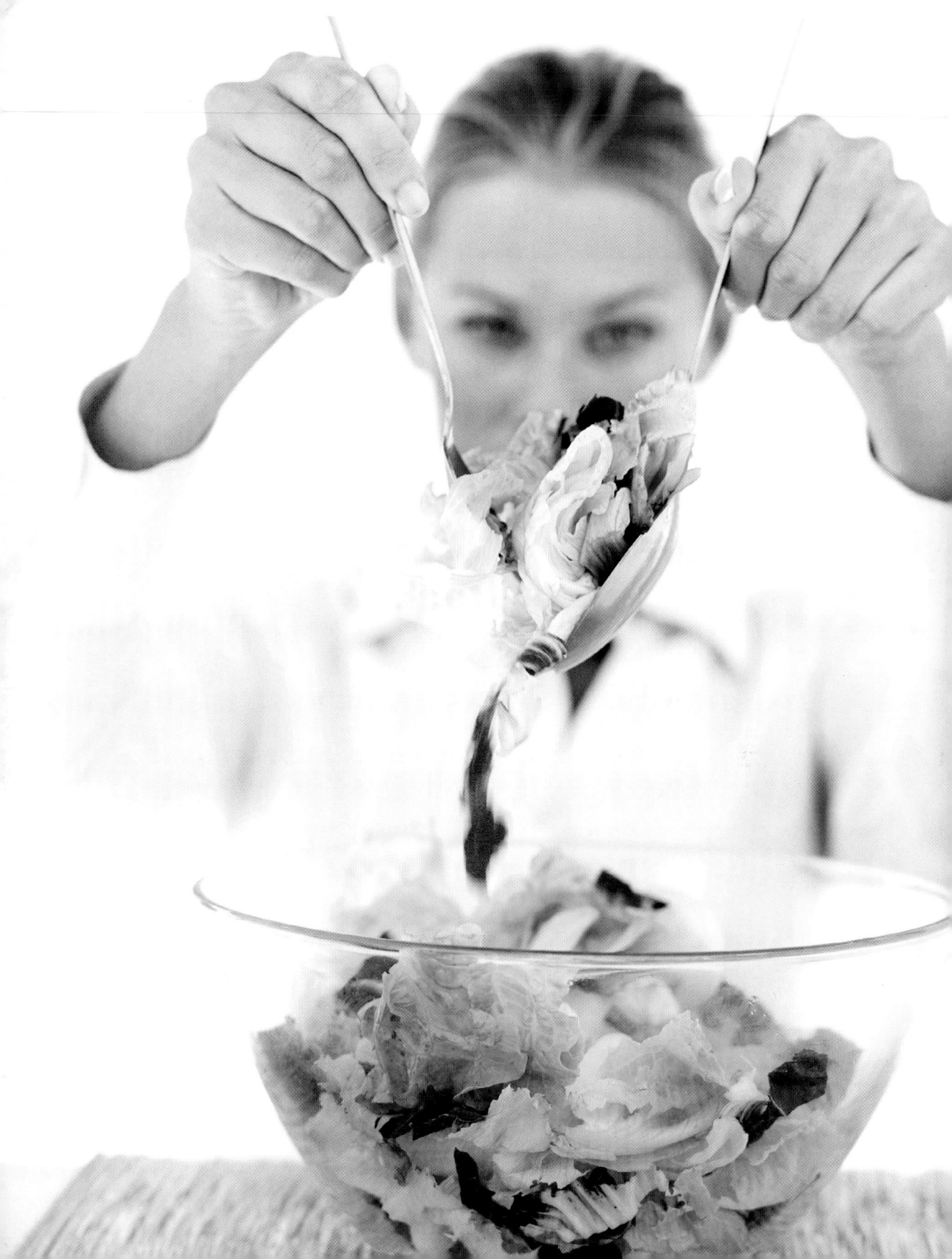

Chapter 11

Green Party

Cast a vote for great nutrition with these five-ingredient salads, all of which are all under 425 calories. Each one is the perfect blend of protein, carbohydrates and fat that will help you reach your goal of building a leaner body without leaving you feeling as though you're starving yourself.

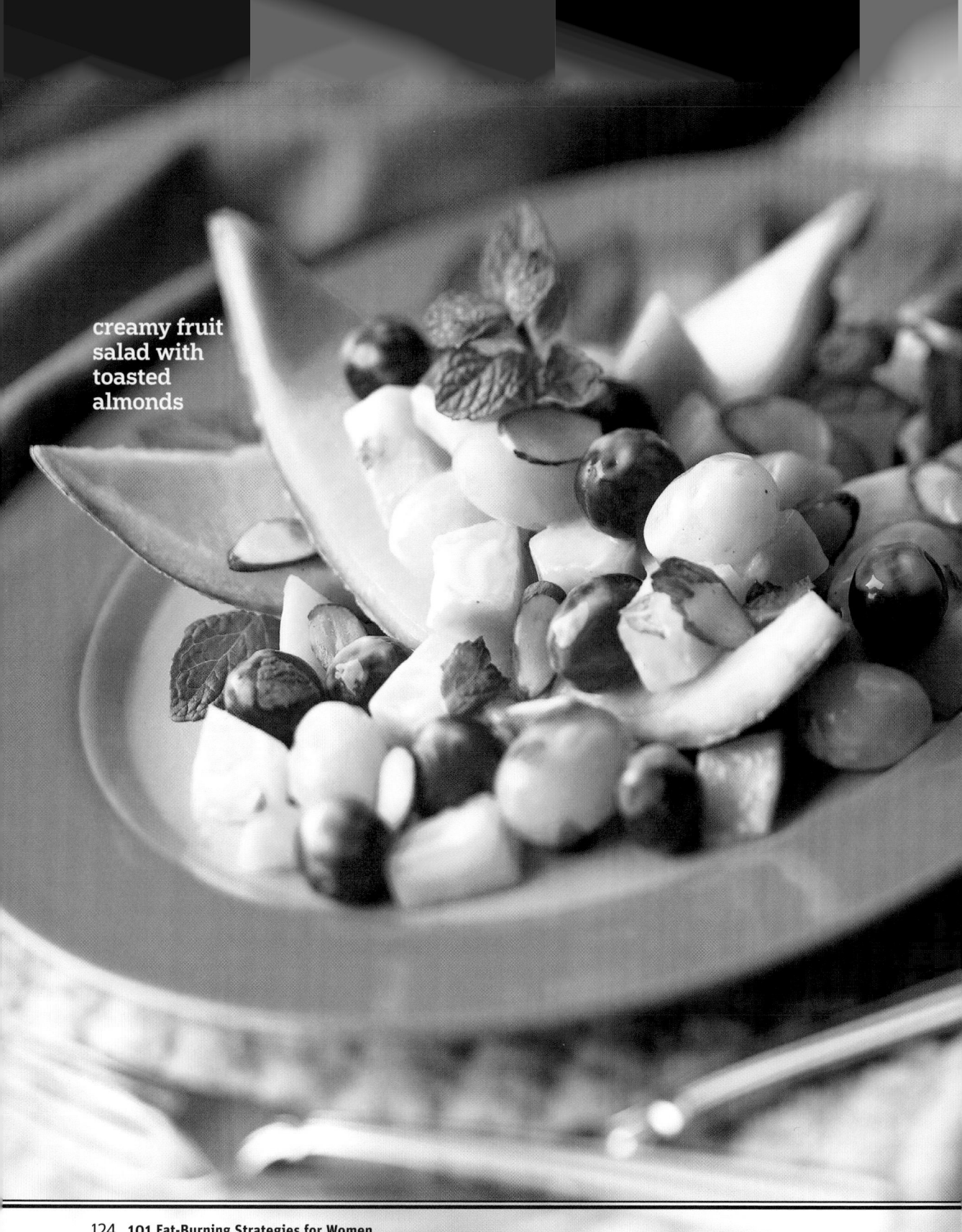

creamy fruit salad with toasted almonds

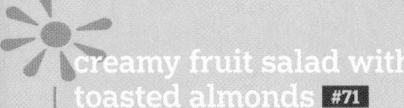

creamy fruit salad with toasted almonds #71

Prep time: 5 minutes
Cooking time: 2-3 minutes

Almonds are a great source of heart-healthy monounsaturated fat, as well as calcium, vitamin E, iron and protein; grapes are jam-packed with flavonoids — unusually potent antioxidants; cantaloupe is an excellent source of vitamins A and C; and yogurt is rich in bone-building calcium.

2 Tbsp. sliced almonds
½ cup each seedless green and red grapes
½ cup cubed cantaloupe melon
½ cup nonfat vanilla yogurt
1 Tbsp. chopped fresh mint

Place almonds in a small skillet and set pan over medium heat. Cook 2-3 minutes, until golden brown, shaking the pan frequently. Remove from heat. In a medium bowl, combine grapes, melon, yogurt and mint. Toss to combine. Top with toasted almonds. **Serves 1**
NUTRITION FACTS (per serving): *297 calories, 10 g protein, 44 g carbohydrates, 9 g fat, 4 g fiber*

*These **5-ingredient salads** are not only nutritious — they're hearty and quick*

japanese noodles with peas and soy nuts #72

Prep time: 5 minutes
Cooking time: 10-12 minutes

Buckwheat noodles are loaded with intestine-friendly insoluble fiber; green peas are a good source of the B vitamin thiamin; and soy nuts are rich in isoflavones — phytoestrogens that maintain strong bones.

2 oz. uncooked soba (Japanese buckwheat) noodles, or whole-wheat spaghetti
2 Tbsp. black bean sauce
¼ cup frozen green peas, thawed
1 scallion, chopped
¼ cup roasted soy nuts

Cook noodles according to package directions, without added fat or salt. Drain and transfer to a medium bowl. Add black bean sauce and toss to coat. Add peas and scallion and toss to combine. Top with soy nuts. **Serves 1**
NUTRITION FACTS (per serving): *401 calories, 19 g protein, 61 g carbohydrates, 9 g fat, 6 g fiber*

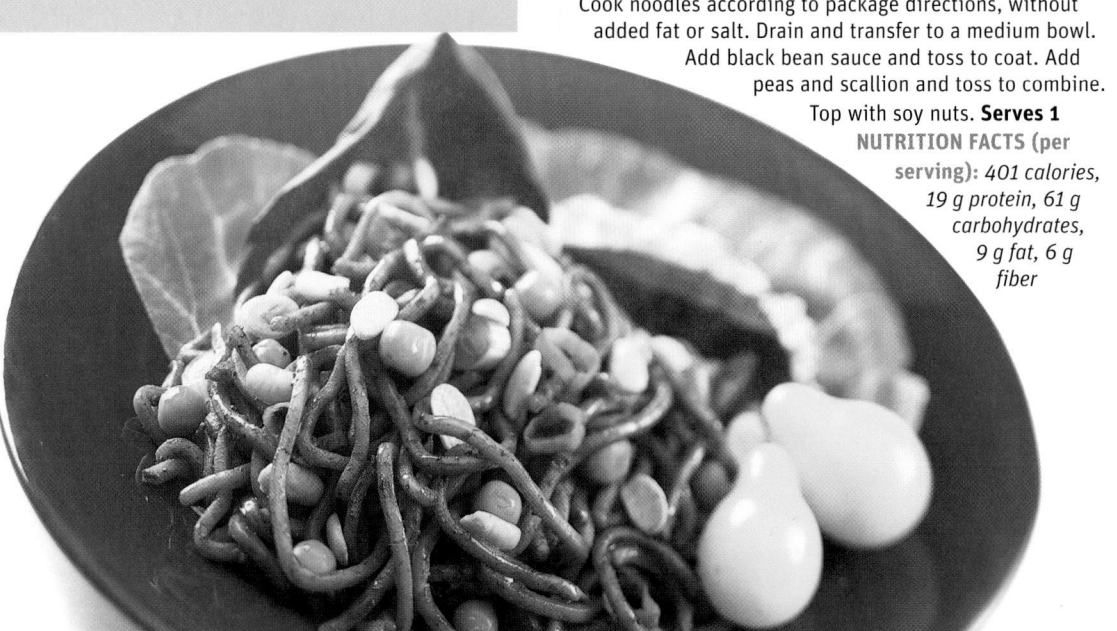

asian slaw with roast beef and swiss #73

Prep time: 5 minutes

Cabbage is rich in indoles, compounds that reduce breast cancer risk; roast beef is an excellent source of iron and high-quality protein; and Swiss cheese is packed with calcium, an important mineral that influences weight loss. Alternate serving suggestion: Roll cheese inside roast beef slices and place atop Asian slaw.

2 cups cole slaw mix (shredded cabbage and carrots)
1/3 cup fat-free Thousand Island dressing
1 tsp. sesame oil
3 oz. lean roast beef, sliced into thin strips
2 oz. reduced-fat Swiss cheese, shredded or sliced
  into thin strips

Combine cole slaw mix, dressing and sesame oil in a medium bowl. Mix well. Transfer mixture to a serving plate and top with roast beef and Swiss. **Serves 1**
NUTRITION FACTS (per serving): *350 calories, 37 g protein, 28 g carbohydrates, 10 g fat, 3 g fiber*

mexican rice and beans with smoked turkey #74

Prep and standing time: 10 minutes
Cooking time: 3 minutes

Brown rice is loaded with B vitamins; turkey is an excellent source of high-quality, low-fat protein; beans dish up lots of cholesterol-lowering fiber and tomatoes are packed with vitamin C — important to aid recovery from exercise.

1/2 cup instant brown rice, uncooked
1 tsp. chili powder
3 oz. smoked, cooked turkey breast, diced
1/2 cup canned black beans, rinsed and drained
1/2 cup diced tomato
Salt and ground black pepper

Combine rice, chili powder and 1/2 cup of water in a microwave safe bowl. Cover and microwave on high 3 minutes. Let stand 5 minutes covered, then fluff with fork. Add remaining ingredients and toss to combine. Season to taste with salt and ground pepper.
Serves 1
NUTRITION FACTS (per serving): *387 calories, 30 g protein, 60 g carbohydrates, 3 g fat, 11 g fiber*

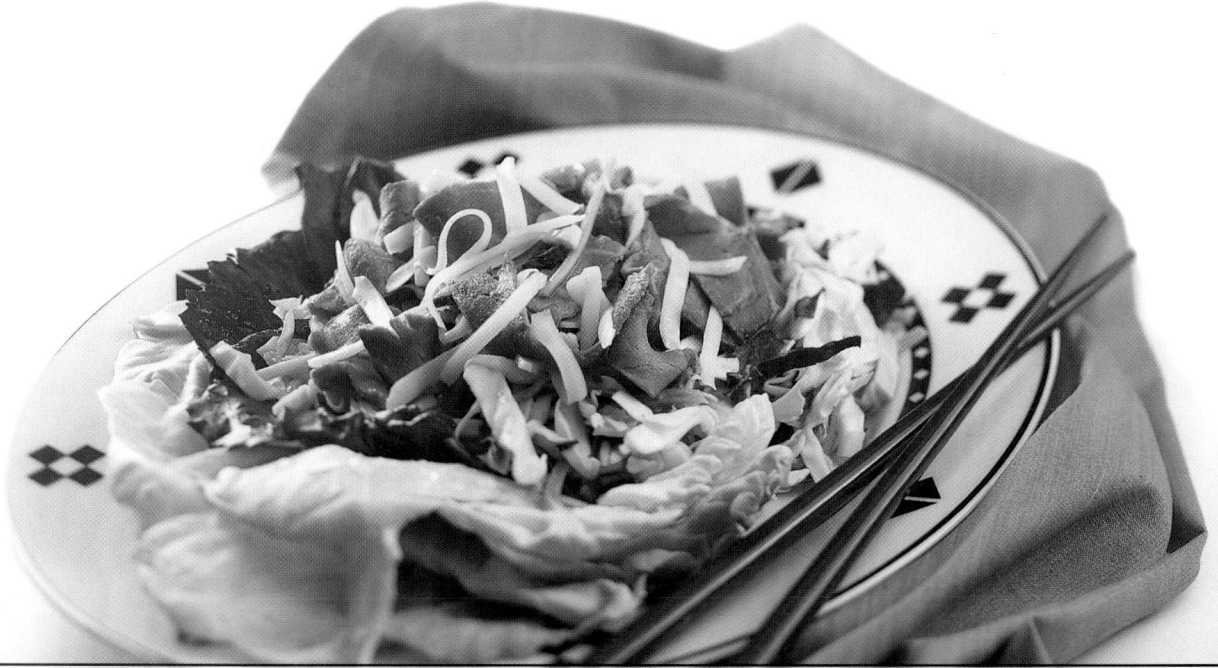

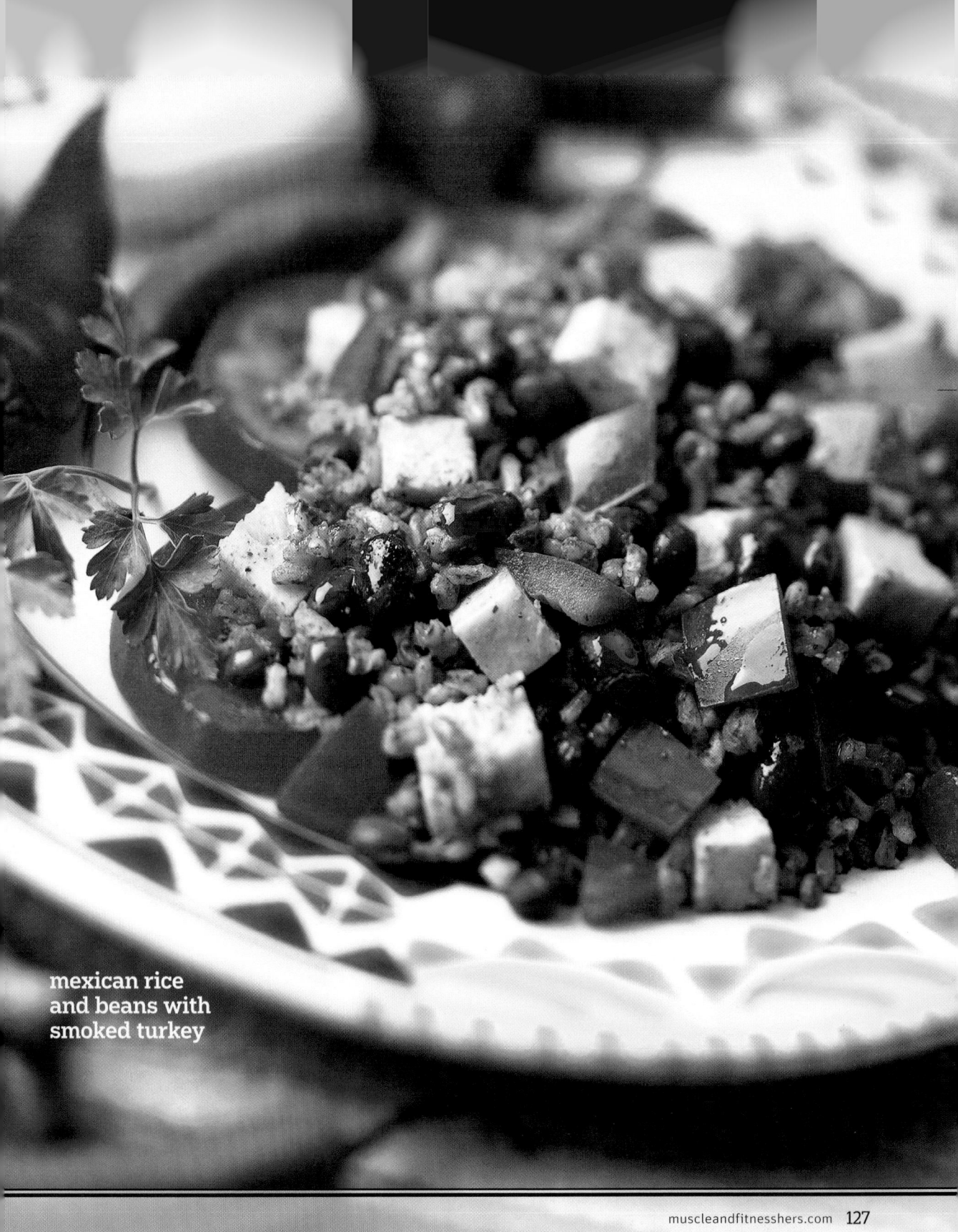

mexican rice
and beans with
smoked turkey

tomato-sourdough salad with mozzarella and basil #75

Prep and standing time: 10 minutes
Cooking time: 10 minutes

Tomatoes are packed with immune-boosting vitamin C; sourdough bread contains complex carbohydrates, which take longer to break down than simple ones and provide a long-lasting fuel source; and mozzarella cheese is rich in weight-loss-inducing calcium.

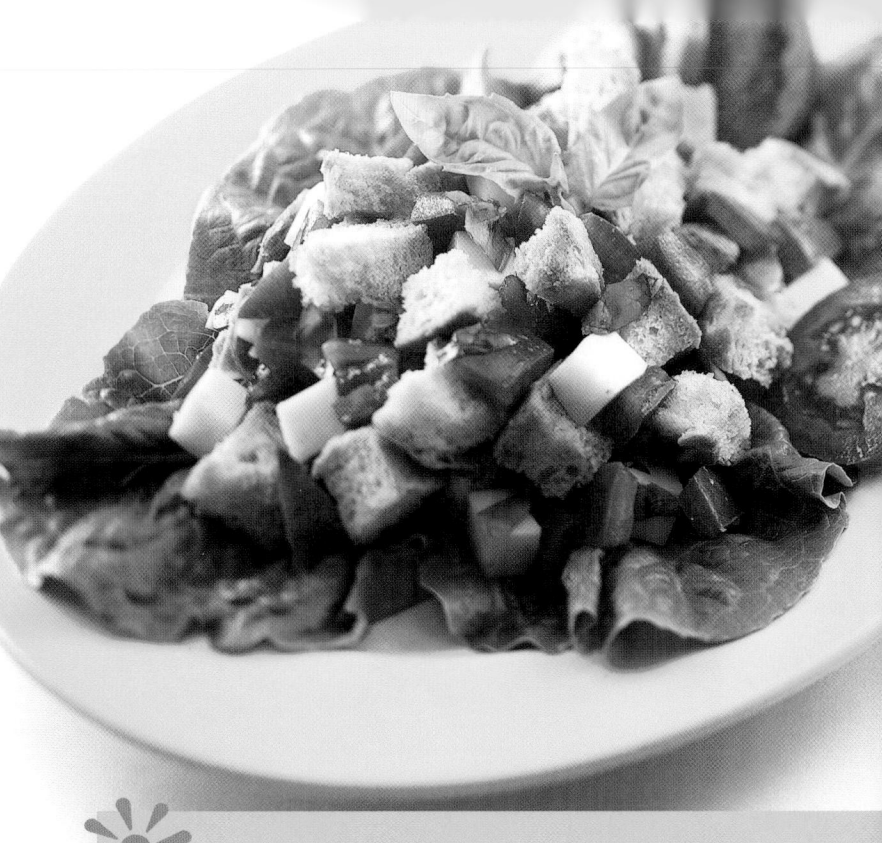

3 cups cubed sourdough bread
1 cup diced tomato
2 oz. fat-free mozzarella cheese, cut into small cubes
3 Tbsp. chopped fresh basil
2 Tbsp. balsamic vinegar
Salt and ground black pepper

Preheat over 400 degrees F. Arrange bread cubes on a baking sheet and bake 10 minutes until golden. Transfer bread to a large bowl and pour over enough water to cover. Let stand 5 minutes. Meanwhile, in a medium bowl, combine tomato, mozzarella, basil and balsamic vinegar. Toss to combine. Drain bread and squeeze bread cubes to remove excess water. Add bread to tomato mixture and toss to combine. Season to taste with salt and pepper. **Serves 1**

NUTRITION FACTS (per serving):
388 calories, 25 g protein, 63 g carbohydrates, 4 g fat, 5 g fiber

taboule with salmon and feta #76

Prep and standing time: 25 minutes
Cooking time: 2 minutes

Bulgur wheat is packed with energizing B vitamins and fiber, white beans are loaded with fiber and folate, and salmon is crammed with heart-healthy omega-3 fatty acids and calcium (especially if the salmon is canned).

½ cup Taboule Wheat Salad mix (Near East brand)
½ cup canned white beans, rinsed and drained
3 oz. canned salmon
1 Tbsp. crumbled feta cheese
1 Tbsp. fresh lemon juice
Salt and ground black pepper

Combine Taboule Wheat Salad mix, half of the seasoning packet, beans and ¾ cup of water in a microwave-safe bowl. Cover with plastic and microwave on high 2 minutes. Let stand for 20 minutes, until liquid is absorbed. Fluff with a fork. Add remaining ingredients and toss to combine. Season to taste with salt and black pepper.
Serves 1

NUTRITION FACTS (per serving): *365 calories, 31 g protein, 40 g carbohydrates, 9 g fat, 9 g fiber*

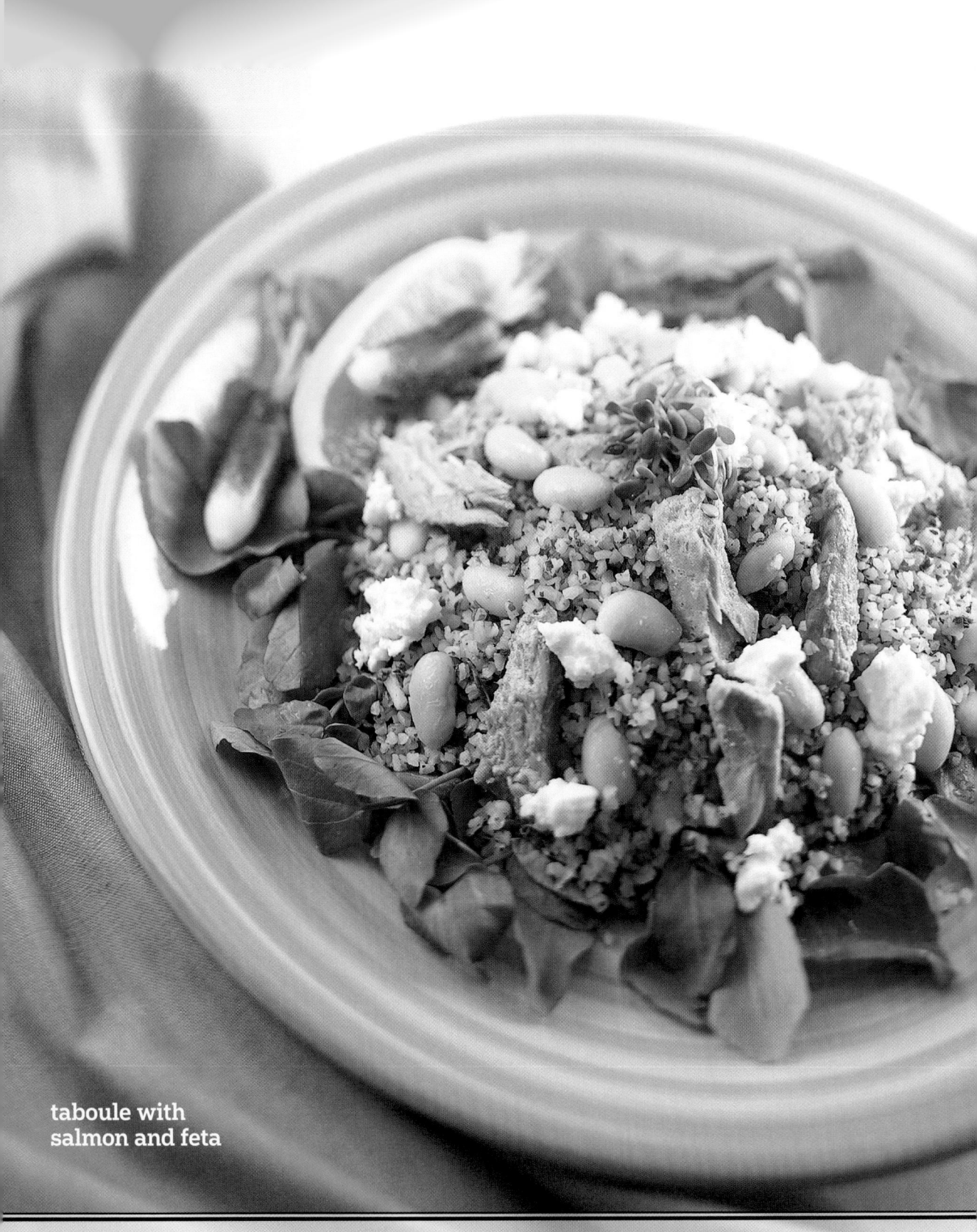

taboule with salmon and feta

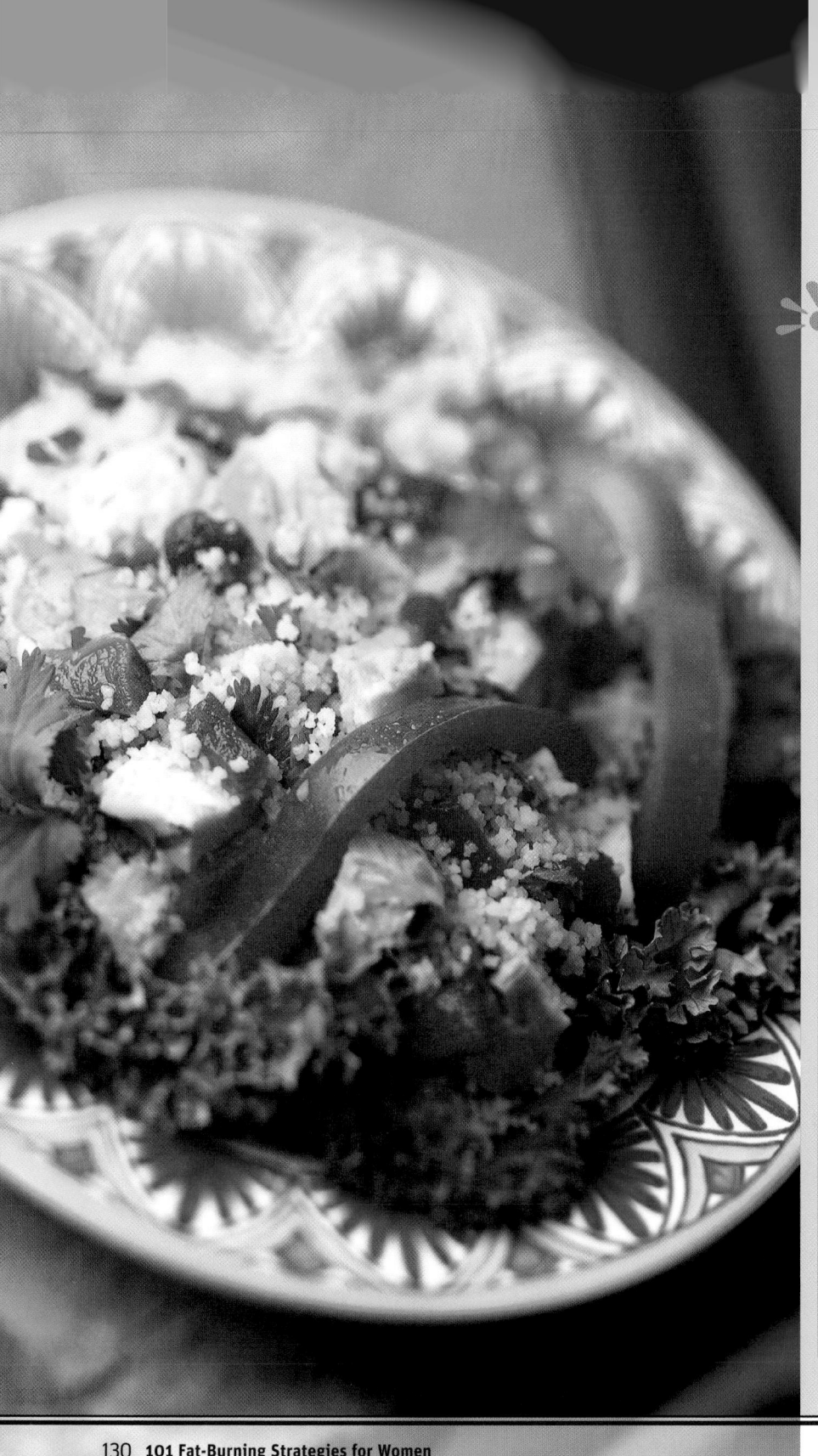

adobo couscous with chicken and roasted peppers #77

Prep and standing time: 10 minutes
Cooking time: 2 minutes

Whole-wheat couscous is a good source of B vitamins; skinless chicken breast dishes up plenty of low-fat protein; and red peppers are packed with vitamin C and beta-carotene.

¼ cup uncooked whole-wheat couscous
2 tsp. adobo seasoning with cumin (or if not available, ½ tsp. cumin)
1 cup cubed, cooked chicken breast
¼ cup diced roasted red peppers (from water-packed jar)
2 Tbsp. chopped fresh cilantro
Salt and ground black pepper

Combine couscous, adobo seasoning and ⅓ cup plus 2 Tbsp. water in a microwave-safe bowl. Cover and microwave on high 2 minutes. Let stand 5 minutes covered, then fluff with a fork. Add chicken, red peppers and cilantro. Toss to combine. Season to taste with salt and pepper.

Serves 1

NUTRITION FACTS (per serving): *373 calories, 35 g protein, 47 g carbohydrates, 5 g fat, 9 g fiber*

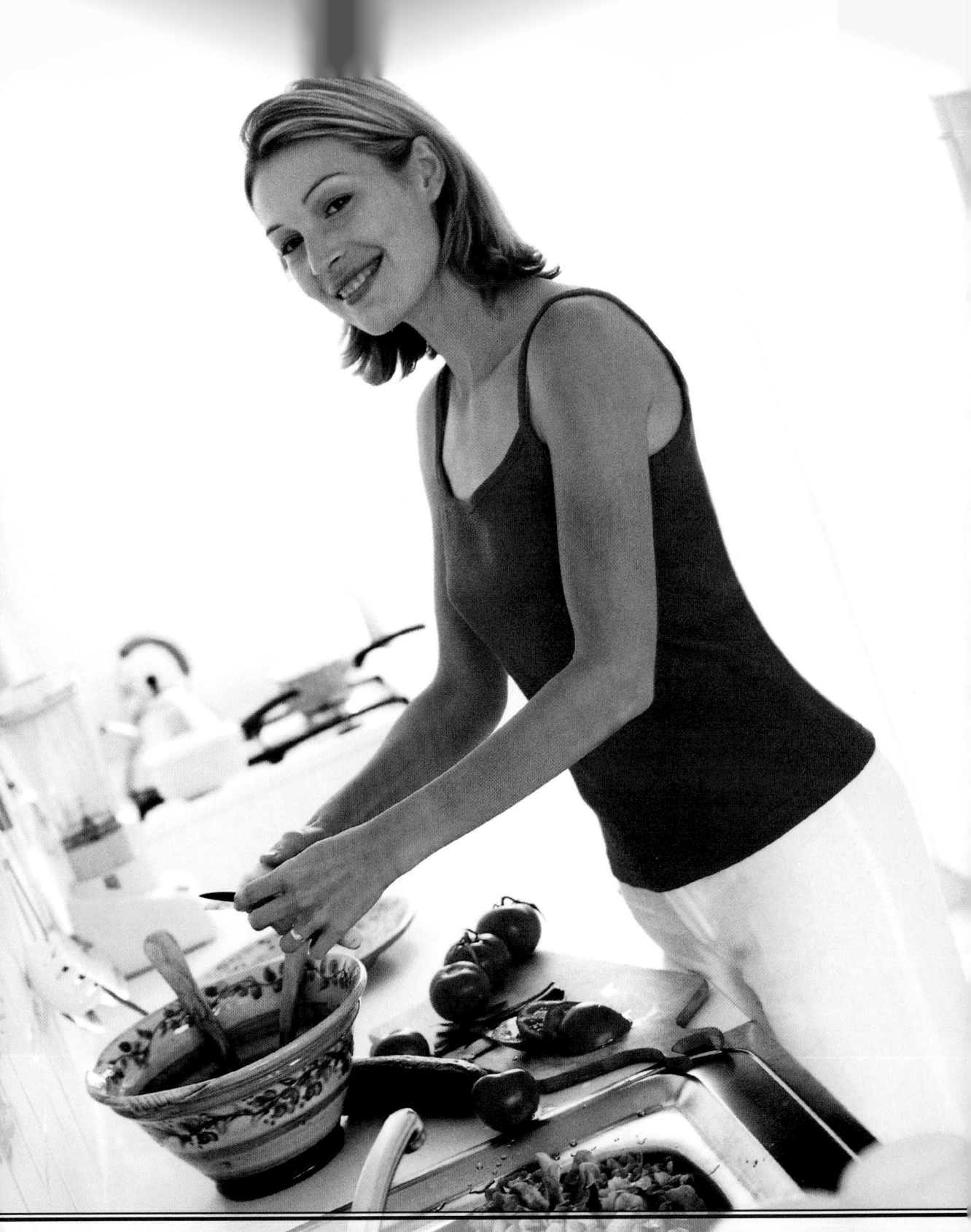

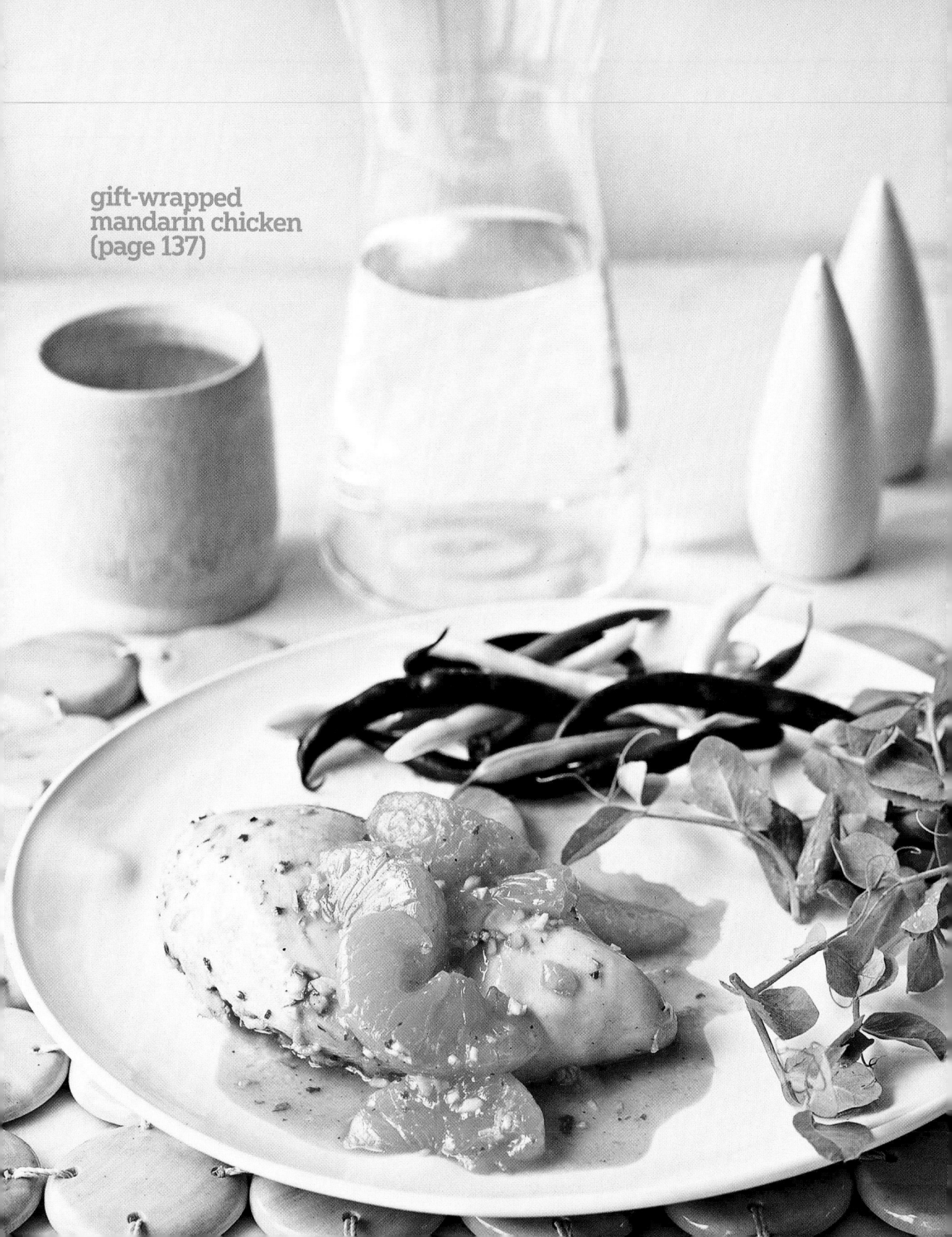

gift-wrapped
mandarin chicken
(page 137)

Chapter 12

Kickin' Chicken

When it comes to lean protein, chicken breast is king. Talk about a low-fat source that won't make you bloat, but *will* fuel your muscles without adding fat to your physique! On the next few pages, you'll not only find delicious recipes, but you'll also learn how to buy and cook the best breast. The result: You can make chicken for dinner night after night, each entrée with its unique taste. Here's how to enjoy a lean staple.

Here's a thought: Next time you make chicken for dinner (and you know it's going to be soon), try something different. We've got pro techniques to make your low-fat, high-protein chicken breasts juicy and flavorful. Behold chicken demystified.

#78
prep step 1:
SMART SHOPPING

Chicken can be purchased frozen, found in bags in the freezer section or fresh (often previously frozen) from the butcher or meat counter. Boneless, skinless breasts, though a bit more expensive, are worth it for their ease of preparation. If you purchase chicken breasts from the freezer, be sure to look at the nutrition label — some frozen varieties are pumped with added fats before they're frozen. A 4-ounce raw, boneless, skinless chicken breast should have only about 1.5 grams of fat.

If you're trying to save money, it's often more economical to buy breasts with the bone and skin. You can easily pull the breast from the skin and bone before cooking it.

#79
prep step 2:
DEFROSTING

If you have chicken breasts in the freezer, remove the amount you need the night before you plan to cook them. Place them in a dish, cover with plastic wrap and let them thaw overnight in the refrigerator. Important safety tip: Make sure juices won't leak out onto other foods as the chicken defrosts.

If you need to defrost quickly, soak the chicken in a bowl of cold water or under cold running water until it's thoroughly defrosted. Make sure the water is cold; if you soak frozen chicken in hot or warm water, the heat will start to cook the chicken ever so slightly. Drain the breasts or pat them with paper towels to remove excess moisture before you cook them.

#80
prep step 3:
READY TO GO

Fresh or defrosted boneless, skinless breasts require little attention. Using a sharp knife (a boning knife is ideal), cut any visible fat from the breasts. At the thicker end of the breast, on the underside, you may notice a shiny, white formation of threads; cut this section out.

Place the trimmed breast flat on a cutting board with the smooth side up. Using the flat side of a meat mallet or the bottom of a heavy skillet, pound the breast so that the thickest portion becomes as thin as the thinnest portion. The meat will cook evenly for a juicier result. Now your chicken is ready for seasoning. Prepare it according to one of the following cooking techniques.

Note: Nutrition calculations for these recipes are based on consuming all the marinade; if you leave some behind, you'll get slightly fewer calories.

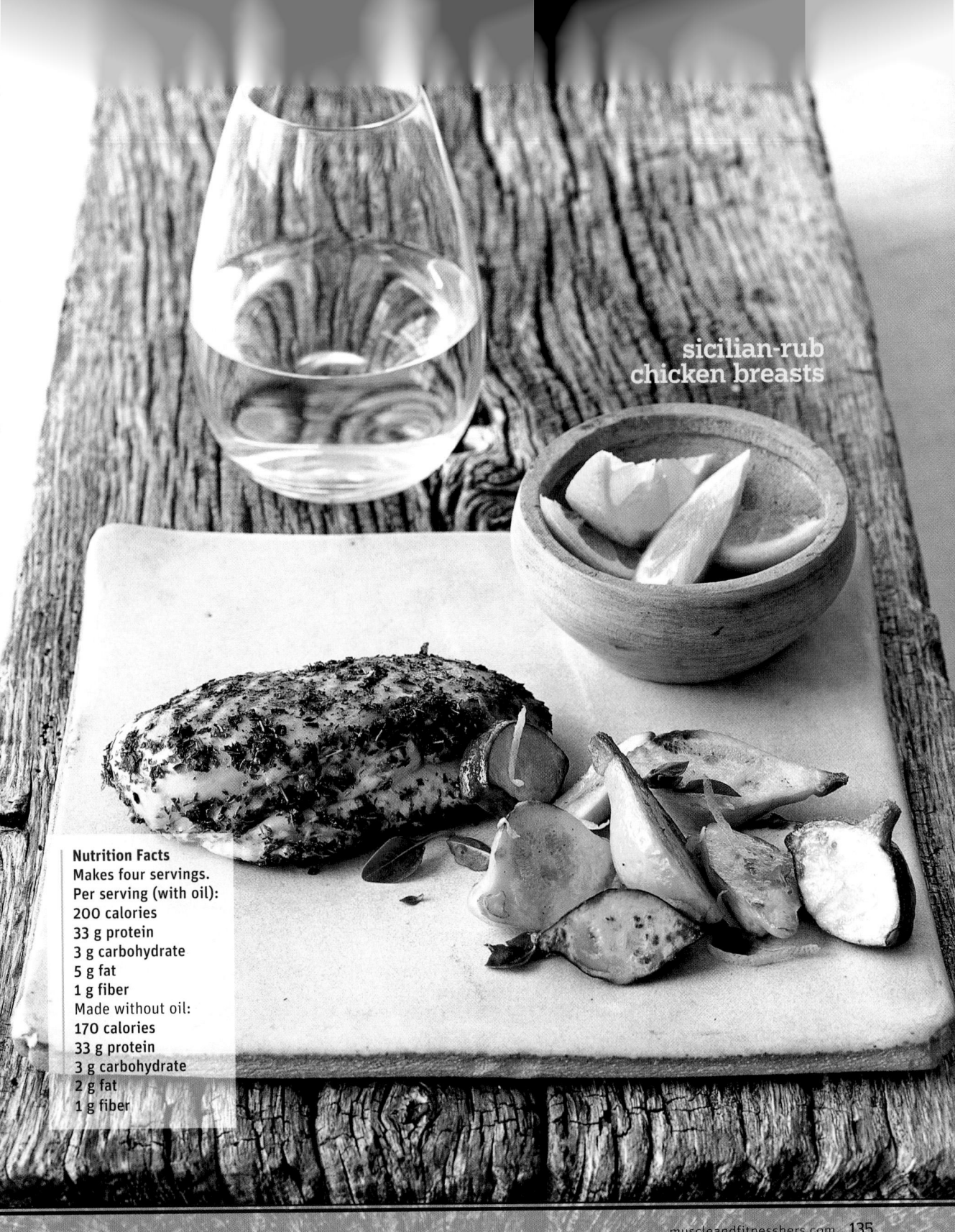

sicilian-rub
chicken breasts

Nutrition Facts
Makes four servings.
Per serving (with oil):
200 calories
33 g protein
3 g carbohydrate
5 g fat
1 g fiber
Made without oil:
170 calories
33 g protein
3 g carbohydrate
2 g fat
1 g fiber

Simple Cooking Technique
No. 1: Grilling

If good health is on your agenda, you definitely can't go wrong by investing in a grill. A gas or charcoal grill adds flavor to your meats and veggies, but an indoor grill is a viable alternative when year-round grilling isn't an option.

Grills allow you to easily cook chicken at a high temperature, sealing in juices that keep it tender without adding much fat. A grill is great if you're in a hurry, and it's versatile enough to use with rubs and marinades.

To Cook: Turn on your grill to the highest heat setting. When hot (chicken should sizzle when placed on it), add rubbed or marinated chicken and turn heat to low. Cook for about five minutes — on a good nonstick grill, the chicken should no longer stick when it's ready to be flipped — then turn and cook another five minutes, until no longer pink inside or a meat thermometer inserted in the center reads 170 degrees F. Don't overcook breast or it'll become tough and dry.

Sicilian-Rub Chicken Breasts

2 Tbsp. dried oregano
1 Tbsp. dried parsley
½ Tbsp. dried basil
½ tsp. onion powder
½ tsp. red pepper flakes
½ tsp. garlic powder
½ tsp. salt
4 boneless, skinless chicken breasts,
  4–6 oz. each
1 Tbsp. extra-virgin olive oil (optional)

Combine all ingredients except chicken and oil in a bowl, mixing well. Place chicken in a large resealable plastic bag. Add rub mix and oil. Shake until chicken is evenly coated. Follow grilling instructions above.

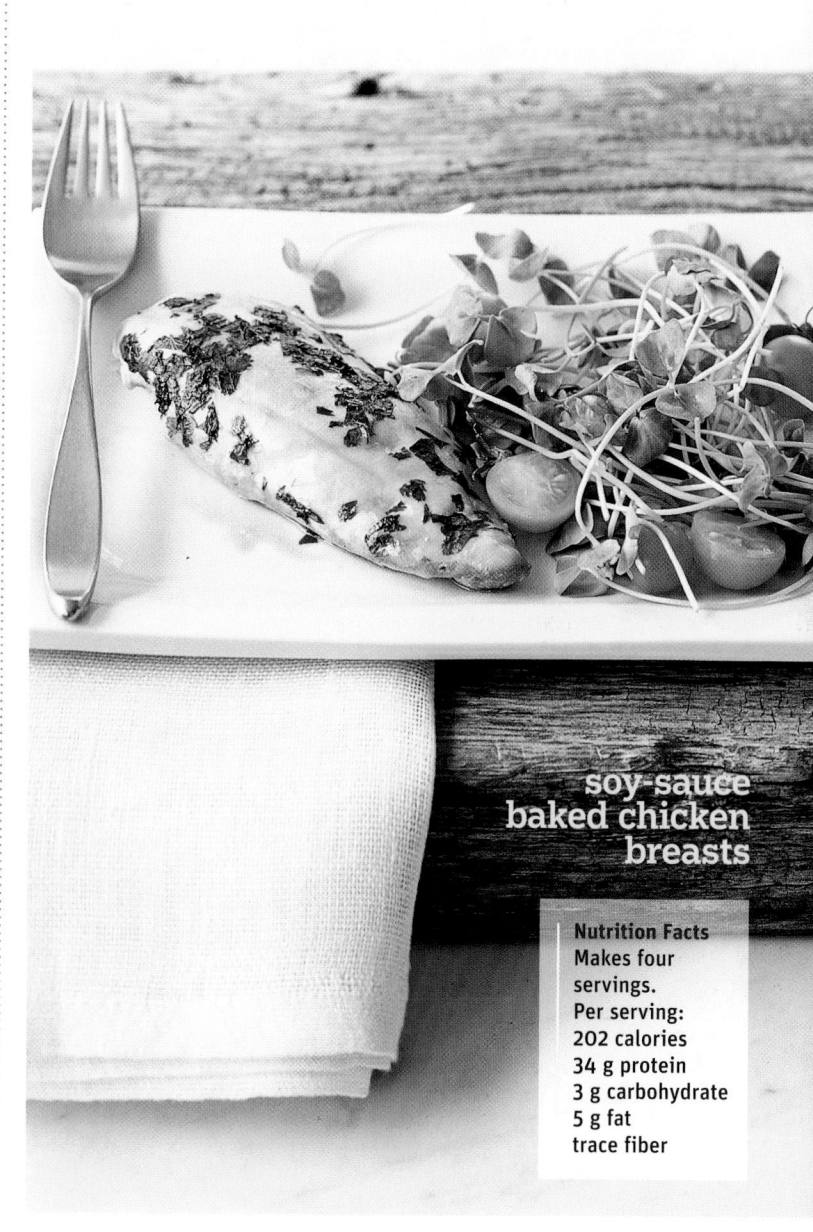

**soy-sauce
baked chicken
breasts**

Nutrition Facts
Makes four
servings.
Per serving:
202 calories
34 g protein
3 g carbohydrate
5 g fat
trace fiber

Simple Cooking Technique
No. 2: Baking

Baking chicken is ideal if you're a big fan of cooking once and eating for days or if you want to throw an easy dinner party that allows time for you to actually enjoy being with your guests. However, baking chicken works best after marinating the meat in the refrigerator for at least six hours or overnight, so you need to plan ahead.

To Cook: In advance, marinate chicken. When ready to cook, preheat oven to 400 degrees F. Remove chicken from marinade and place breasts in a baking dish large enough to lay them flat, but not so big that there's a lot of space between them. Ideally, they'll still be somewhat swimming in the marinade while being cooked. Cover the dish with aluminum foil and bake approximately 30 minutes, until chicken is no longer pink inside or a meat thermometer inserted in the center of the breasts reads 170 degrees F. Serve with a bit of remaining cooked sauce. If entertaining, you can take an attractive dish from oven to table and serve it family-style.

Soy-Sauce Baked Chicken Breasts

¼ cup fat-free chicken broth
¼ cup low-sodium soy sauce
1 Tbsp. toasted (or roasted) sesame oil
4 cloves garlic
1½ Tbsp. chopped fresh cilantro leaves
4 boneless, skinless chicken breasts, 4–6 oz. each

Combine all ingredients in a medium plastic container with a lid or resealable plastic bag and marinate in refrigerator at least six hours or overnight. Follow directions for baking chicken at left.

Simple Cooking Technique
No. 3: Foil Wrap

To impress your guests (or yourself), bake your chicken in individual foil-wrapped packets. This creates very tender pieces of chicken, easy to serve and clean up.

To Cook: If you wish to marinate chicken, do so in advance. When ready to cook, preheat oven to 400 degrees F. Tear a piece of aluminum foil large enough to create a tent around each chicken breast, about a 12x18-inch sheet of foil for each breast. Place foil flat and put a chicken breast in the center. Spoon one-fourth of remaining marinade over breast and fold sides up over breast so they meet. Fold the ends over twice, leaving space inside for air circulation. Then fold top and bottom of packet together, double-folding the ends again. Repeat with remaining breasts. Place packets on a cookie sheet or baking pan and bake 20–25 minutes or until breasts are no longer pink inside.

Gift-Wrapped Mandarin Chicken

3 medium garlic cloves, minced
½ cup canned mandarin oranges with juice (unsweetened)
3 Tbsp. frozen orange juice concentrate, thawed
2 Tbsp. low-sodium soy sauce
1 Tbsp. orange honey (or any honey)
2 tsp. chili-garlic sauce (found in international section of most major grocery stores)
½ Tbsp. roasted sesame oil
4 skinless, boneless chicken breasts, 4–6 oz. each

In a medium plastic or glass container with a lid, whisk together all ingredients except the chicken. Add chicken, submerging it in marinade. Cover and marinate in refrigerator at least six hours or overnight. Follow instructions for foil-wrap cooking at left.

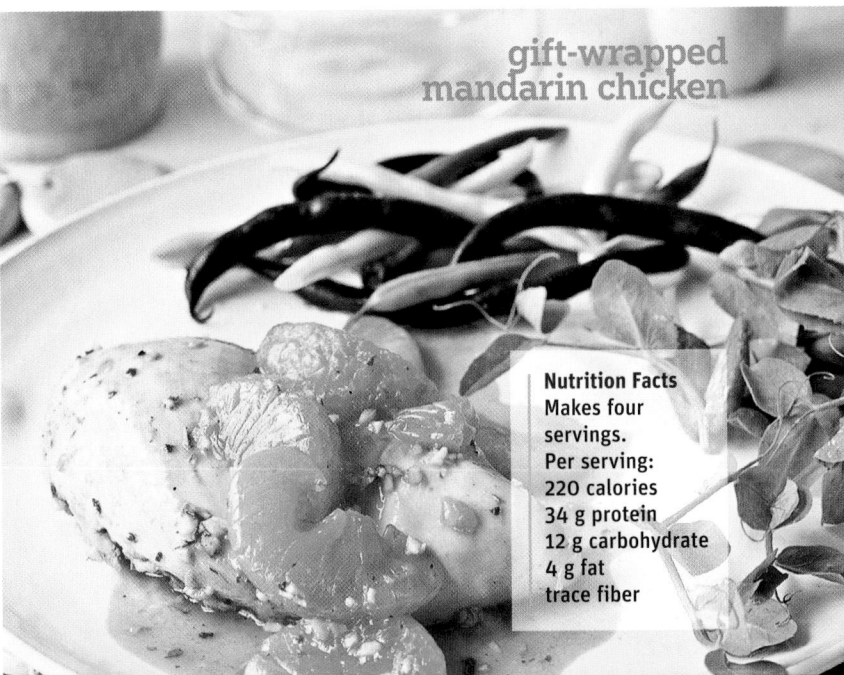

gift-wrapped
mandarin chicken

Nutrition Facts
Makes four servings.
Per serving:
220 calories
34 g protein
12 g carbohydrate
4 g fat
trace fiber

Simple Cooking Technique
No. 4: Ground and Sautéed

Ground chicken breast offers endless options for seasonings, cooking methods and recipe combinations. Butchers at most major grocery stores will grind boneless, skinless breasts for you for free; just ask. Or you can do it yourself, cutting breasts into 1-inch chunks, then grinding them in seconds in a food processor fitted with a chopping blade.

To Cook: If you're craving tacos or chili, simply spray a nonstick frying pan with cooking spray and cook the meat, chopping it apart as it cooks, then season it. If a burger is your preference, add your favorite ingredients to ground chicken and cook it over medium-high heat in a nonstick skillet sprayed with cooking spray. You can even make a mouthwatering ground-chicken "steak" like the one below.

Chicken-Peppered "Steak"

6 oz. ground chicken breast
¼ cup cooked brown rice
5 tsp. minced fresh parsley, divided
½ tsp. salt
1 tsp. freshly ground black pepper
¼ cup burgundy or other red wine
1 Tbsp. fresh-squeezed lemon juice
Nonstick cooking spray

In a large bowl, mix the chicken, rice, 4 tsp. parsley and salt. Form a 1-inch-thick, oval-shaped steak. Season with pepper and press it into steak on all sides. Spray a small nonstick pan with cooking spray and place over high heat. When hot, add steak. Sear steak on one side until browned, then flip and sear the other side. Reduce heat to medium and continue cooking until no longer pink inside (approximately 4–5 minutes per side). Remove steak from pan; cover to keep warm. Add wine to the pan and increase heat to high, scraping any pan drippings as liquid begins to boil. Continue to boil the wine until it is reduced by half. Stir in lemon juice, then pour mixture over steak (not shown). Top the meat with the remaining parsley and serve while hot.

Marinades

Whenever possible, a homemade marinade is the way to go. Not only can you control the chemical and sodium content and opt for more natural ingredients, but they also tend to taste better. Besides, store-bought marinades are often loaded with fat and sodium or are full of sugar, as our test shoppers found. We purchased several that seemed nutritionally sound, but when we returned to our test kitchen, we were highly disappointed with the results. After trying more than 20 varieties, we found only three tasty enough to mention:

Consorzio Jamaican Jerk 10-Minute Marinade (we thought it tasted much better marinated overnight)

Classico Italian Garlic & Herb EZ Marinader (marinade in a bag)

Jack Daniel's Mesquite EZ Marinader (marinade in a bag)

Rubs

Though less prevalent than marinades at most grocery stores, rubs deliver a greater success rate.

With the exception of a few that listed salt as the first ingredient, we found a number that were great. When choosing a rub, read the ingredient list and search for herbs that you know you like. To add extra moisture to chicken, rub each breast with about ½ teaspoon extra-virgin olive oil before seasoning it with rub. Our testers really liked:

Emeril's Chicken Rub

McCormick Rotisserie Chicken Seasoning (this one has salt as the first ingredient)

Stubb's Rosemary-Ginger Spice Rub

Food Safety

1) Never eat or even taste an uncooked marinade that contains or has had any contact with uncooked chicken (or any raw meat). Discard any remaining marinade that isn't cooked.

2) Be sure to wash your hands and all cutting boards, plates, utensils, etc., that have touched raw chicken or its juices. Never return cooked chicken to the plate that held raw chicken without washing the plate first.

chicken-peppered "steak"

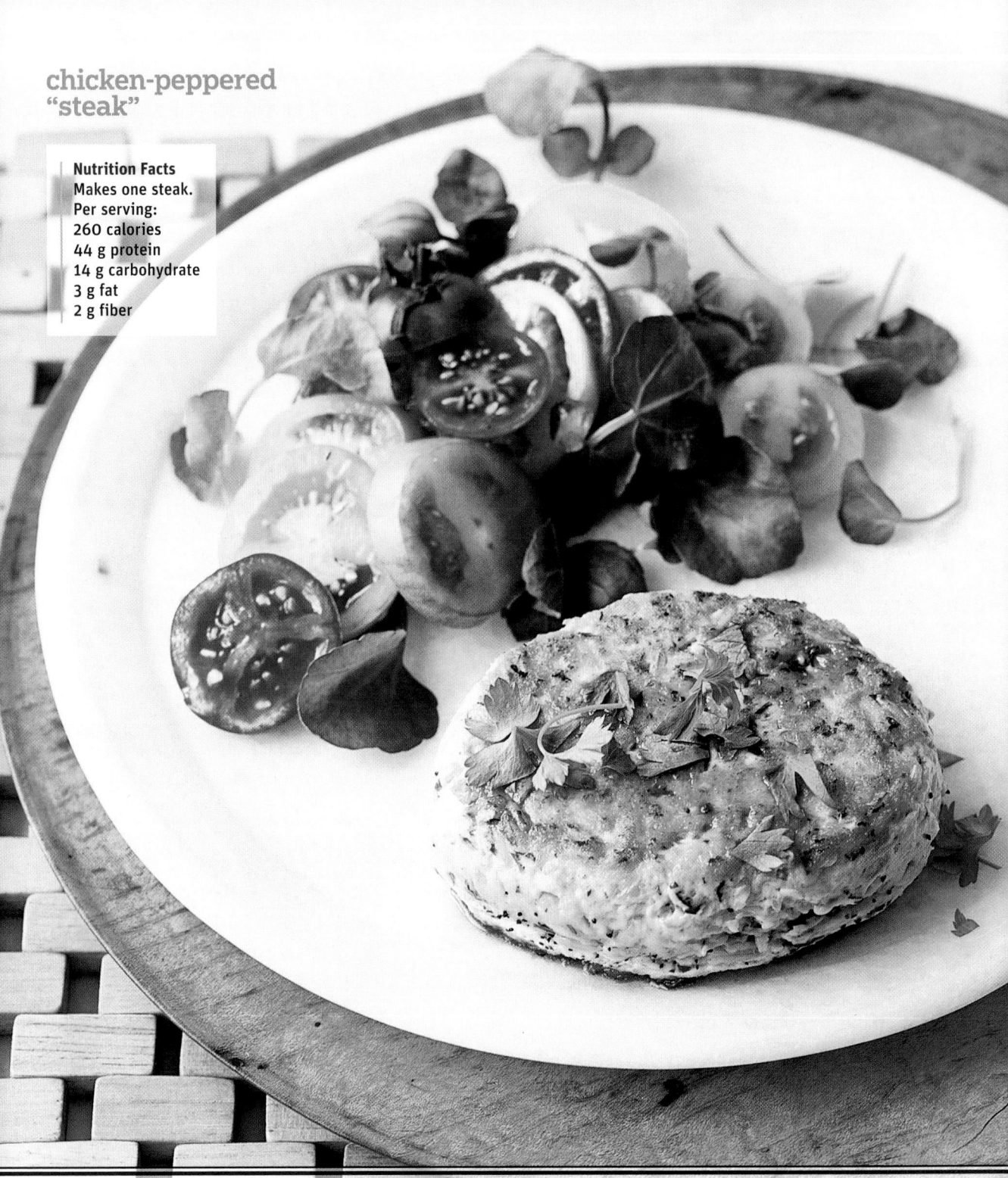

Nutrition Facts
Makes one steak.
Per serving:
260 calories
44 g protein
14 g carbohydrate
3 g fat
2 g fiber

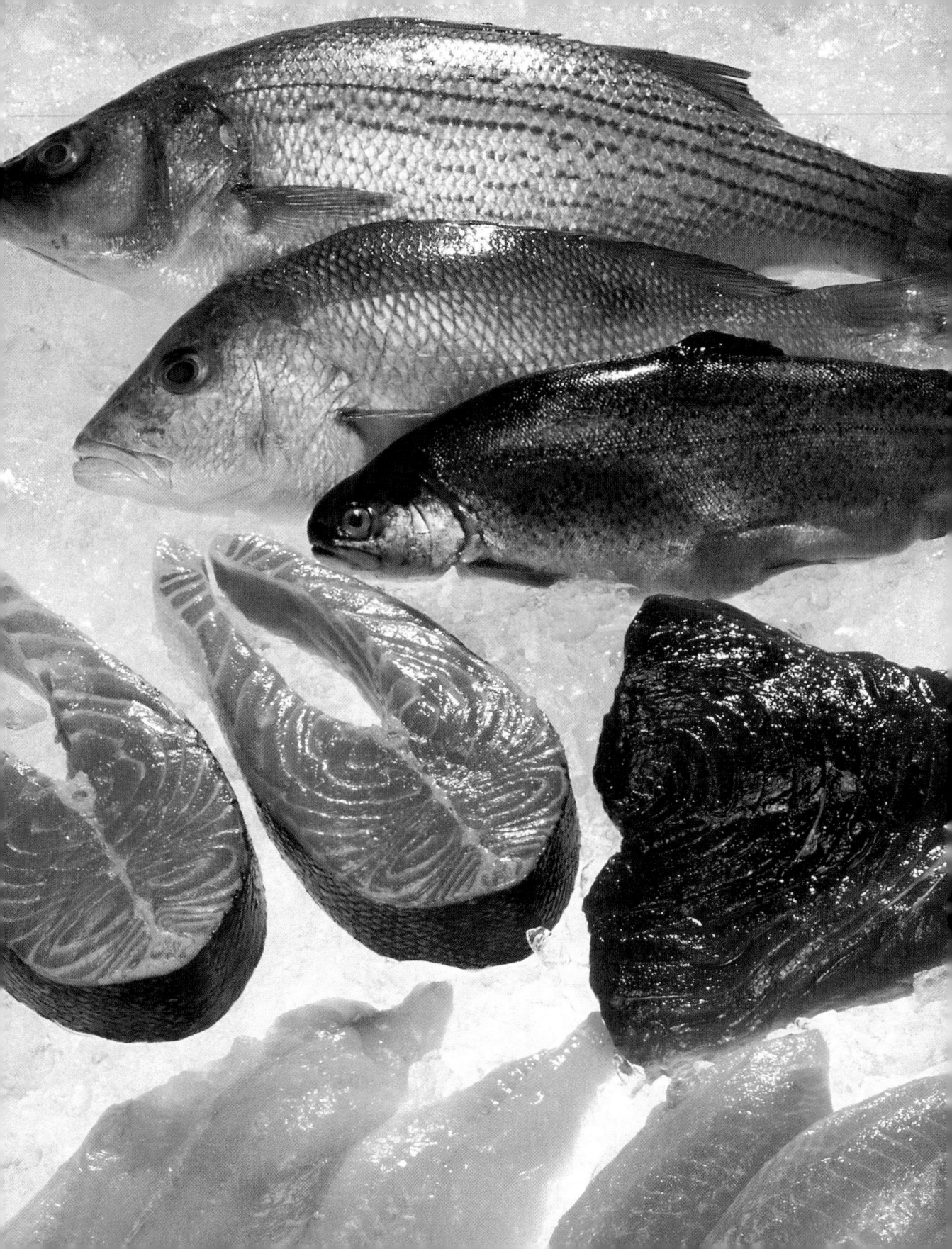

Chapter 13

Under The Sea

M**any** people don't eat fish because they don't know how to prepare it or just don't care for the taste. Maybe they tried fish that wasn't fresh or was poorly cooked. Yet, fish is so healthy that experts are telling us to eat more of it. You can start enjoying the health benefits that come with getting more of your menus from the sea by trying four tasty, quick-fix recipes.

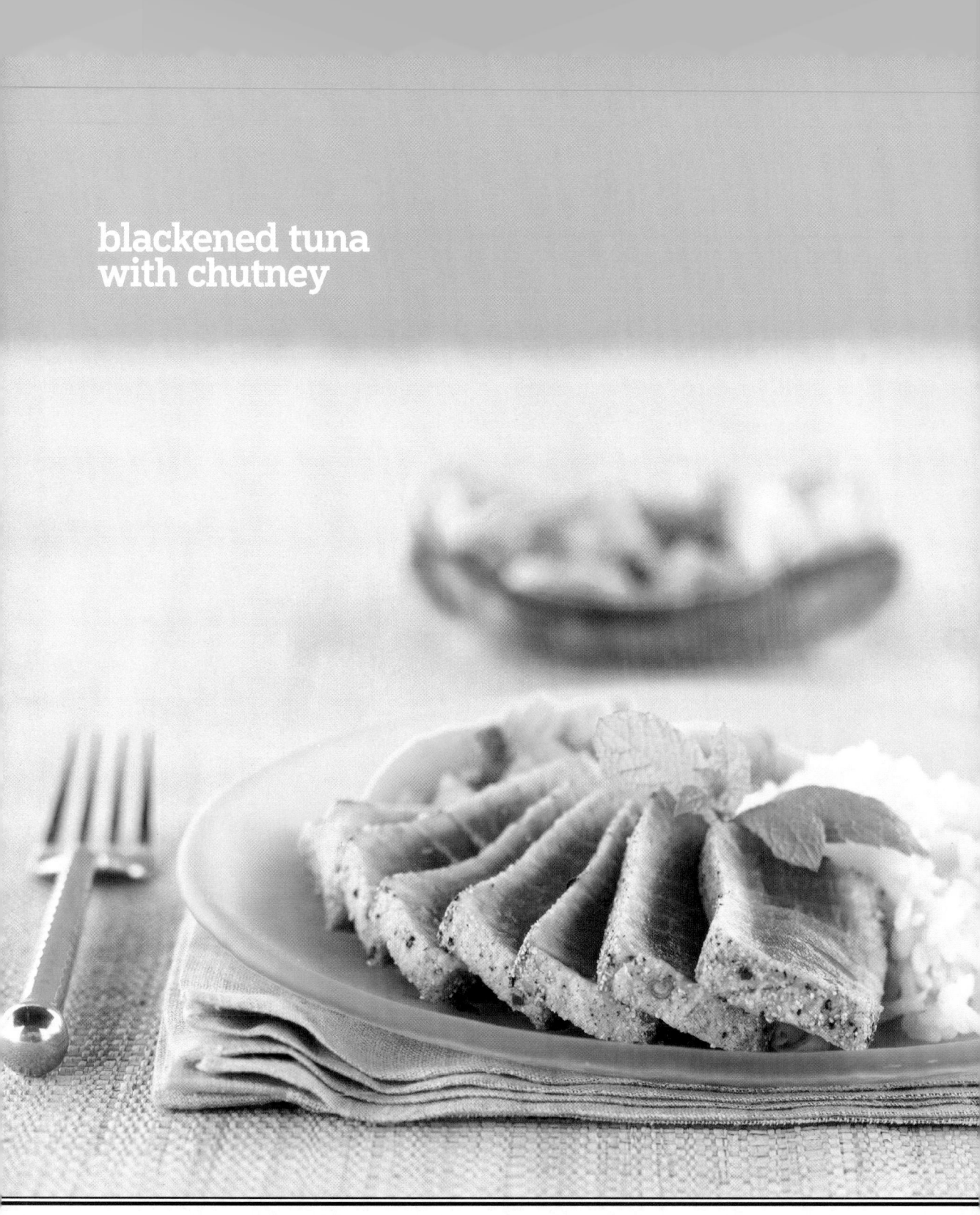

blackened tuna
with chutney

Taking a page from our favorite restaurant menu items, we've created healthy recipes with a gourmet flare. Use them as a jumping-off point to suit your own tastes. Part of the fun of cooking is personalizing a recipe by adding a touch of something here or omitting an ingredient there.

One piece of advice about preparing fish is to err on the side of under-cooking. Dry fish never tastes good, and a medium-rare temperature is preferred to well-done. Remove fish from heat when it just starts to flake.

blackened tuna with chutney

Fruit chutney is wonderful with blackened fish — it adds a sweet taste to a spicy dish. This homemade chutney recipe is delicious; however, many great chutneys can be purchased at your grocery store if you don't have time to make this from scratch. Our favorite tuna is sushi-grade ahi, cooked rare. You can purchase a blackening seasoning, such as Cajun's Choice, but most of these are very salty. If you have time, make your own seasoning instead.

Blackened Tuna

1 lb. fresh tuna fillet
1 Tbsp. cornmeal
½ tsp. black pepper
1 tsp. white pepper
1 tsp. red pepper flakes
⅛ tsp. garlic powder

Mix seasoning ingredients together and coat both sides of fish with mixture. Preheat a nonstick skillet over very high heat. Reduce heat to medium and place fish in skillet. Cook fish, uncovered, for 4–5 minutes on each side, depending on desired degree of doneness. Serve with favorite chutney.
Serves 4

Peach Chutney

4 cups peach slices, fresh or frozen
1 onion, finely chopped
¼ cup white wine vinegar
2 Tbsp. granulated sugar
¼ cup golden raisins
2 Tbsp. fresh ginger, minced
2 Tbsp. garlic, minced
2 Tbsp. curry powder
½ tsp. salt
3 Tbsp. fresh mint, chopped

In a non-aluminum saucepan, combine all ingredients except fresh mint. Bring to a slow boil over medium heat. Reduce heat and cook gently until onions are cooked and chutney is thickened (about 25 minutes). Remove from heat and cool. Add mint and stir. **NUTRITION FACTS (per serving w/ chutney):** *322 calories, 30 g protein, 46 g carbohydrate, 2 g fat, 7 g fiber*

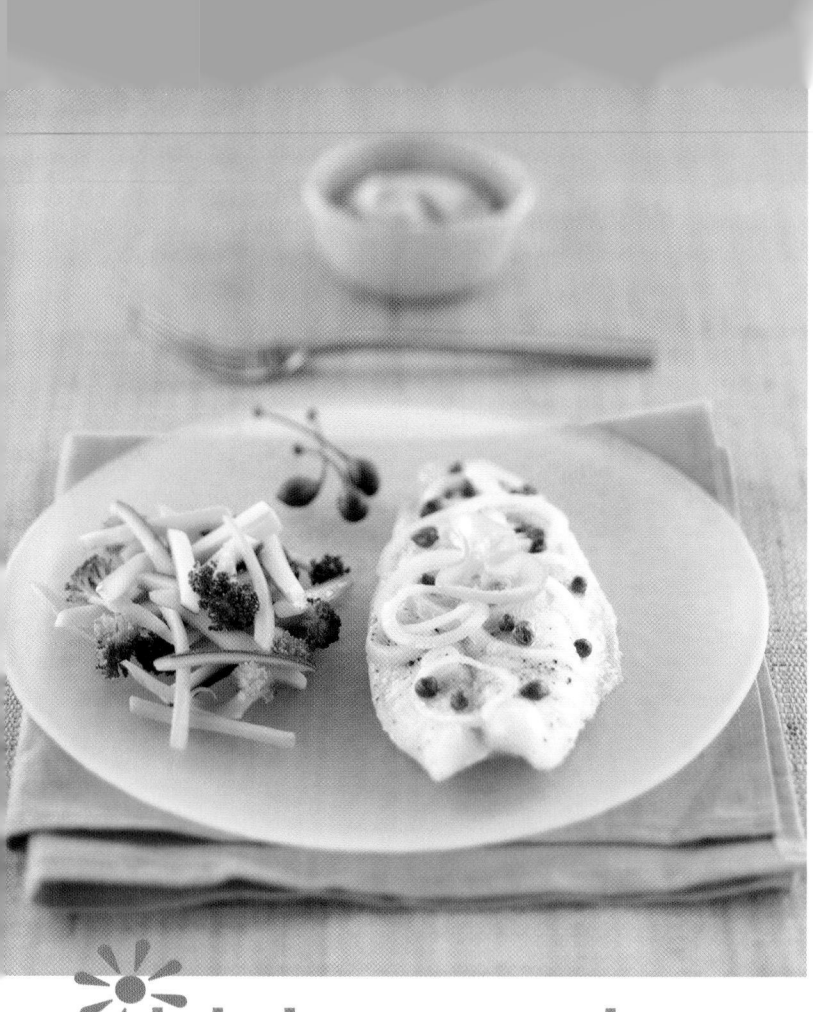

baked orange roughy

½ pound orange roughy (or cod)
Garlic powder, to taste
Black pepper, to taste
½ lemon, sliced very thinly
2 thin slices sweet onion
1 tsp. capers
1 Tbsp. light margarine or light butter

Preheat oven to 350 degrees F. Place a large piece of aluminum foil or parchment paper on a baking sheet. Place fish fillet in center of foil. Sprinkle garlic powder and pepper over fillet. Place 4–5 lemon slices on fillet and top that with thinly sliced onions. Sprinkle capers over onions. Break margarine or butter into pieces and place on top of fish. Wrap prepared fish in the foil, bringing ends of foil together and folding to seal. Place the baking sheet in oven and bake for 20 minutes. Serve with fresh lemon wedges or tartar sauce.

Serves 2 NUTRITION FACTS (per serving): *200 calories, 17 g protein, 3 g carbohydrate, 13 g fat*

#86

BUYING AND STORING FISH

Without a doubt, the best fish is purchased fresh at the local market and cooked the same day. Frozen fish is a good alternative and might be easier to find in many areas.

Some tips for buying fish:

>> Shop for fresh fish where turnover of product is high.

>> Make sure fish is packed on ice and nicely displayed.

>> The fish market should smell like the sea, but not foul.

>> When buying steaks or fillets look for firm flesh, a moist appearance and a fresh smell.

For storing fish:

>> Keep fresh fish in refrigerator and use within two days.

>> If buying fresh fish for cooking in more than two days, use a vacuum pack or place in freezer bags and freeze.

>> Thaw frozen fish in the refrigerator the day of cooking, or carefully defrost in the microwave shortly before cooking. Do not refreeze.

>> Immediately place frozen fish in freezer if not using the same day of purchase.

grilled salmon with dill sauce

1 lb. salmon fillet
2 tsp. minced garlic
2 Tbsp. golden brown sugar
¼ cup orange juice

Turn grill on high to preheat. Place salmon skin-side down in 9x11-inch pan. Mix garlic and brown sugar together in small bowl. Rub garlic/brown sugar mixture into salmon flesh, coating whole piece. Pour orange juice gently over fillet and let sit 20–30 minutes while grill is heating up. Place salmon on hot grill flesh-side down and sear 2–3 minutes on high. Turn fillet over and reduce heat to medium. Cook salmon to medium, being careful not to dry out fish. Cooking time will vary depending on thickness of fish, but estimate about 5 minutes total for a 1-inch fillet. Skin will stick to the grill. Slide spatula between fillet and skin to remove salmon from grill. Top with dill sauce and serve. **Serves 4**

This recipe also is good broiled.

dill sauce

2 Tbsp. reduced-fat mayonnaise
1 Tbsp. plain fat-free or low-fat yogurt
1 tsp. lemon juice
1 tsp. spicy brown mustard
1 Tbsp. finely chopped fresh or dried dill

Place first 4 ingredients into small bowl and stir until well blended. Add chopped dill. If using fresh dill, serve immediately. When using dried dill, let the sauce sit for 15 minutes before serving.

NUTRITION FACTS (per serving w/ sauce):
200 calories, 23 g protein, 8 g carbohydrate, 8 g fat

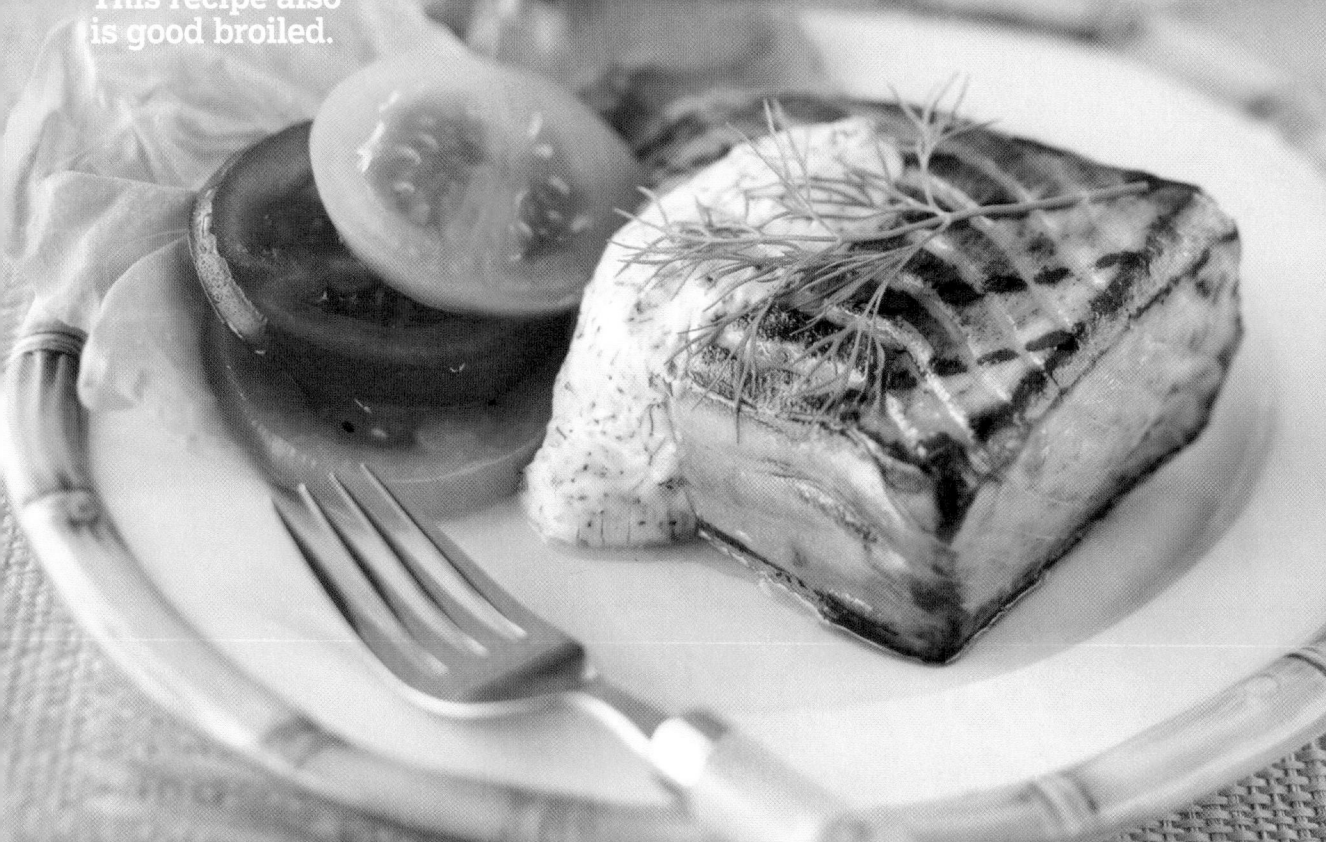

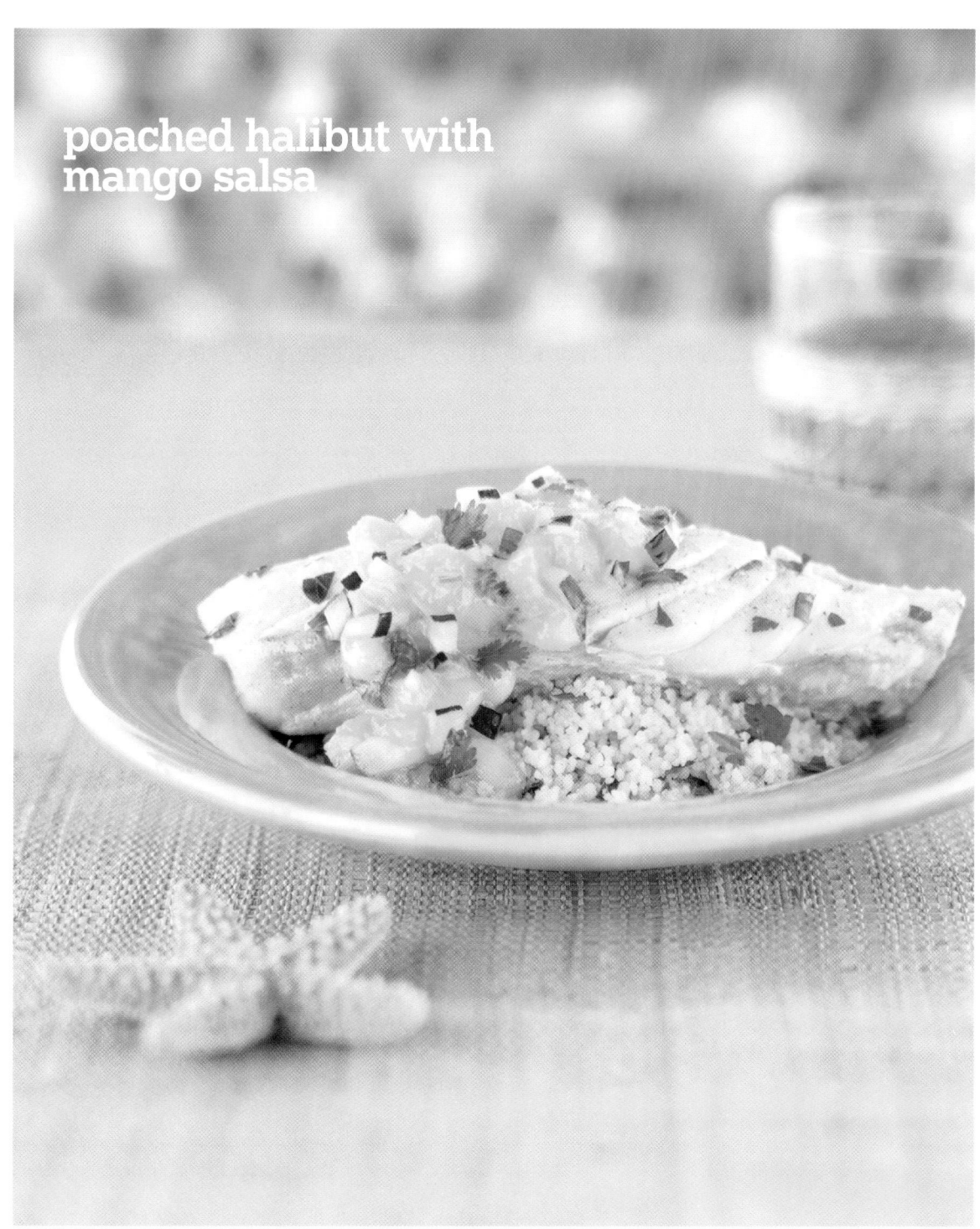

poached halibut with
mango salsa

poached halibut with mango salsa

Poached Halibut

1 lb. halibut, either fresh or frozen and thawed
½ tsp. garlic powder
Pinch salt
¼ tsp. white pepper
1 Tbsp. light margarine or light butter
1–2 cups skim or low-fat milk

Coat a sauté pan with nonstick spray. Place halibut in pan. Lightly sprinkle garlic powder, salt and pepper on fillet. Put margarine on top of fillet. Pour milk into pan until all but the very top of fish is covered. Turn heat to medium and cover pan, bringing milk to a slow simmer. Poach fish for about 20 minutes or until fish flakes, occasionally lifting the lid to spoon milk over top of fish. Remove fish from pan with a slotted spatula and serve topped with mango salsa.
Serves 3

Mango Salsa

2 cups diced fresh or frozen mango
½ cup fresh cilantro, chopped
¼ cup sweet red onion, finely diced
2 cloves garlic, crushed
Juice of one lime

Mix mango, cilantro, onion and garlic together in small bowl. Pour lime juice over salsa and toss. Set aside while preparing halibut.
NUTRITION FACTS (per serving w/ salsa): *319 calories, 36 g protein, 28 g carbohydrate, 7 g fat, 2 g fiber*

#87

HOW MUCH FISH SHOULD YOU EAT?

According to the American Heart Association's recent dietary guidelines, a minimum of two 3-oz. servings of fish is recommended per week for all Americans. Fatty fish such as salmon, trout, mackerel, herring and anchovies are highest in omega-3 fatty acids.
Note: *Three ounces of fish is about the size of a deck of cards.*

SAFETY CONCERNS

Because fish comes from lakes, rivers, streams and the sea, it can pick up both natural and unnatural contaminants. In particular, the mercury level in some fish concerns health officials. If mercury is found in local soil, it can contaminate the fish supply. Toxicity from consuming high levels of mercury is rare, but the USDA recommends that pregnant women and children use caution when consuming certain kinds of fish highest in mercury, as this neurotoxin has a potentially negative effect on the developing brain.
Fish with the highest of mercury include:

- Fresh tuna
- Swordfish
- Shark
- Tilefish
- King mackerel

Pregnant women and young children should avoid the above fish and should eat no more than two cans of tuna per week. Older children, men and women above childbearing age should limit the above fish to one serving per week.
Fish with the lowest levels of mercury include:

- Salmon
- Trout
- Flounder
- Haddock
- Catfish (farmed)
- Shrimp

Note: *If eating locally caught fish, check with the department of fish and wildlife about mercury levels in rivers, streams and bays.*

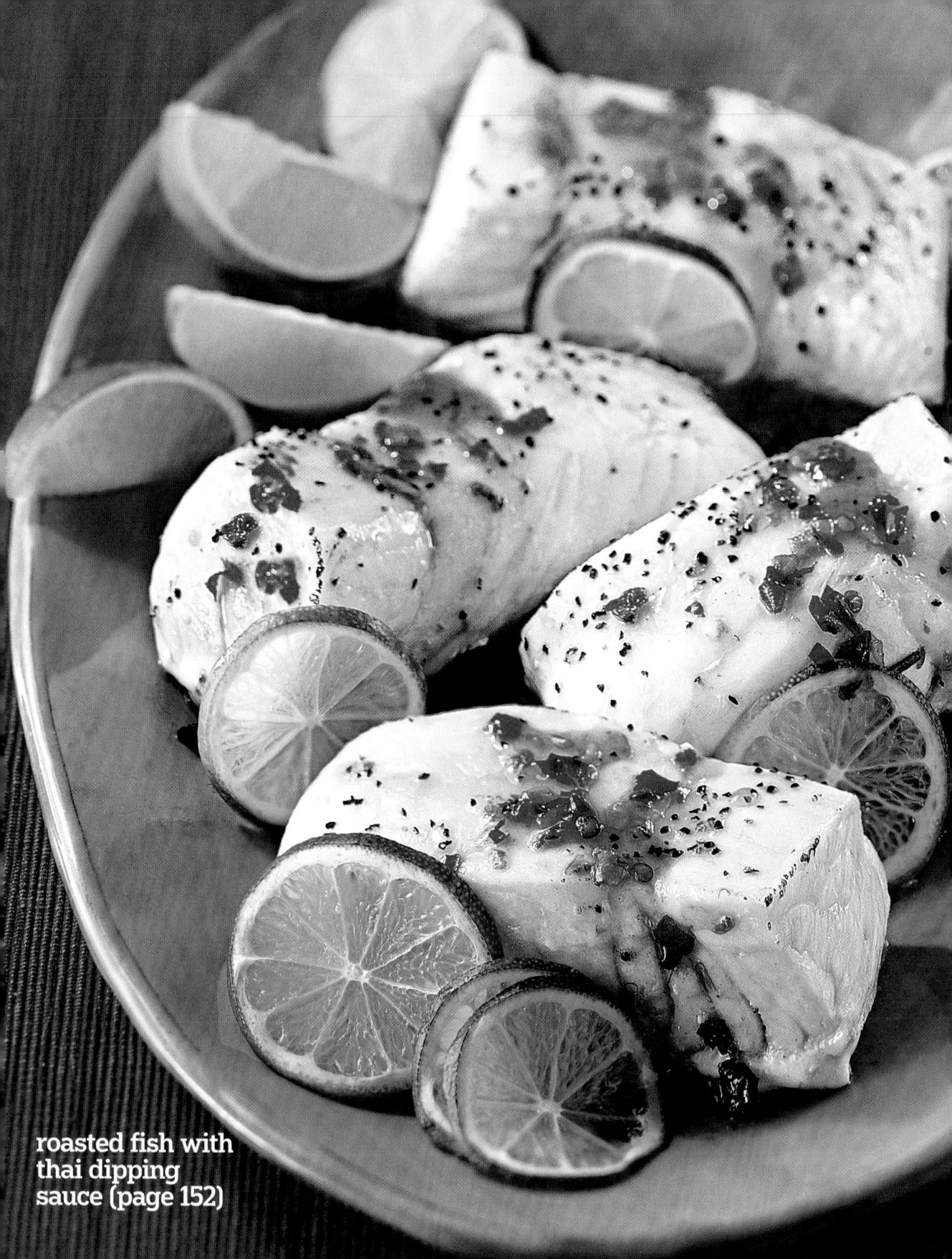

roasted fish with thai dipping sauce (page 152)

Chapter 14

Fire & Spice

Some people love to torture themselves with the mouth-burning, eye-watering, sinus-clearing effects of chili peppers. From super-hot habañeros to the more mild paprika, they all contain capsaicin, the fiery substance that gives chilies their zing and also puts a zip into your metabolism — actually helping your body burn calories by temporarily increasing your metabolic rate for up to four hours after you eat.

whole-wheat tomato basil pasta #88

This quick, fresh pasta sauce showcases late summer's ripe tomatoes accented with basil and a bite of red pepper.

8 oz. whole-wheat fettuccine
2 Tbsp. olive oil
1 small onion, chopped
2 cloves garlic, minced
½ tsp. crushed red pepper flakes
½ tsp. oregano
3 medium ripe tomatoes, chopped
1 tsp. salt
3 Tbsp. chopped fresh basil
¼ cup grated Parmesan cheese

1. Cook whole-wheat fettuccine according to package directions.
2. Meanwhile, heat oil in a large skillet over medium heat. Sauté onion until tender (about five minutes). Add garlic, pepper flakes and oregano; cook one minute.
3. Add tomatoes and salt to skillet and cook until tomatoes are soft and hot, about five minutes more.

4. Place fettuccine in a large serving bowl and top with sauce. Sprinkle with basil and Parmesan cheese. Dish should be served immediately.
Serves 4

NUTRITION FACTS (per serving):
334 calories, 12 g protein, 49 g carbs, 10 g fat, 13 g fiber, <1 g sugar, 712 mg sodium

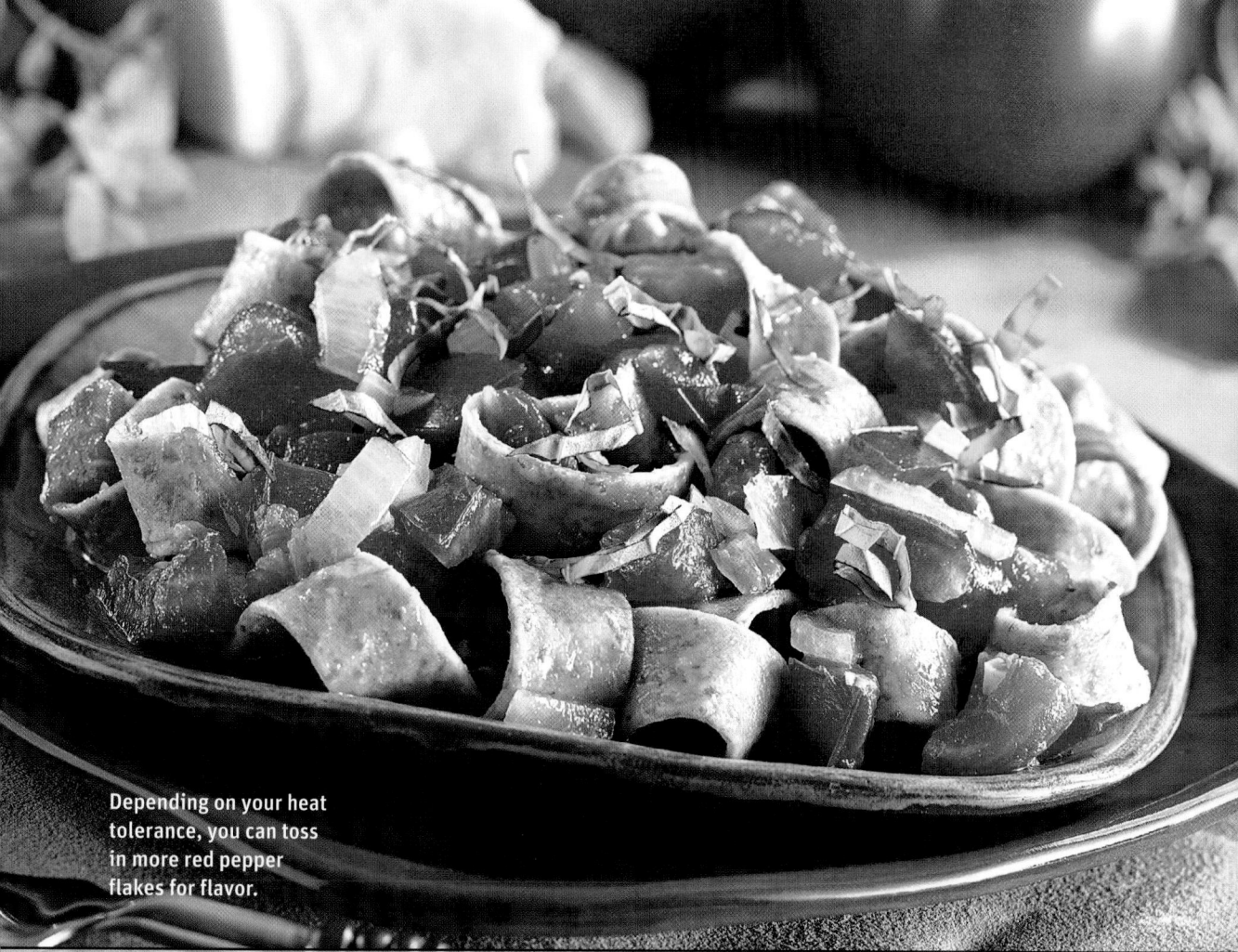

Depending on your heat tolerance, you can toss in more red pepper flakes for flavor.

ginger-chili chicken stir-fry #89

The key to a good stir fry is prepping all the ingredients, then cooking the food quickly. Start by making the rice and chopping the veggies, and this meal will be on the table in minutes.

2 Tbsp. oil (divided)
1 lb. boneless, skinless chicken breasts, cut into ½-inch pieces
2 Tbsp. fresh minced ginger
1 fresh Serrano chili, seeded and sliced into strips
1 medium onion, halved lengthwise and sliced into strips
1 small red bell pepper, seeded and julienned
1 small green bell pepper, seeded and julienned
1 small yellow bell pepper, seeded and julienned

Sauce

¼ cup reduced-sodium soy sauce
2 Tbsp. water
2 cloves garlic, minced
2 tsp. cornstarch
1 tsp. sugar

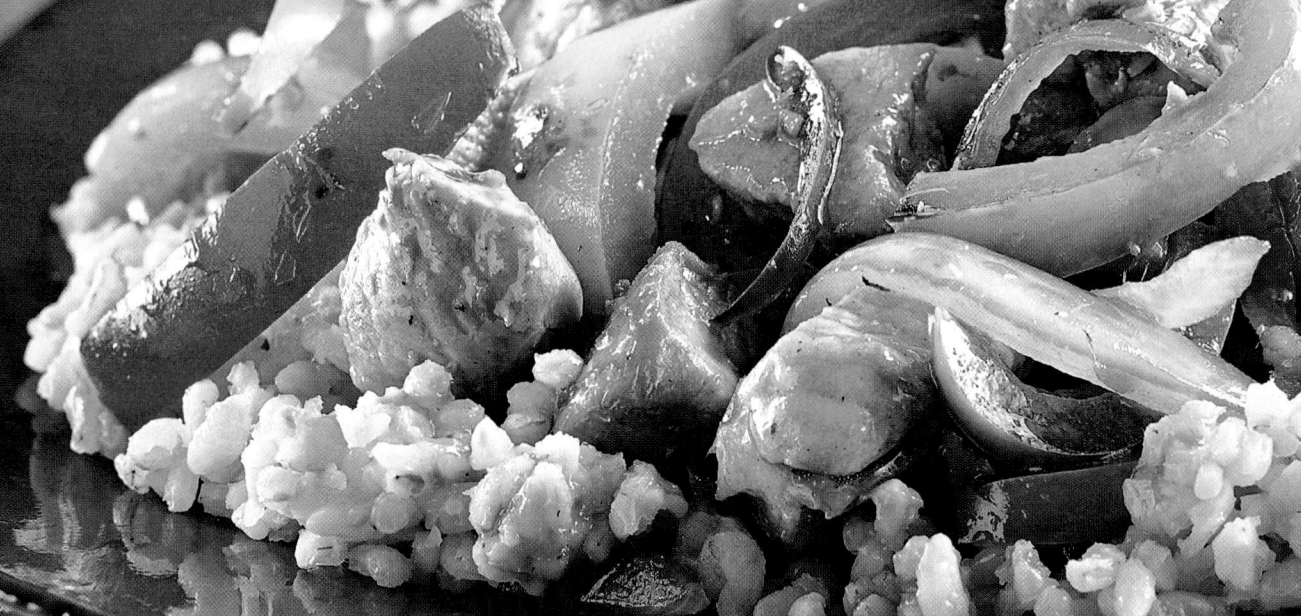

1. Heat 1 Tbsp. oil in a wok or large skillet over medium-high heat. Add chicken and stir-fry until almost cooked through. Remove chicken to a plate; cover to keep warm.
2. Heat remaining oil in wok. Add ginger, chili, onion and bell peppers; stir-fry five minutes or until peppers are crisp-tender. Return chicken to wok.

3. Mix sauce ingredients together in a small bowl. Pour into wok and cook until sauce is thick and bubbly, about two minutes. Serve over rice. **Serves 4**

NUTRITION FACTS (per serving): *260 calories, 27 g protein, 22.5 g carbs, 7 g fat, 2 g fiber, 4 g sugar, 608 mg sodium*

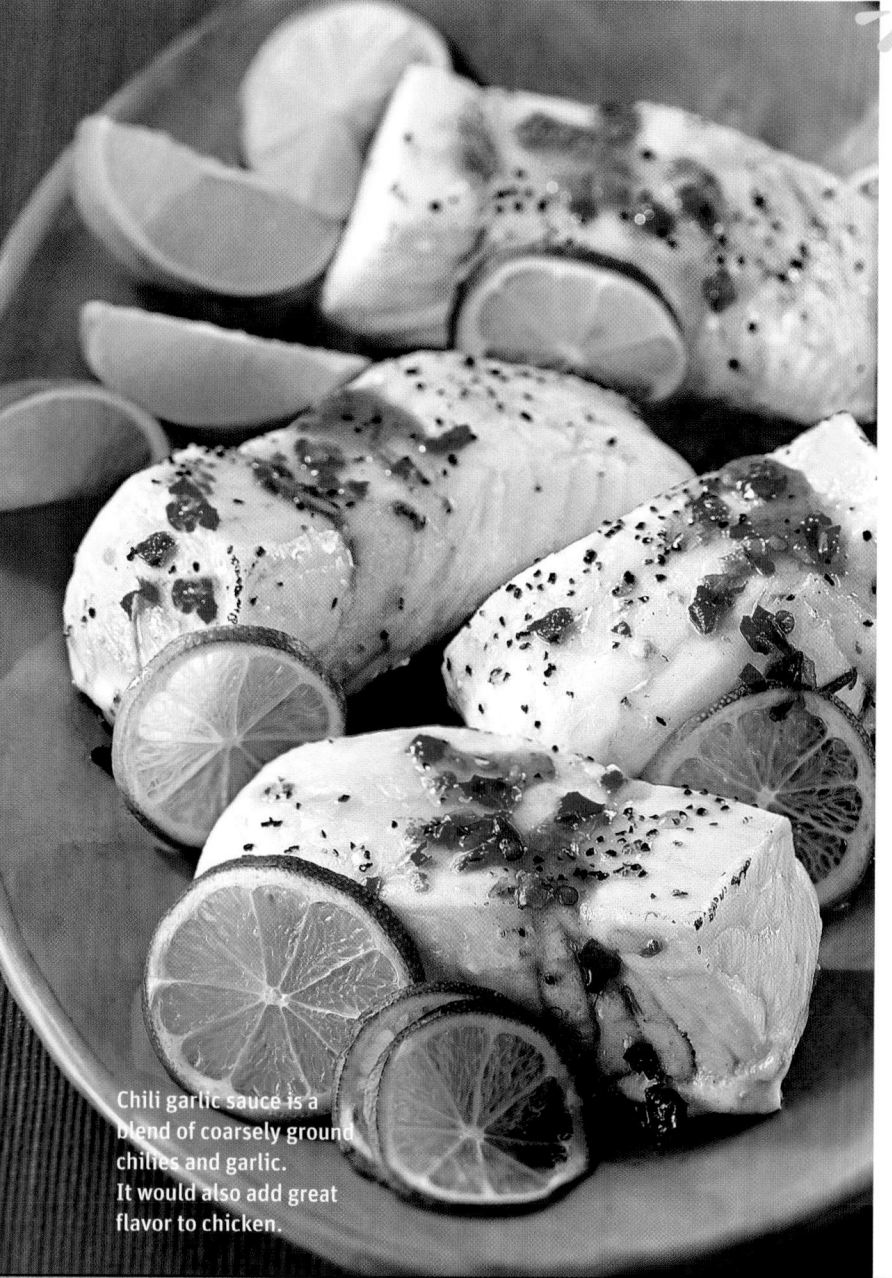

Chili garlic sauce is a blend of coarsely ground chilies and garlic. It would also add great flavor to chicken.

roasted fish with thai dipping sauce #90

You can find fish sauce and chili garlic sauce in the Asian section of your supermarket.

1 lb. mild white fish fillets
    such as halibut,
    cod or tilapia (4 oz. each)
½ tsp. freshly ground black pepper

Dipping sauce
2 Tbsp. lime juice
2 Tbsp. fish sauce
1 Tbsp. brown sugar
1 tsp. chili garlic sauce

1. Preheat oven to 400 degrees F. Line a baking sheet with aluminum foil. Place fish on foil, skin side down. Sprinkle with pepper and gently pat into flesh.
2. Roast fish for 10–15 minutes or until it's opaque in the center and flakes easily.
3. Meanwhile, whisk dipping sauce ingredients together in a small bowl. Serve in individual bowls for dipping, or drizzle over fish on a platter. **Serves 4**

NUTRITION FACTS (per serving):
130 calories, *25 g protein, 5 g carbs, 0 g fat, 0 g fiber, 4 g sugar, 782 mg sodium*

red-hot oven-fried potatoes #91

These spicy potatoes are easy to make and much better for you than deep-fried potato chips. Use half the cayenne for less heat.

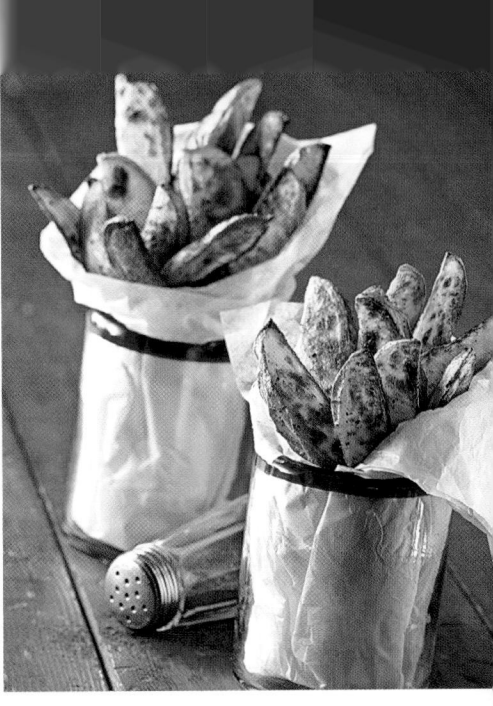

4 medium red potatoes
½ Tbsp. olive oil
½ tsp. garlic powder
¼ tsp. onion powder
¼ tsp. cayenne pepper
¼ tsp. salt
¼ tsp. black pepper

1. Preheat oven to 475 degrees F. Slice potatoes in half, then into thin wedges. Place in a medium bowl and drizzle with olive oil. Toss until evenly coated.

2. In a small bowl, combine garlic powder, onion powder, cayenne, salt and pepper. Sprinkle evenly over potatoes and toss to coat. Place potatoes on a rimmed baking sheet.
3. Roast 15–20 minutes, turning potatoes occasionally, until they are are golden brown and fork-tender. **Serves 4**

NUTRITION FACTS (per serving): *187 calories, 4 g protein, 35 g carbs, 3.5 g fat, 4 g fiber, 2 g sugar, 159 mg sodium*

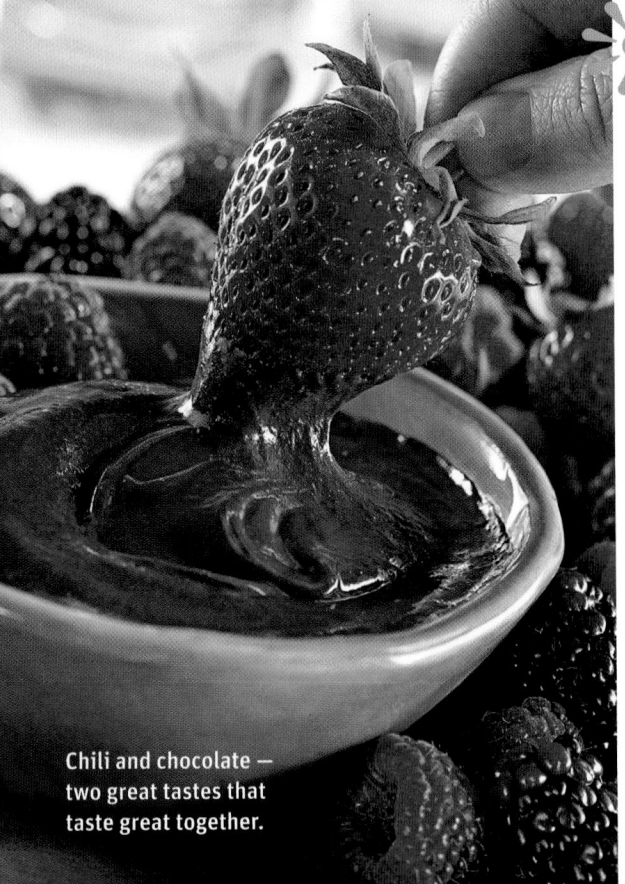

Chili and chocolate — two great tastes that taste great together.

chili chocolate sauce #92

This sauce spiked with sweet-hot ancho chilies combines fat-free cocoa powder and antioxidant-rich bittersweet chocolate. Enjoy with fresh fruit, over low-fat ice cream or frozen yogurt, or stirred into coffee.

¼ cup unsweetened cocoa powder
¼ cup sugar
½ Tbsp. cornstarch
1 cup evaporated skim milk
2 oz. bittersweet chocolate, coarsely chopped
2 tsp. vanilla
½ tsp. cinnamon
1½ tsp. ancho chili powder
Dash salt

1. Combine cocoa powder, sugar and cornstarch in a small saucepan. Whisk in evaporated milk. Bring to a simmer over medium heat; reduce heat to low and simmer two minutes or until thickened, stirring constantly. Remove from heat and add chocolate. Let sit three minutes; whisk until smooth.
2. Stir in vanilla, cinnamon, chili powder and salt. Serve warm or at room temperature; will keep in refrigerator for one month. **Serves 8**

NUTRITION FACTS (per serving): *102 calories, 3 g protein, 17 g carbs, 2.5 g fat, 1.5 g fiber, 14 g sugar, 38 mg sodium*

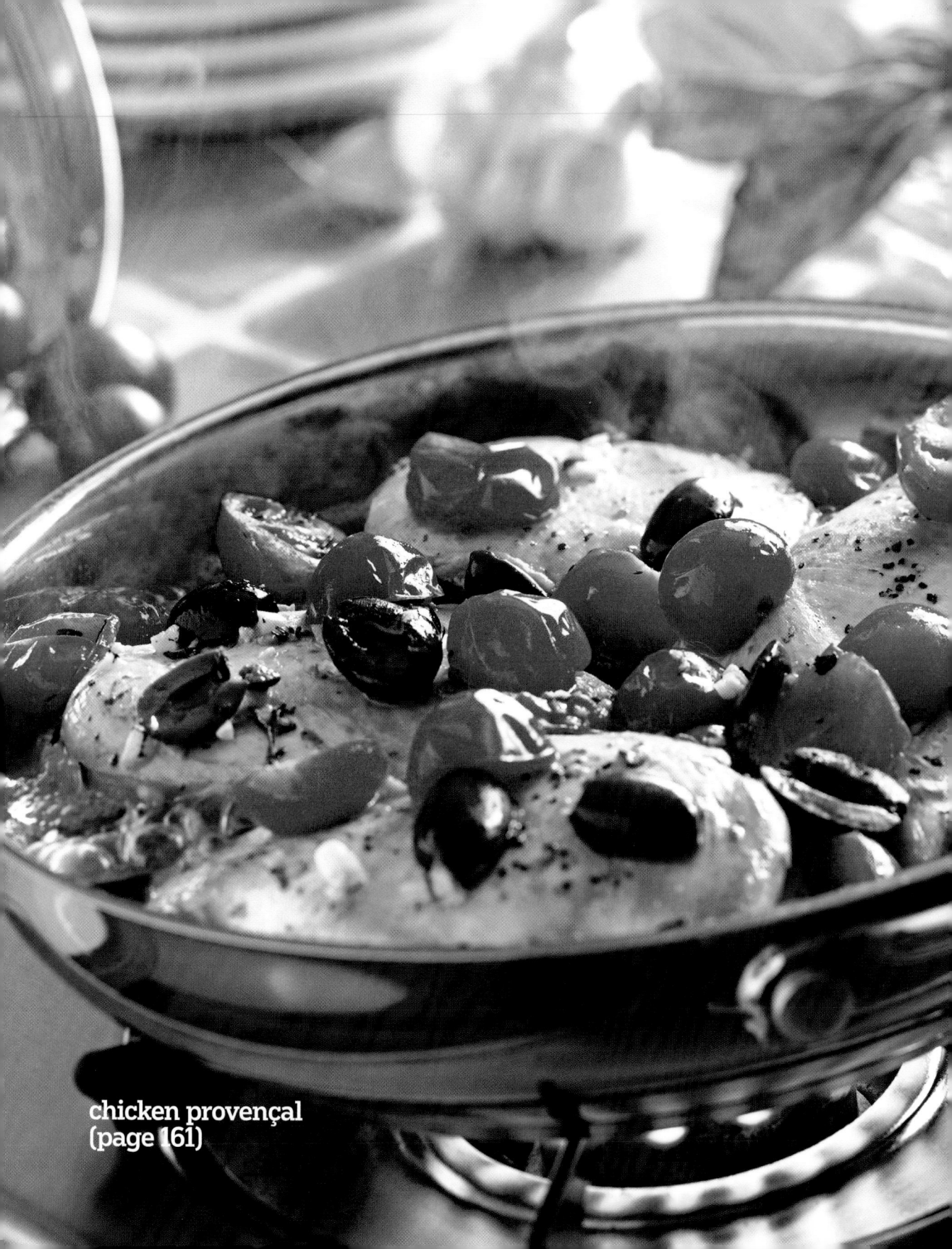

chicken provençal
(page 161)

Chapter 15

One-Pot Wonders

These quick, fitness-friendly dishes are chock-full of veggies and lean protein, perfect for fueling your trips to the gym or for an easy meal on your rest days. The best part? Prep and cleanup are a breeze. These recipes leave you with no excuses for not fueling up your fat-burning efforts, especially since these meals require only a minimal amount of your time. So what are you waiting for? Get cooking.

lentil stew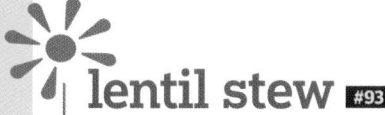

This hearty, nutritious stew takes the chill off a breezy spring day, and it tastes even better as leftovers. Make it on a Sunday, since it needs to simmer for a couple of hours, and eat it during the week. Serve with a slice of hearty whole-grain bread to soak up the juices.

½ lb. extra-lean (5% fat)
 ground beef
46-oz. can low-sodium tomato
 or V8 juice
4 cups water
1 cup brown lentils, rinsed and
 picked over
1 cup diced carrots
1 cup chopped celery
1 cup chopped cabbage
1 medium onion, chopped
1 tsp. salt
½ tsp. black pepper
⅛ tsp. cayenne pepper
1 bay leaf
½ cup shredded low-fat
 cheddar cheese

1. Brown ground beef in a large soup kettle, then drain. Add tomato juice and water; bring to a boil.
2. Add lentils, carrots, celery, cabbage, onion, salt, black and cayenne peppers, and bay leaf.
3. Return to boil; reduce heat and simmer 1½–2 hours or until lentils are just tender, stirring occasionally. Remove bay leaf and discard. Serve in individual bowls with cheese sprinkled on top. **Serves 6**
NUTRITION FACTS (per serving): *225 calories, 19 g protein, 32 g carbs, 2.3 g fat, 12 g fiber, 25 mg cholesterol, 660 mg sodium, 11 g sugar*

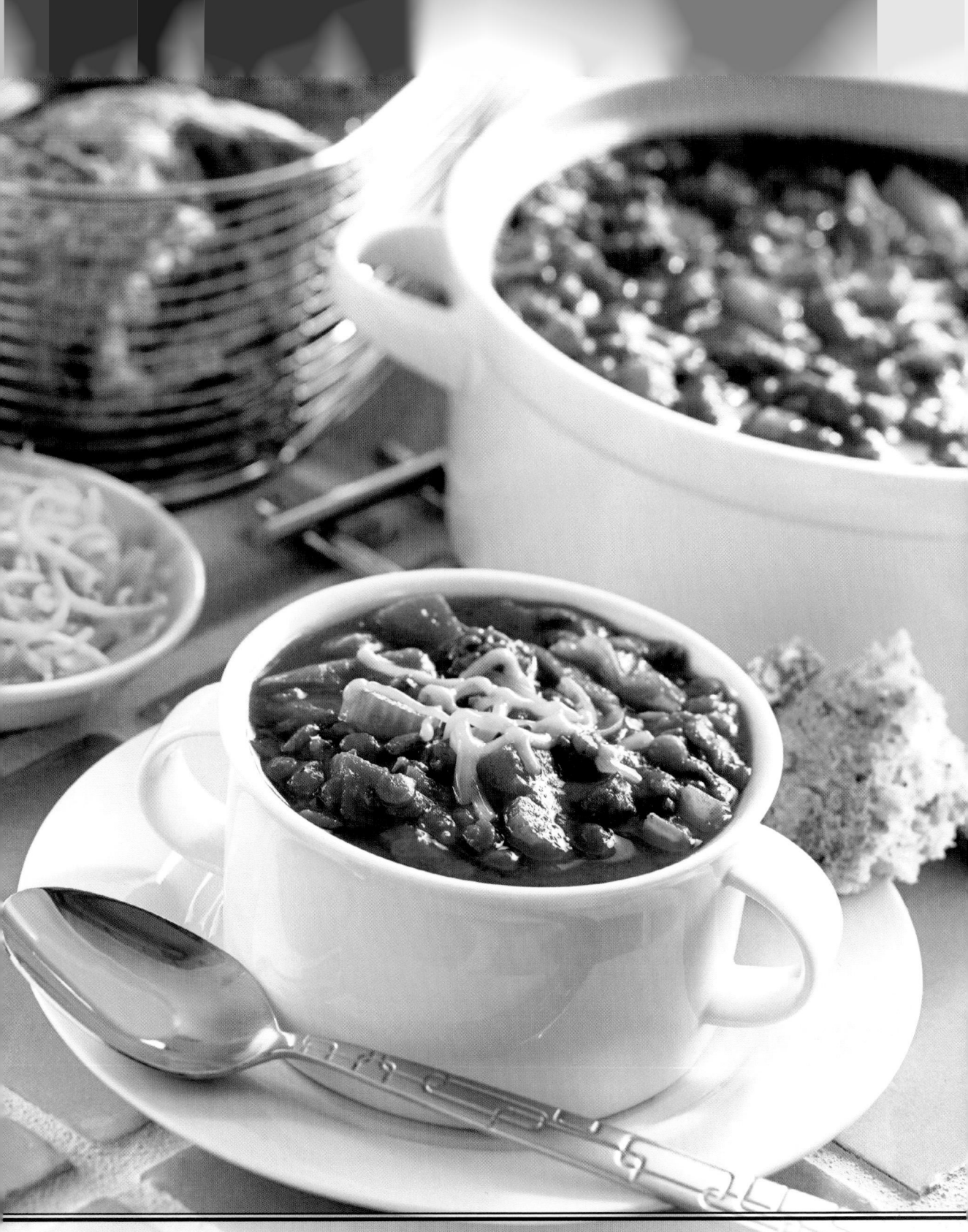

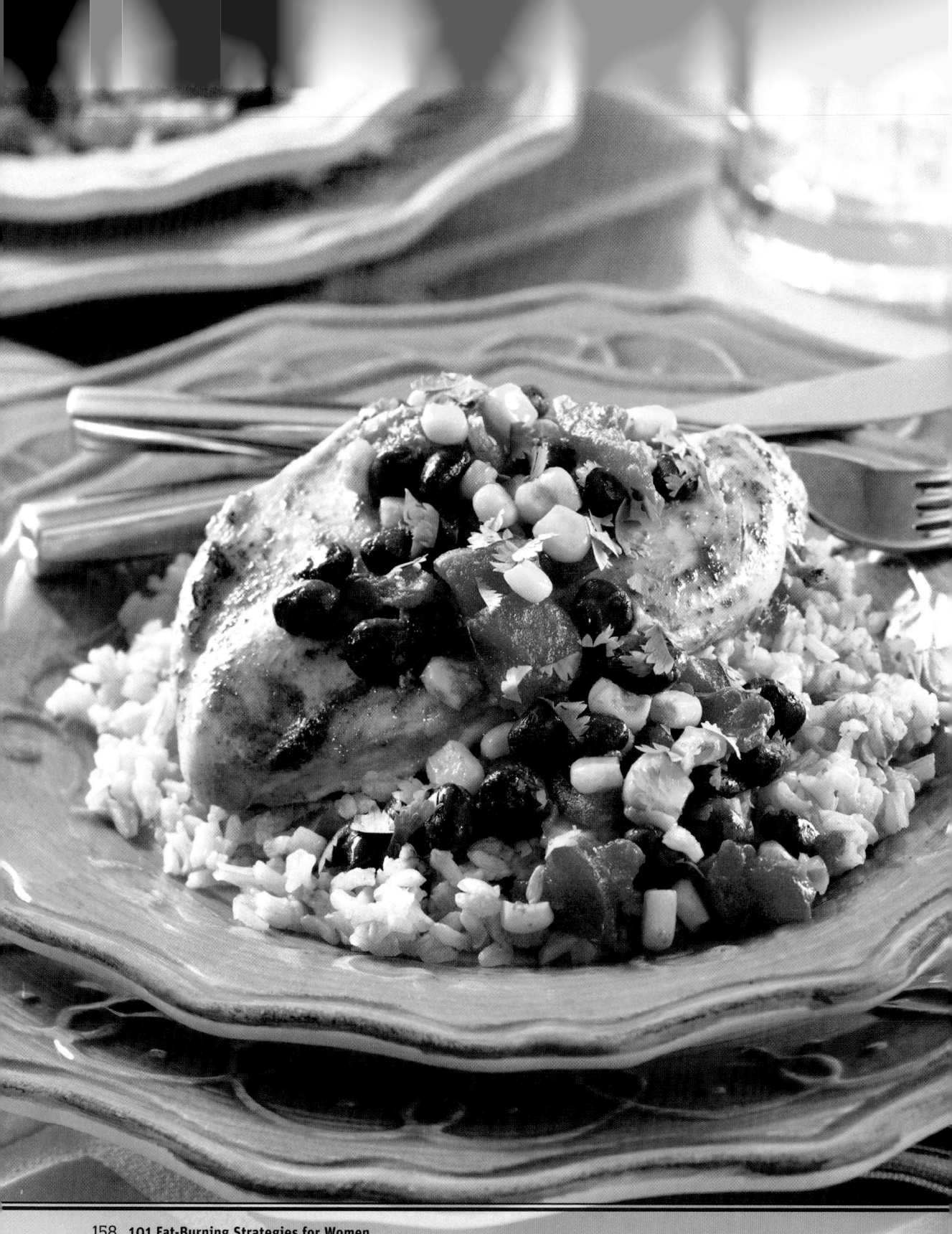

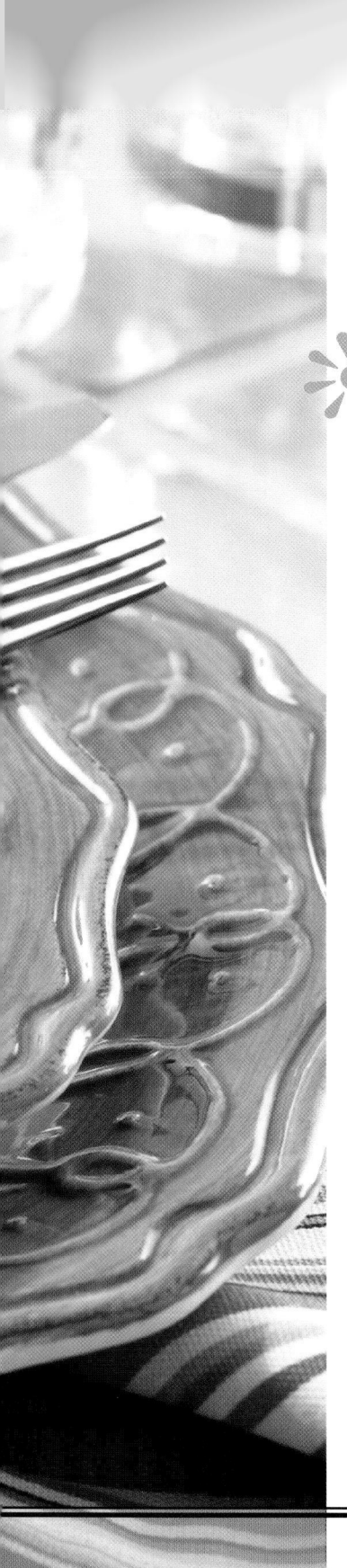

southwestern chicken with black beans and brown rice #94

This dish can easily be made vegan. Just omit the chicken and oil, and add spices to the bean mixture.

1 Tbsp. canola oil
1 lb. boneless, skinless chicken breasts
½ tsp. chili powder
½ tsp. cumin
⅛ tsp. cayenne pepper
1 cup brown rice
2 cups water
15-oz. can black beans, rinsed and drained
15-oz. can diced tomatoes with jalapeño peppers
15-oz. can no-salt-added corn, drained
2 garlic cloves, minced
Chopped fresh cilantro (optional)
½ cup low-fat sour cream (optional)

1. Heat oil in a large pot over medium-high heat. Season chicken with chili powder, cumin and cayenne on both sides. Add chicken to pot and brown quickly (two minutes per side).
2. Remove chicken, then add rice and water to pot. Bring to a boil; reduce heat to medium, cover and simmer 20 minutes.
3. Meanwhile, mix beans, tomatoes (including juices), corn and garlic in a medium bowl.
4. Layer chicken atop rice mixture, and top chicken with bean mixture. Cover and turn heat to medium-high until mixture begins to bubble; reduce heat and simmer 15–20 minutes more or until rice is tender and chicken is cooked through. Serve topped with cilantro and sour cream, if desired. **Serves 6**
NUTRITION FACTS (per serving): *358 calories, 25 g protein, 52 g carbs, 5.5 g fat, 6 g fiber, 25 mg cholesterol, 588 mg sodium, 2 g sugar*

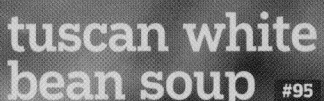

tuscan white bean soup #95

This easy-to-make, fragrant soup comes together quickly, so it's perfect for a weeknight.

2 medium leeks, white and
  light-green parts
2 Tbsp. olive oil
1 cup sliced celery
1 cup chopped carrots
3 cloves garlic, minced

2 15-oz. cans white beans
  (such as cannellini or great
  northern), drained and rinsed
4 cups (1 quart) low-sodium
  vegetable broth
1 sprig fresh rosemary
  (or ½ tsp. dried)
⅓ cup grated Parmesan cheese

1. Quarter leeks lengthwise and chop. Wash well in a sinkful of water; change water several times. Drain and pat dry with paper towels.

2. Heat oil in a large soup kettle over medium heat. Add leeks, celery and carrots; cook for five minutes, stirring frequently, until vegetables are crisp-tender. Add garlic; cook one additional minute.

3. Add beans, vegetable broth and rosemary. Bring to a boil; reduce heat to low, cover and simmer for 15 minutes or until vegetables are tender. Remove rosemary sprig and discard.

4. Season with salt and pepper, if desired. Serve in individual bowls with cheese sprinkled on top. **Serves 6**
NUTRITION FACTS (per serving): *380 calories, 13 g protein, 40 g carbs, 19.3 g fat, 7 g fiber, 4.8 mg cholesterol, 490 mg sodium, 4 g sugar*

tip: To make a creamy soup without adding fat, purée half of the soup in a blender and then return it to the kettle.

chicken provençal #96

A dish prepared in the style of Provence — a region in southeastern France — often focuses on fresh ingredients such as olive oil, tomatoes and garlic.

1 Tbsp. olive oil
4 boneless, skinless chicken breast halves
¾ tsp. salt, divided
½ tsp. pepper
½ cup dry white wine
1 pint cherry tomatoes, halved
¼ cup pitted, halved black olives (such as kalamata)
2 garlic cloves, minced
½ tsp. dried thyme
2 Tbsp. fresh minced basil

1. Heat oil in a large, deep skillet over medium-high heat. Season chicken with 1/2 tsp. each of salt and pepper. Place chicken in skillet and cook for 2–3 minutes per side. Add wine and cook one minute.

2. Add tomatoes, olives, garlic, thyme and remaining salt. Bring to a simmer; turn heat to medium-low. Cook uncovered, turning chicken once, for 10 minutes or until chicken is cooked through. Serve topped with fresh basil. **Serves 4**

NUTRITION FACTS (per serving): *190 calories, 27.5 g protein, 6 g carbs, 5.5 g fat, 2 g fiber, 68 mg cholesterol, 644.5 mg sodium, 2 g sugar*

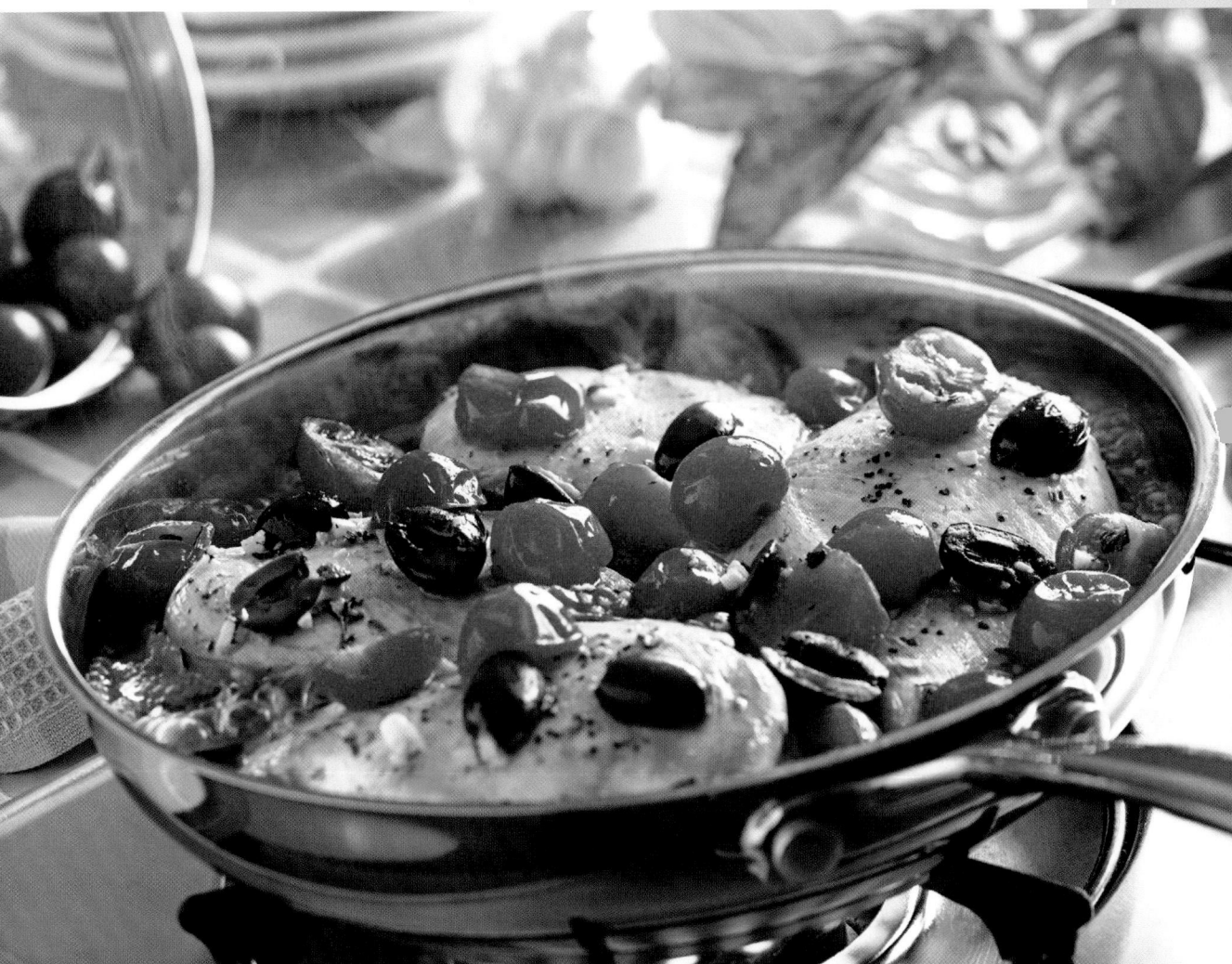

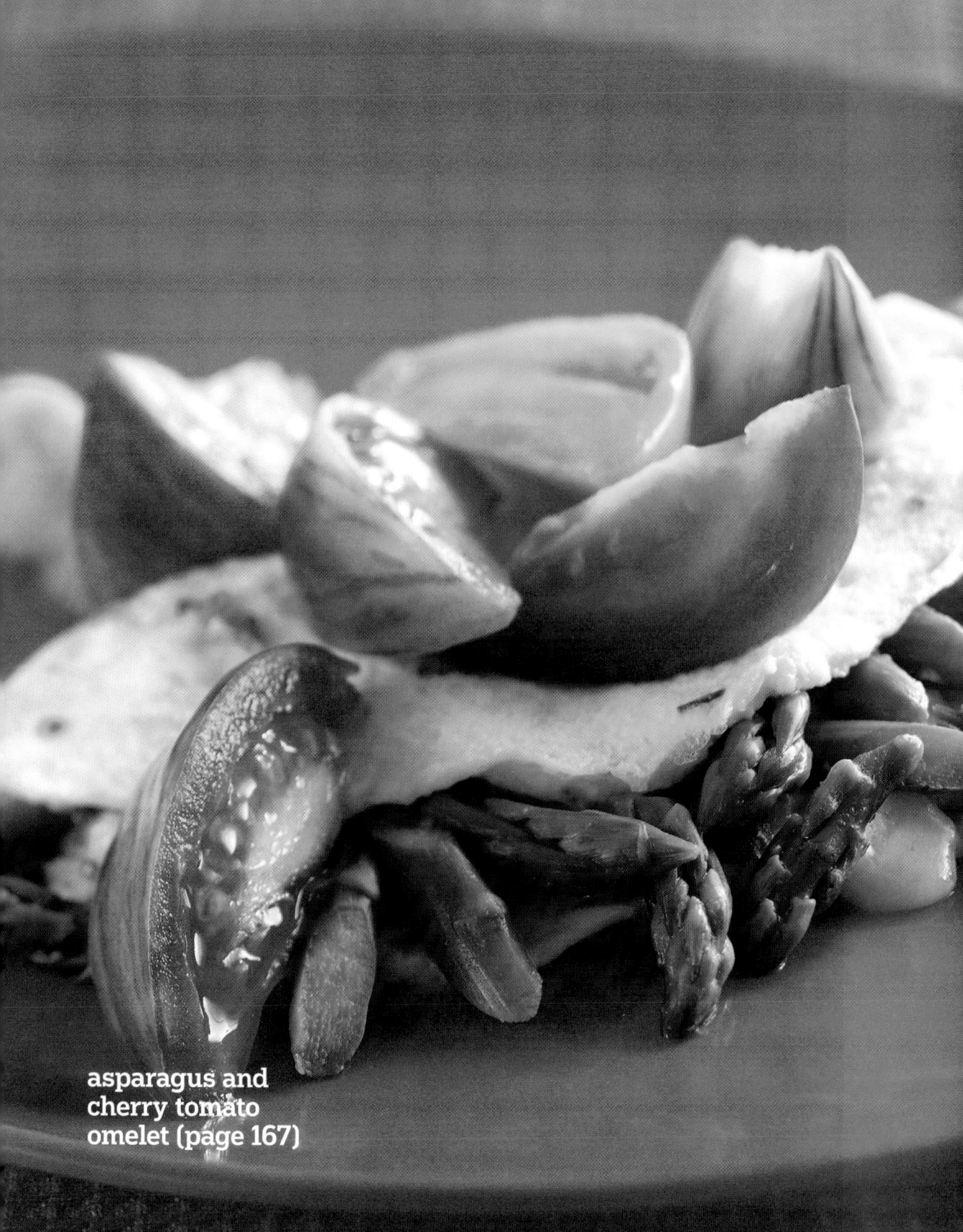

asparagus and
cherry tomato
omelet (page 167)

Chapter 16

Dishes For The Active Veg

If you're vegetarian or vegan, dreaming up tasty, nourishing meals that fuel your workouts and keep your muscles strong is a challenge. These high-protein, low-fat vegetarian dishes will make eating for performance easier — even if you just like to eat meatless once in a while. In addition, eating fruits and vegetables keeps the pounds off, as you'll stay fuller longer without consuming lots of calories.

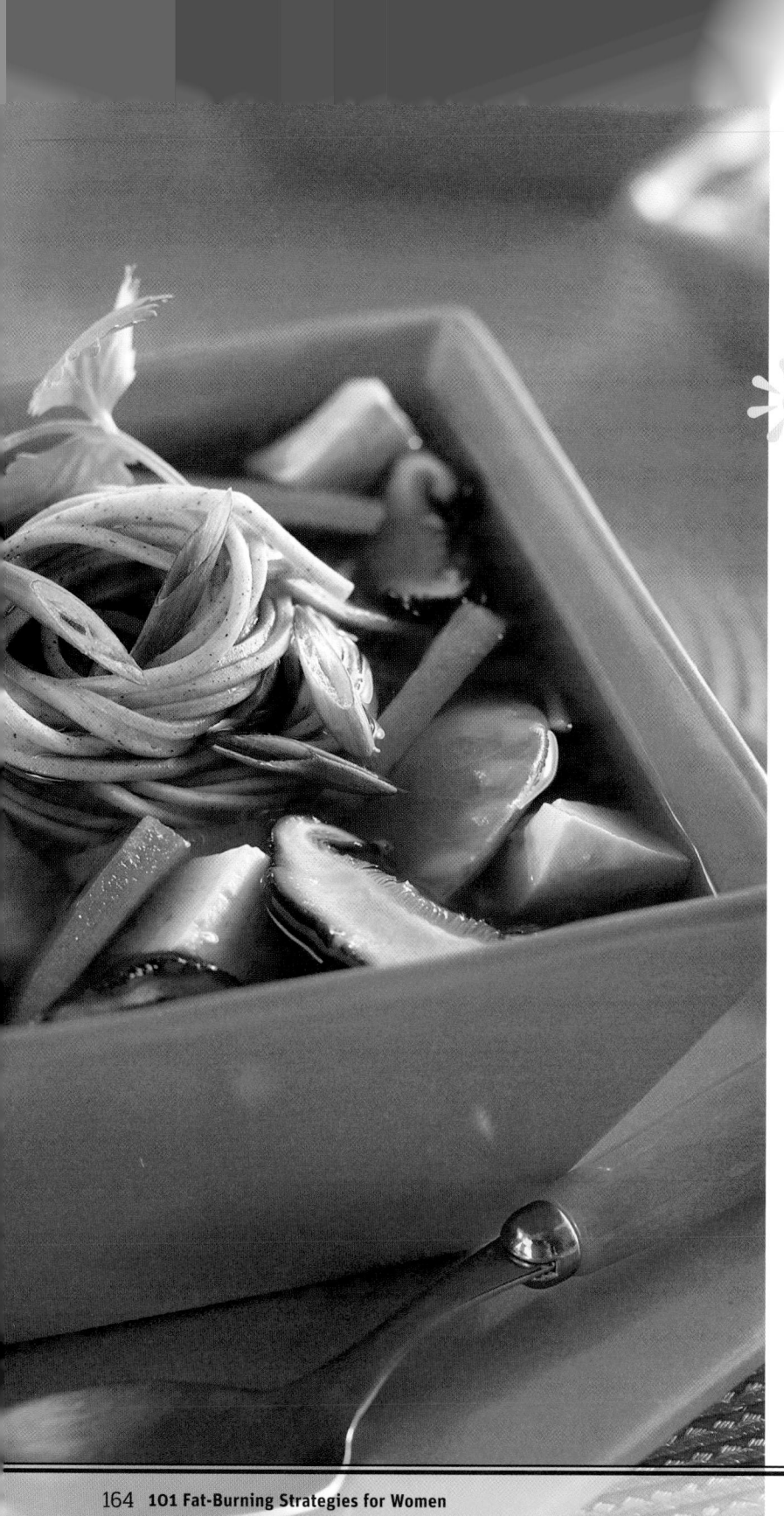

tofu noodle bowl #97

Spice up your meal plans with a bowl of warm noodles topped with fresh veggies and tofu simmered in broth.

8 oz. soba noodles
12 oz. light firm tofu, drained and
    cut into ½-inch cubes
4 cups low-sodium vegetable broth
2 cups snow peas, ends trimmed
8 oz. mushrooms, sliced
2 carrots, julienned
2 Tbsp. low-sodium soy sauce
½ jalapeño pepper, seeded
    and minced
2 tsp. minced fresh ginger
2 Tbsp. chopped fresh cilantro
2 green onions, sliced

1. Bring a large pot of water to a boil and cook soba noodles according to package directions. Meanwhile, in another large pot, bring tofu, vegetable broth, snow peas, mushrooms, carrots, soy sauce, jalapeño and ginger to a boil; reduce heat and simmer 5–7 minutes or until vegetables are soft.
2. Divide cooked noodles into four bowls and ladle soup mixture over noodles. Sprinkle cilantro and green onions over each serving. **Serves 4**
NUTRITION FACTS (per serving):
390 calories, 22 g protein, 59 g carbs, 7 g fat, 5 g fiber, 8 g sugar, 892 mg sodium

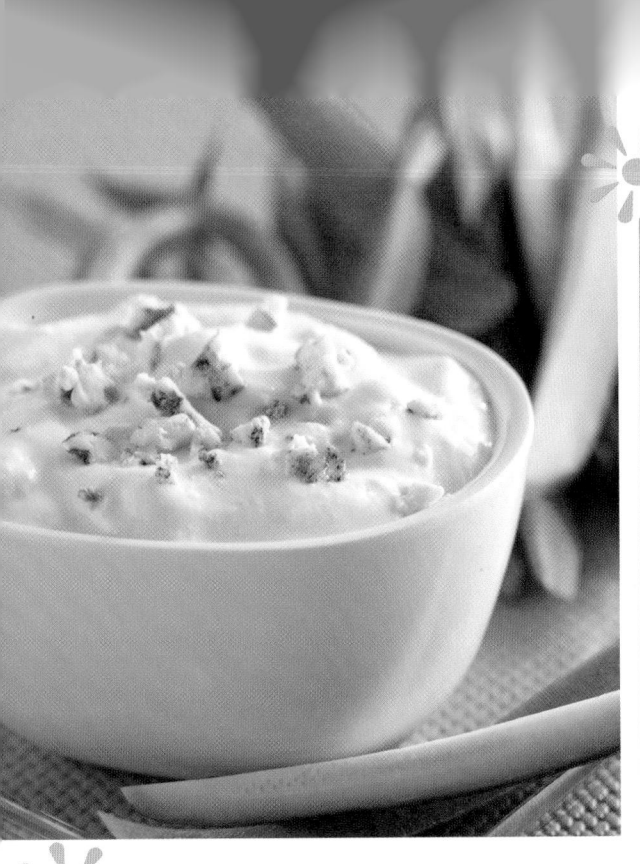

blue cottage cheese dip #98

Serve this dip with an assortment of fresh vegetables (such as celery, bell peppers and carrots) and wedges of whole-wheat pitas.

1½ cups fat-free small-curd cottage cheese
3 Tbsp. fat-free milk
2 tsp. finely chopped onion
1 tsp. lemon juice
¼ tsp. salt
⅛ tsp. pepper
Pinch cayenne pepper
½ cup crumbled vegetarian blue cheese (such as Point Reyes Original Blue Cheese)

1. Place cottage cheese, milk, onion, lemon juice, salt and peppers in a blender. Cover and blend on medium until smooth. Pour into a bowl and stir in blue cheese; if you prefer a smooth dip, blend the blue cheese with other ingredients.
2. Cover and refrigerate at least one hour to blend flavors. Serve chilled. **Makes about 2 cups**
NUTRITION FACTS (per 1/4-cup serving): *68 calories, 9 g protein, 1 g carbs, 3 g fat, 0 g fiber, 1 g sugar, 199 mg sodium*

slow-cook bean bourguignonne #99

Bourguignonne means "in the style of Burgundy," one of France's most famous food and wine regions. Most bourguignonne dishes are beef braised in red wine, which intensifies other flavors in the dish, but we've substituted beans for the beef in this easy-to-assemble slow-cooker meal.

2 cans (15 oz. each) great northern beans, drained and rinsed
8 oz. mushrooms, quartered
1 onion, chopped
1 large or 2 medium potatoes, unpeeled, cut into ½-inch chunks
2 carrots, sliced into ½-inch rounds
2 celery ribs, sliced ½-inch thick
2 cloves garlic, minced
1 tsp. dried thyme
1 tsp. salt
½ tsp. black pepper
1 bay leaf
1½ cups dry vegan red wine (such as Frey Cabernet Sauvignon)
6 oz. canned tomato paste
½ cup water

1. Place beans, mushrooms, onion, potatoes, carrots and celery in a 4-quart slow cooker. Sprinkle with garlic, thyme, salt and pepper; add bay leaf. Stir to coat vegetables.
2. Pour wine over mixture in cooker. In a small bowl, mix tomato paste and water; pour into cooker and stir.
3. Cover and cook on low 8–10 hours or high 4–5 hours, or until vegetables are tender. Remove bay leaf and serve.
Serves 6
NUTRITION FACTS (per serving):
230 calories, 12 g protein, 44 g carbs, 0 g fat, 11 g fiber, 10 g sugar, 992 mg sodium

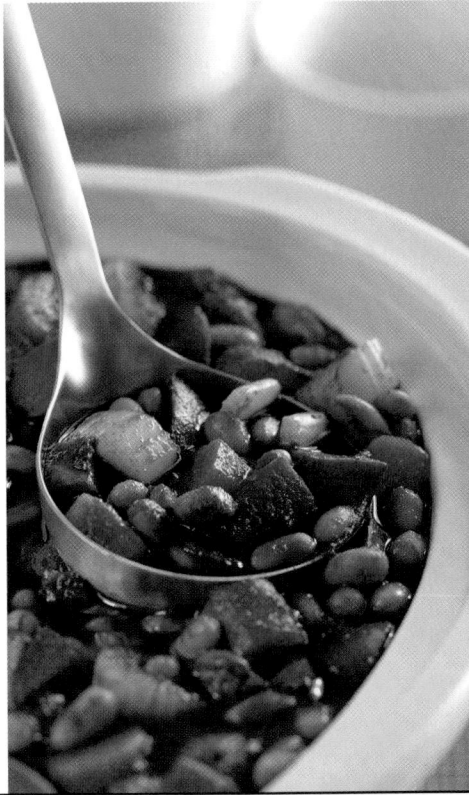

lettuce rolls with peanut sauce #100

These spicy lettuce rolls are great for a quick lunch, especially if you use leftover rice.

1 carrot, shredded
½ cup bean sprouts
½ small cucumber, cut into matchsticks
3 green onions, sliced
¼ cup chopped fresh cilantro
1½ cups cooked jasmine rice
7 oz. (½ package) light firm tofu, drained and cut into matchsticks
12 Boston lettuce leaves

12 tsp. low-fat, low-sodium bottled peanut sauce (such as Mr. Spice Thai Peanut Sauce), divided, plus extra for serving

1. Combine carrot, bean sprouts, cucumber, green onions and cilantro in a medium bowl. Divide vegetable mixture, rice and tofu evenly among lettuce leaves. Drizzle filling with

1 tsp. peanut sauce each.
2. Fold the top and bottom of lettuce leaves, roll and place seam-side down on a serving plate.
3. Serve with additional peanut sauce for dipping, if desired. **Serves 4 NUTRITION FACTS (per three-roll serving):** *158 calories, 8 g protein, 24 g carbs, 3 g fat, 2 g fiber, 3 g sugar, 345 mg sodium*

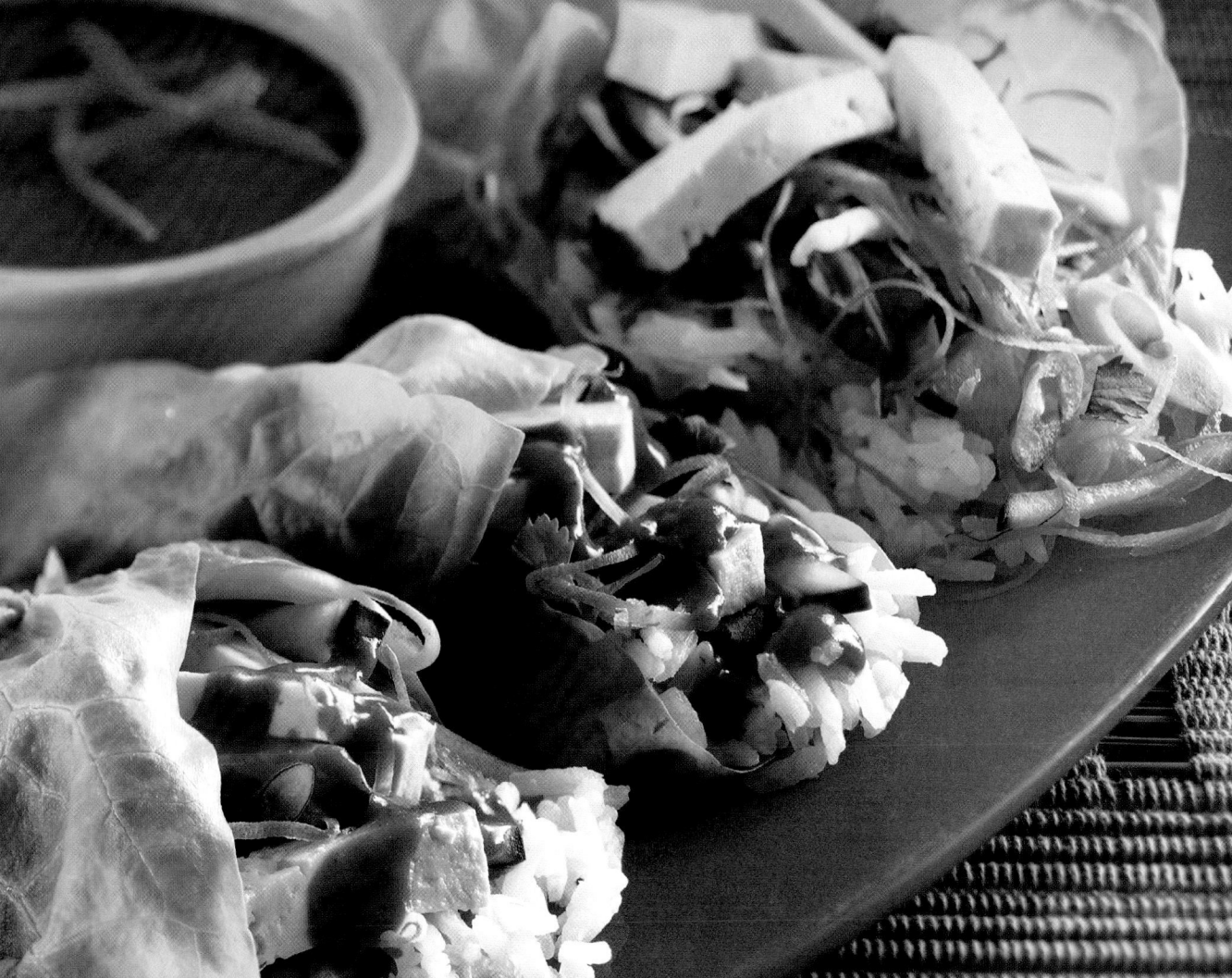

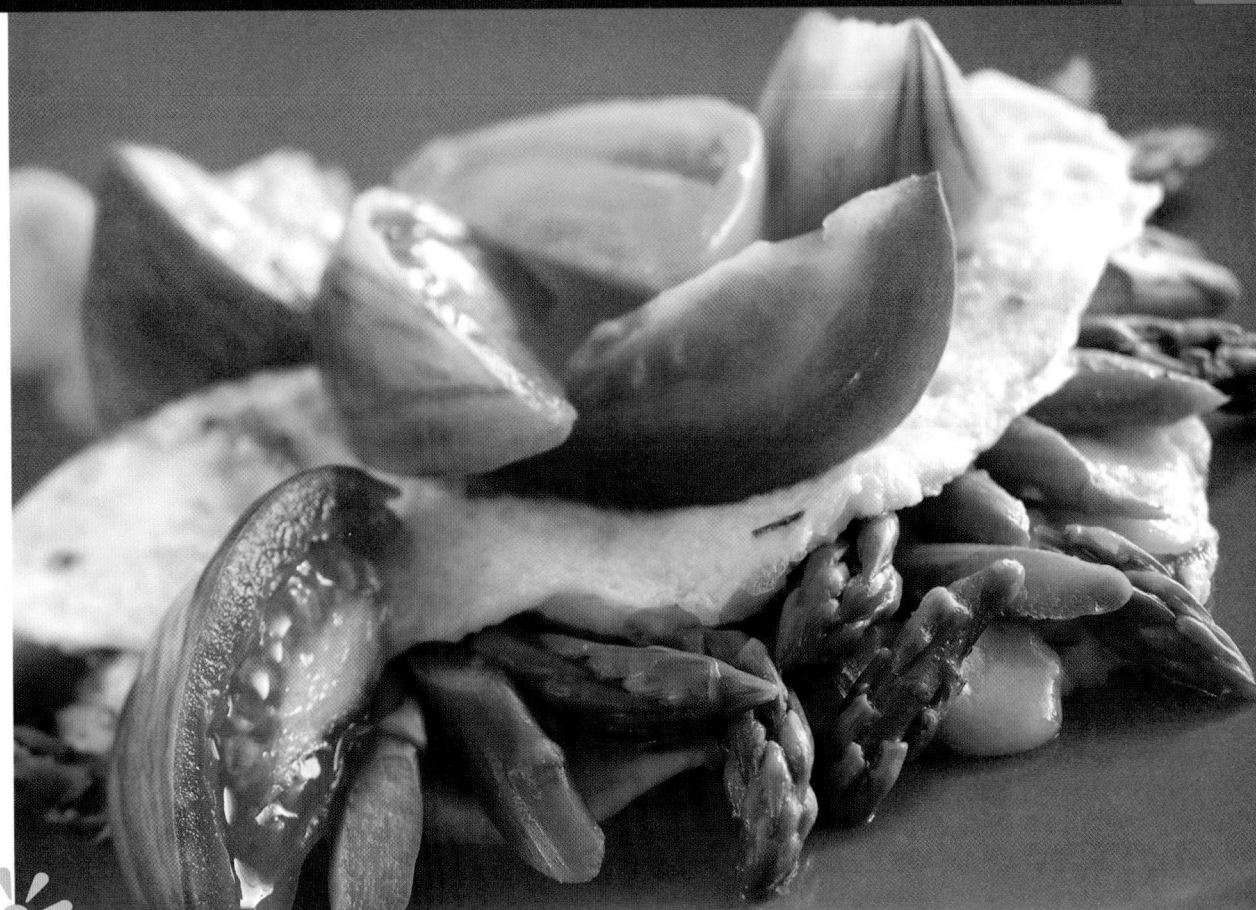

asparagus and cherry tomato omelet #101

This easy omelet is ideal for any meal of the day. If you can find heirloom cherry tomatoes, they will make the perfect topping for a touch of color, flavor and antioxidant variety.

½ lb. asparagus, woody ends snapped off, cut into 1-inch pieces

8 large egg whites (or 1 cup egg substitute)

2 Tbsp. fat-free milk

2 Tbsp. chopped chives

¼ tsp. salt

¼ tsp. pepper

⅓ cup grated Gruyère cheese, divided

½ cup cherry tomatoes, halved

Nonstick cooking spray

1. Bring a small saucepan of water to a boil; add asparagus and cook three minutes or until tender. Drain and set aside.

2. Lightly coat a small nonstick skillet with cooking spray and preheat over medium heat. Whisk egg whites, milk, chives, salt and pepper in a small bowl until soft peaks form.

3. Pour half of egg mixture into skillet; cook three minutes or until almost cooked through. Place half the asparagus and cheese onto half the omelet. Fold omelet in half and cook two minutes more.

4. Place omelet on a plate and garnish with cherry tomatoes. Repeat Steps 3 and 4 with remaining egg mixture, vegetables and cheese. **Serves 2**

Tip: If desired, sauté tomatoes for 3–4 minutes in 1 tsp. olive oil before topping the omelet.

NUTRITION FACTS (per serving):
190 calories, 23 g protein, 11 g carbs, 6 g fat, 4 g fiber, 6 g sugar, 579 mg sodium

Index Of Exercises

Below is a listing of exercises broken down by bodypart; if listed here,
the movement is described, and in most cases pictured, on the listed page.

Index Of Recipes

101 FAT-BURNING WORKOUT CHART

MONDAY EXERCISE	SET 1 REPS / WEIGHT		SET 2 REPS / WEIGHT		SET 3 REPS / WEIGHT		SET 4 REPS / WEIGHT		SET 5 REPS / WEIGHT	

TUESDAY EXERCISE	SET 1 REPS / WEIGHT		SET 2 REPS / WEIGHT		SET 3 REPS / WEIGHT		SET 4 REPS / WEIGHT		SET 5 REPS / WEIGHT	

WEDNESDAY EXERCISE	SET 1 REPS / WEIGHT		SET 2 REPS / WEIGHT		SET 3 REPS / WEIGHT		SET 4 REPS / WEIGHT		SET 5 REPS / WEIGHT	

THURSDAY EXERCISE	SET 1 REPS / WEIGHT		SET 2 REPS / WEIGHT		SET 3 REPS / WEIGHT		SET 4 REPS / WEIGHT		SET 5 REPS / WEIGHT	

FAT-BURNING WORKOUT CHART

FRIDAY EXERCISE	SET 1 REPS / WEIGHT		SET 2 REPS / WEIGHT		SET 3 REPS / WEIGHT		SET 4 REPS / WEIGHT		SET 5 REPS / WEIGHT	

SATURDAY EXERCISE	SET 1 REPS / WEIGHT		SET 2 REPS / WEIGHT		SET 3 REPS / WEIGHT		SET 4 REPS / WEIGHT		SET 5 REPS / WEIGHT	

SUNDAY EXERCISE	SET 1 REPS / WEIGHT		SET 2 REPS / WEIGHT		SET 3 REPS / WEIGHT		SET 4 REPS / WEIGHT		SET 5 REPS / WEIGHT	

CARDIO	EXERCISE	TIME	NOTES
MONDAY			
TUESDAY			
WEDNESDAY			
THURSDAY			
FRIDAY			
SATURDAY			
SUNDAY			

MEALS — DATE:

QUANTITY	FOOD/LIQUIDS/SUPPLEMENTS	TIME	CALORIES	PROTEIN	CARBS	FAT
	TOTALS					

LIQUIDS: 8 OZ = 1 CUP | 4 CUPS = 1 QUART | 4 QUARTS = 1 GALLON
WEIGHT: 16 OZ = 1 LB | 1 LB = 454 GRAMS | 1 OZ = 28.35 GRAMS

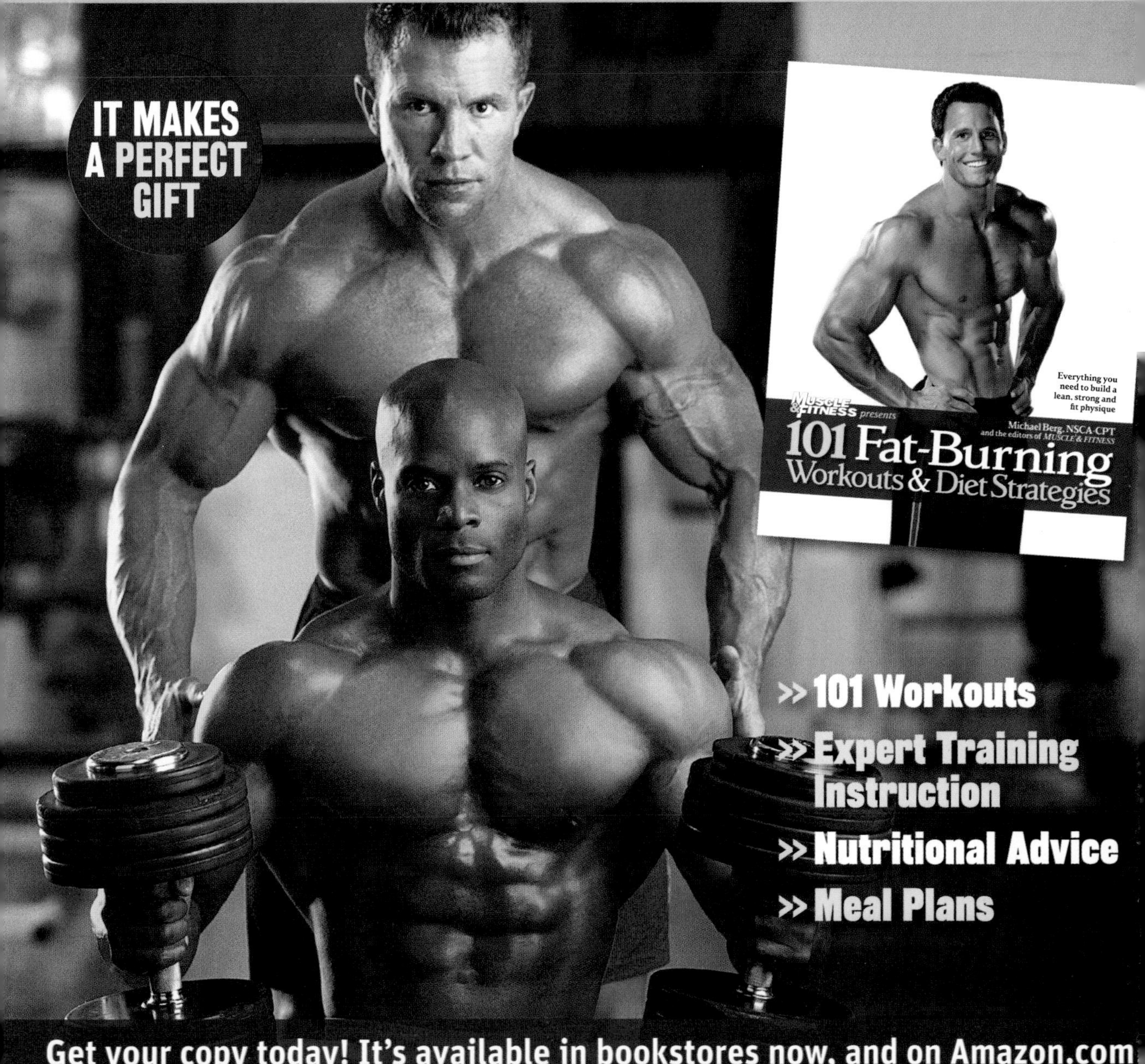